BECOMING WHO WE ARE

Becoming Who We Are

TEMPERAMENT AND PERSONALITY IN DEVELOPMENT

MARY K. ROTHBART

THE GUILFORD PRESS
New York   London

© 2011 The Guilford Press
A Division of Guilford Publications, Inc.
72 Spring Street, New York, NY 10012
www.guilford.com

Printed in the United States of America

This book is printed on acid-free paper.

Last digit is print number: 9   8   7   6   5   4   3   2   1

Library of Congress Cataloging-in-Publication Data

Rothbart, Mary Klevjord.
  Becoming who we are: temperament and personality in development /
Mary K. Rothbart.
    p. cm.
  Includes bibliographical references and index.
  ISBN 978-1-60918-069-0 (hbk.: alk. paper)
  1. Temperament in children.   2. Personality in children.   3. Child
development.   I. Title.
  BF723.T53R68 2011
  155.4′1—dc22

                                                      2010049002

About the Author

Mary K. Rothbart, PhD, is a Distinguished Professor Emerita of Psychology at the University of Oregon. Her research has focused on temperament, attention, emotion, and social development, and she has developed several widely used measures of temperament, including parent and self-report questionnaires, home observations, and laboratory observations. In recent years, Dr. Rothbart's work with Michael Posner has explored the cognitive skills, attention networks, and attention genes that support effortful control in children. She has coauthored or coedited numerous books, including *Attention in Early Development: Themes and Variations* (with Holly Ruff in 1996), *Educating the Human Brain* (with Michael Posner in 2007), and *Temperament in Childhood* (with Gedolph Kohnstamm and John E. Bates in 1989). Dr. Rothbart also coauthored (with John E. Bates) two important reviews of temperament research in the *Handbook of Child Psychology* (2006) and *Child and Adolescent Development* (2008). She has received numerous awards, including the Gold Medal for Life Achievement in the Science of Psychology from the American Psychological Foundation, the G. Stanley Hall Award for Distinguished Contribution to Developmental Psychology from the American Psychological Association, and the Award for Distinguished Scientific Contribution to Child Development from the Society for Research in Child Development. One of the offshoots of her early temperament research was the founding of Birth to Three, a parent support and education program that has reached thousands of families in the United States and abroad, and which recently celebrated its 30th birthday. Dr. Rothbart is most pleased to have received Birth to Three's Champion of Children award.

Acknowledgments

When a book reflects the learning of a lifetime, as this one does, the number of people to thank would make a large volume in itself. Nevertheless, I especially wish to recognize, from the early years, my parents and sisters; at Reed College, Carol Creedon and William Wiest; at Stanford University, Eleanor Maccoby and Robert Sears; and at the University of Oregon, the students, research assistants and coordinators, psychology faculty, and all the families who have come to our laboratory and allowed us into their homes over years of research.

The book takes particular inspiration from the ideas of Doug Derryberry, Diane Pien, Jack Bates, Myron Rothbart, and Mike Posner. In addition, Myron Rothbart and Mike Posner read each chapter as it was written, offering invaluable commentary and advice and giving me the courage to finally complete the project. The book's readers, Jack Bates, Grazyna Kochanska, and Rebecca Shiner, improved all aspects of the manuscript. Seymour Weingarten, Editor in Chief of The Guilford Press, waited patiently for the book beautifully to be begun, and then read and shaped the book throughout its development. My sincere gratitude to all.

Chere' DiValerio typed the manuscript, and the book would not have been completed without her skilled assistance. Dr. Cody Wasner cared for my rheumatoid arthritis, and helped to keep me going. My teacher Sadhviji Vrnda Chaitanya and the Vedanta tradition have helped immensely in allowing me to step back from the writing effort and let what I have learned come forward in this book.

Finally, as the reader will discover, the inspiration for this study of the development of individual differences came from my husband, Myron (Mick), and our two sons, Daniel and Michael. For this and all the meaning they bring to my life, I am deeply grateful, and to them I dedicate this book.

Contents

Introduction

There is an order to who we are. It is not a simple order; many factors affect our lives, and they are played out in the course of our development. Those of us who study temperament and social development are privileged to study this order, and findings from our work are presented in this volume. This book is about the development of the person, beginning with individual differences in temperament. Temperament is a term used since ancient times, but only in recent years have we come to better understand its nature. In this book, I begin by considering temperament in infancy, but throughout the volume, it will be clear that temperament applies to each of us daily, and contributes in important ways to our lives.

Temperament has many applications, and they range across a broad set of topics. Recently, temperament was an important factor in the outcome of the 2008 U.S. presidential election. At the time of the election, the country faced the prospect of a huge financial crisis and was involved in two wars, in Iraq and Afghanistan. At the polls, a calm and deliberate Barack Obama, who seemed temperamentally suited to addressing these problems, defeated the more impulsive and quick-to-anger John McCain.

Temperament is a term also used to describe individual differences among nonhuman animals such as dogs, horses, and mice. This book considers aspects of temperament we share with other animals and aspects of temperament and personality we do not share with them. Individual differences in temperament are also critical to the child's development, although adults have been most often interested in how the children's differences affect us as parents or teachers. Is the infant difficult? Easy? Slow to warm

1

up? In this book, I argue that these social judgments are less important than identifying the structure of temperament, its links to biology, and its applications to the child's developing personality.

Within the past 80 years, many researchers have discovered temperament in infants. One of the earliest systematic observers of infant development, Arnold Gesell (1928, cited by Kessen, 1965), followed the development of hundreds of children, filming their behavior at the Yale Laboratory for the Study of Human Development. He described individual differences in temperament and upbringing that together would influence the emerging personality. He also recognized that many outcomes are possible for any infant or child, depending on the child's history. Here, he describes a little girl, CD, who grew up in a variety of nonfamily settings, and whose temperament had been observed in the Yale laboratory from infancy:

> This girl exhibited a striking degree of amenability, sociality, and good nature as early as the age of nine months. . . . She is now five years of age, and in spite of a varied experience in boarding homes and institutions, she has not lost these engaging characteristics. They are part and parcel of her make-up quite as much as the lowered tempo and the lowered trend of her general development. It can be predicted with much certainty that she will retain her present emotional equipment when she is an adolescent and an adult. But more than this cannot be predicted in the field of personality. For whether she becomes a delinquent, and she is potentially one, will depend upon her subsequent training, conditioning, and supervision. She is potentially also a willing, helpful, productive worker. Environment retains a critical role even though heredity sets metes and bounds. (Gesell, 1928, as cited in Kessen, 1965, p. 223)

Temperament refers to the biologically based individual differences shown in infants and young children, but through the study of temperament we have also identified the processes we all share and from which personality develops. Although we differ in the functioning of temperamental processes, they are qualities common to all of us. As personality grows out of temperament, it is continually under revision as the child gains new experiences, ways of understanding, and strategies for coping with the social and physical world. As children develop in their capacities for self-regulation, they will be able to shape their own behavior, thoughts, and lives.

Personality development can be defined as "an orderly sequence of change, with the individual's location at a later point in the sequence being related to location at an earlier point in the sequence" (Kohlberg, 1969, p. 371). And to describe a sequence of change, we need a starting point: What is the initial state of individual differences among infants and young children? Are all infants basically the same, or can we also see the kinds of temperamental characteristics observed by Gesell? Temperament qualities of arousability, emotionality, and self-regulation can be studied from infancy to adulthood, and from the start they form the initial building blocks of personality. Cognitive aspects of personality (our thoughts about ourselves, others, and events) will be added throughout development as children construct mental models of who they are; experience the feelings, thoughts, and actions linked to their concept of self; and develop narratives describing the self and others. These differences go beyond temperament to personality, although temperament is likely to influence them.

In this book, I consider these important questions:

1. What are the basic dimensions of temperament and how do they relate to the biology of the person?
2. How do we describe the initial state and its variations, and what is their contribution to temperament?
3. How does temperament influence our adjustment to others and the physical world?
4. Finally, all of us, from the youngest to the elderly, live lives full of possibilities. To what degree can temperament and personality change or contribute to change in the person?

Temperament has an ancient history in medical and psychological thought, but has been most often directed toward understanding individual differences in adults. Only recently has temperament been scientifically applied to infant and child development. Over the past three decades, however, there has been an explosion of research on temperament in childhood (Rothbart & Derryberry, 2002). This has been possible because researchers have created new tools for measuring temperament. These measures allow us to study stability and change in children as they develop, and to examine the role of temperament in shaping children's experiences of the social and physical world.

Findings from this research have come as a surprise to some people. Even a few short years ago, differences among children, even infants, were thought to result chiefly from social rewards and punishments—that is, how parents, teachers, and peers treated their children and shaped their adaptations to life. We now realize, however, that temperament influences the development of social traits of major importance to the person and society, including empathy, conscience, and the prevention of aggression and behavior problems. In fact, there is now a danger that the pendulum will swing too far on the genetic side; my hope is that this book will follow a middle road, recognizing influences of both genes and experience.

The temperament traits discussed in this book are also basic psychological processes that underlie the functioning of all of us, providing the initial state from which social and personality dispositions develop. Temperament is related to underlying biological processes and to social interchanges. On the biological side, temperament makes links to animal studies, genes, and neuroscience; on the social side, the child's temperament both influences and is influenced by the social environment. Advances in neuroscience, such as neuroimaging and genetic analysis, and advances in the study of social and personality development further our understanding of what temperament is and its role in our lives.

From ancient times, ideas about temperament have also been directed toward answering practical questions, such as how temperament is related to social interaction and maladjustment. More recently, concepts of temperament have helped parents and educators to better understand a wide range of children, and to encourage their healthy development. One goal of this book is to allow parents, clinicians, and teachers to deal more effectively and humanely with children, giving both children and our society more positive futures. A second goal is to use the study of temperament and personality to understand better who we are and who we might be in the future.

A major theme of the book is that the effects of a given childrearing and environmental event often depend on the temperament of the child. In the home, children's temperament influences their everyday activities, their reactions to challenge, and their coping and adaptation to new situations. How the child acts influences the actions and thoughts of the parent, and vice versa. In the classroom, teaching methods that work well with one child may not work with another. Temperament concepts remind teachers and parents to respect and speak to *all* children, including those who do not fit our models of the ideal child or the ideal student.

Although temperament theorists sometimes think of temperament as being stable and unchanging across development (see, e.g., Buss & Plomin, 1975, 1984), careful observations of infants and young children have made it clear that temperament itself develops over time, and that new temperament traits emerge with development. In addition, one temperament system can influence the expression of another temperament system, and the balance between the two will also change over time (Rothbart, 1989b; Rothbart & Bates, 2006; Rothbart & Derryberry, 1981). These observations inspire a second set of questions:

1. When and how do changes in temperament occur?
2. How does the balance between different aspects of temperament change with development?
3. How does temperament affect children's coping and adaptations to environmental challenges? This book addresses these questions in addition to those offered above.

Genetic inheritance plays an important role in temperament throughout life, and with recent advances in molecular genetics, exciting new research questions are currently being addressed. Although temperament and personality are influenced by the genetic code, they are also influenced by variations in the child's experience, which typically occur in a social context. In animal research, we have found that individual temperament can be influenced by extreme or repeated stressors and by the quality of maternal care. High levels of stress can lead to heightened emotional reactivity, especially in animals who were more fearful and stress prone to begin with. Developmental psychologists have also known for many years that "gentling," or handling laboratory animals early in their development, can lead to lower levels of temperamental reactivity later in life. In human infants, children's early reactions may also influence the stimulation that the mother or other caregiver offers the child, further shaping children's experiences.

In recent years, researchers have studied children's temperament, environment, and developmental outcomes over long periods of time in longitudinal research. These studies reflect contributions of researchers from many countries, including Australia, China, Finland, France, Greece, Japan, the Netherlands, New Zealand, Norway, Spain, Sweden, and the United States. Results from several of these studies are discussed in this book, but a comprehensive review of longitudinal temperament research is not attempted. Indeed, an overall review of the field is not possible, at least for this author. A comprehensive review could have been done 20 years ago, but now the field has expanded so greatly that multiple reviews are necessary. Instead, I present some of the ideas and research findings that have advanced my own understanding of temperament and development with the hope they will be of value to the reader, while realizing that due to oversight, many fine studies will not be reviewed.

Overall, I hope to introduce readers to the field of temperament and to important concepts and ideas related to it, with the goal of inspiring others to continue work in this area. Pete Seeger has said that with aging, we have the good fortune of going to seed, and I like this metaphor. Seeds

are a product of the mature organism and when they come to rest on prepared ground, new structures can develop. In this book, I offer ideas that
I hope might become the seeds for new explorations. The overall structure
of the book traces the remarkable history of temperament as a set of ideas
and a topic of research, describing the search for the structure of temperament and offering a model of how temperament provides the material from
which personality and adjustment develop. I try in the last chapter to pose
some of the many unanswered questions available to younger scholars and
researchers.

Is there a specific audience for this book? I hope it will be helpful
to undergraduate and graduate students in the areas of clinical psychology; social, cognitive, and personality development; as well as researchers
in all of these areas. In addition, parents, teachers, and students of self-
understanding can also benefit, although it will require getting used to the
way psychologists cite references in the text using parentheses. These cita-
tions are of interest chiefly if the reader would like to seek more information on a topic, and they refer the reader to full references at the back of the
book.

If readers are interested in some of the additional work that underlies this book, it can be partnered with any of the following three books I
have previously coauthored or coedited. The first, *Temperament in Childhood*
(Kohnstamm, Bates, & Rothbart, 1989), is now out of print and expensive,
but the later two books, *Attention in Early Development* (Ruff & Rothbart,
1996), and, most recently, *Educating the Human Brain* (Posner & Rothbart,
2007a), are good sources. Two other sources at a more technical level are
the Rothbart and Bates (2006) chapter on temperament in *Handbook of Child
Psychology* and the Rothbart and Posner (2006) chapter on temperament and
the development of psychopathology in *Developmental Psychopathology*. For a
brief psychological introduction to temperament research, see my paper in
the journal *Current Directions in Psychological Science* (Rothbart, 2007a), and
for a brief introduction to our attention work, our paper in *Child Development
Perspectives* (Rothbart, Sheese, & Posner, 2007).

THE BOOK IN A NUTSHELL

This book traces the remarkable history of temperament as a set of ideas and
a topic of research, describing the search for the structure of temperament
and offering a model of how temperament dispositions can lead to patterns
of personality and adjustment. In the first chapter, definitions of temperament and personality are offered and I describe some of the historical roots

of temperament, ancient and modern. In Chapter 2, new findings on the structure of temperament in infancy are presented, along with a discussion of their importance for understanding early development. In Chapter 3, the biological bases of temperament and developmental change in temperament are discussed, with reviews of findings from animal research and neuroscience. In Chapters 4 and 5, I offer an account of how temperament and the child's developing cognitions about the self provide a basis for the development of personality.

In Chapter 6, the child's development of coping strategies is described and the influence of culture on development is considered. Chapter 7 discusses connections between temperament and the development of competence, including the development of moral character as seen in empathy and conscience. In Chapter 8, I consider the stability and instability of temperament, and its influence on behavior, emotions, and our cognitive models. Chapters 9 and 10 discuss temperament's contributions to understanding the development of behavior problems and psychopathology. Finally, in Chapter 11, the questions posed in this introduction are revisited, temperament is placed within a larger framework including multiple levels of analysis, and new questions are raised for future work.

I would also like to add a few words about the title of this book, *Becoming Who We Are: Temperament and Personality in Development*. This title emphasizes the idea that all development, including the development of personality and social adjustment, is a continuing process of specification, repetition, and change. The adaptive or more maladaptive patterns we develop at one age may be repeated in later times and places or they can be transformed into more healthy ones. Ultimately, we can use the potential for change built into temperament and the organism to better understand who we are and how we can influence ourselves for the future.

Starting at the beginning, however, temperament describes our early emotional, motor, and attentional equipment, along with the regulative capacities that allow us to control our reactions and put them to good use. Part of becoming who we are involves recognizing and freeing human capacities for affiliativeness, service, and contributions to others. Before we reach this point, however, and beginning with Chapters 1 and 2, respectively, we consider definitions of temperament and personality and describe how, through recent research, we have gained important information about the structure of temperament.

CHAPTER 1

Definition and Historical Roots

There are many ways for a person to discover temperament in children. One way is to be exposed to a wide range of children. Another is to intensively study of a smaller number of children in different situations and over time. The third involves observing the differences between one's own children. My discovery of temperament came from observing differences between our two sons, and it led to the exciting challenge of studying the development of individual differences. This book will be in part a story of my studies at Oregon and those of my temperament colleagues, and in part a description of contributions from other areas that can shed light on temperament and vice versa. I begin, however, with some of the differences between our two sons.

My husband and I had thought that after our first child's infancy we had learned what the basic infant was like. It would then be a simple matter of applying the principles of parenting we had learned from the first child to the second one. Like so many parents of two children, we were in for a big surprise. One of the children was easily upset, but his upset was mild, and he could soothe himself. He often seemed to prefer that we did not try to soothe him. His level of activity was moderate. The other child was quite active, positive, and slow to distress, but when he became upset, he required a major effort at soothing. One child was very oriented toward people and sensitive to their reactions to him; the other was chiefly interested in excitement, wherever it could be found. Sitting on the parent's lap did not provide enough excitement for him; he wished to be off and about.

9

As a psychologist, I was not ready for these observations. I had studied social development in the 1960s at Stanford University's graduate program, and at that time the primary shaper of individual differences in children was seen to be social rewards and punishments. The differences between our sons, however, had shown up well before a history of rewards. In graduate school, I had studied how mothers treat their children depending on whether the child is the first- or second-born child in the family. I had carefully reviewed the research literature at the time, and expected our firstborn to be more attuned to his parents than the second, as described in these studies. In our family, however, the differences we observed were actually reversed. I believe that if our two sons had differed as the birth-order research had predicted, I would probably still be studying birth order. If one had been a girl and the other a boy, I would probably be studying gender differences, but since both were boys, gender was ruled out.

Our sons' differences also mapped in uncanny ways onto differences between me and my husband. Up until then, I had assumed these differences were the result of his growing up in Chicago in a Jewish family and my growing up in the west in a family with Scandinavian roots. These quite different environments no doubt affected us, but it was a good deal less likely that they could account for the early differences between our children. The way our sons' differences corresponded to differences between my husband and me led me to look for their more biologically based sources. This turned out to be the area of *temperament*. The temperament differences between our two sons have persisted: as adults, one works as an artist and the other as a computer software architect. In many ways, however, especially in their character and values and their connections to others, they have become more alike than they were as children.

My study of individual differences in temperament has now lasted over 4 decades. In its course, my colleagues and I have defined temperament, measured it, and studied its relation to personality. In this chapter, I begin by considering definitions of temperament and personality, followed by a brief account of temperament's ancient and more recent history.

DEFINING TEMPERAMENT

What is temperament? Doug Derryberry and I defined temperament as constitutionally based individual differences in reactivity and self-regulation (Rothbart & Derryberry, 1981). The term "constitutional" refers to the biological bases of temperament. By reactivity, we meant how disposed we are to emotional, motor, and attentional reactions. One's disposition to a reaction can be measured by the latency, intensity, peak intensity of reaction, and recovery of the reaction. How quick, for example, are we to anger, to fear, to approach? How intense is our reaction? How long does it take us to calm down and recover from the reaction? By self-regulation, we meant processes that regulate our reactivity. These include our tendency to approach or withdraw from a stimulus, and to direct our attention toward or away from it. They also include the ability to control our actions and emotions.

In the mid-20th century, many definitions of temperament stressed the emotions. Valentine (1951), for example, defined temperament as individual differences in emotions and the child's susceptibility to them. Temperament in his view also included "innate tendencies to various kinds of action" (p. 67). By innate tendencies, Valentine meant dispositions toward and away from an object that are built into the structure of the emotions and emotional reactivity. In Valentine's view, individual differences are not only determined by temperament tendencies acting alone, "but by the relative strengths of one (tendency) compared with another, and by the general balance of all the various tendencies" (p. 67). These ideas may seem strange to the reader now, but I hope that in the course of this book, their importance will become clear.

Valentine (1951) recognized that temperament included individual differences in motivations for actions that are part of the organized emotions, such as fighting, fleeing, freezing, avoiding, seeking, and approaching. He also emphasized the importance of a balance among temperamental tendencies. At times, for example, a child can have both strong avoidance *and* strong approach tendencies to the same object or person. In the past, researchers created measures of temperament with high approach at one pole and high avoidance at the other. In these models, a child high in approach would necessarily be low in avoidance, and there would be no conflict between one temperament tendency and another. However, if these tendencies are considered separately, we can accept the possibility of two conflicting or complementary tendencies. The child's reactions in a given situation will then be influenced by the strength of these tendencies and by the child's past experiences in that situation. Reactivity, however, does not provide the full story of temperament; we also need to study individual difference in self-regulation and effortful self-control. Even young infants regulate themselves, and their signals serve to regulate the behavior of their caregivers by leading the caregiver to offer regulation for the infant, as we see in Chapter 4.

Temperament and Personality

Temperament is part of the broader domain of individual differences in personality, defined by Allport (1937) as the organization of "systems that determine his [the person's] unique adjustment to his environment" (p. 48). Personality traits in Allport's view are patterns of thoughts, emotions, and behavior that show consistency across situations and stability over time. Temperament traits, a subset of personality traits, include the emotional, motor, and attentional tendencies and regulative capacities. These also show consistency across situations and stability over time. They are seen early in life and form the earliest individual differences in personality.

Unlike other personality traits, however, temperament traits do not include specific thoughts or cognitions, such as concepts about the self and others (e.g., high self-esteem or paranoia). A number of temperament traits also describe nonhuman animals as well as humans. Temperament is present in infancy and early childhood, and forms the biologically based core from which personality develops. In Michael Rutter's (1987) terms, personality represents the projections of temperament tendencies out into the world, and, as I argue, it also involves the specification of temperament tendencies to particular situations. Temperament will also influence specific cognitions about the social and physical world: what is bad and what is good, what is scary and what is benign. In addition to temperament traits, the larger domain of personality includes attitudes; cognitive coping strategies and defense mechanisms; self-concept and self-related emotions such as pride, guilt, and shame; views of others and the physical world; values; morals; and beliefs. Temperament influences the development of these qualities but can be differentiated from them.

A Thought Experiment

Based on these descriptions, try this thought experiment. If a person is described as both fearful and arrogant, which of these traits would you see as temperamental and which as involving personality? If you chose fear as the temperament trait, and arrogance as the personality trait, you may have applied one or more of the following criteria: (1) fear, but not arrogance, is present in infants and young children; (2) fear, but not arrogance, is present in many nonhuman animals; (3) arrogance seems to be more a product of the person's social and life experience; and (4) arrogance is related to the specific content of thought, that is, thinking one is better than others.

Although any given instance of fear will also be influenced by experience, fear is a biologically based system linked to the functioning of neural structures and circuits that we all inherit (LeDoux, 1989). The objects of fear in older children and adults are often taught by others, but they can also occur without tuition, and they can be self-taught. Differences in the trait of fearfulness or behavioral inhibition also appear early in life, and have roots in biological systems (Kagan, 1994; Kagan & Fox, 2006). We do not inherit arrogance directly but may inherit a social environment and set of experiences that promote it.

Temperament in Nonhuman Animals

Although some researchers have called individual differences in nonhuman animals "personality" (e.g., Gosling & John, 1999), I believe it is important to separate the more biologically based processes that we share with other animals (chiefly temperament) from those we do not (chiefly personality). Temperament is part of our basic biological equipment and has evolved to provide behavioral solutions to expectable problems, that is, problems likely to be posed by the environment. Temperament constructs are thus closely linked to research in neuroscience. Strelau (1983) also separates temperament and personality. In his view, temperament results from biological evolution, and is "peculiar to *both* [emphasis added] humans and animals, which cannot be said of personality" (p. 258). In addition, "The individual has a temperament from the moment of birth, since it is determined by inborn physiological mechanisms which, in turn, may be modified under environmental influences" (p. 258). We return to studies of temperament in nonhuman animals in Chapter 3.

Our Definition of Temperament

We have defined temperament as individual differences in reactivity and self-regulation (Rothbart & Bates, 1998, 2006; Rothbart & Derryberry, 1981). By *reactivity*, we mean how easily our emotions, motor activity, and attention are aroused. Part of this reactivity includes tendencies toward, away from, or against novel or challenging stimuli. Reactivity also refers to the orienting of attention to internal and external stimulation. Temperamental reactivity is seen in broad tendencies, such as negative reactivity or distress proneness, and it is also seen in more specific reactions, such as tendencies to fear or anger, and aspects of physiological reactivity, such as heart rate or galvanic skin response. Reactive temperament can be measured by how rapidly the reaction begins after the occurrence of an arousing event, the intensity of the reaction, its duration, and the nature of its offset and recovery (Rothbart & Derryberry).

Self-regulatory aspects of temperament serve to act upon reactive tendencies, increasing or moderating them. Self-regulation includes individual differences in effortful control operating through attention. Effortful control can serve to decrease or increase the onset, intensity, or duration of temperament reactions. When I discuss temperamental reactivity, I am referring to individual differences in patterns of emotional reaction such as those described for our two sons. At an underlying level, however, I will also be referring to the organization and function of emotion processing and the attentional networks in the human brain that support it (Posner & Rothbart, 2007a, 2007b). The emotions also include motivation and action tendencies that serve a regulatory function. Fear carries with it dispositions toward freezing, withdrawal, or attack; anger carries dispositions toward aggression. In turn, each emotional reaction can feed back to influence the person's future experience. Executive attention and effortful control are more purely self-regulatory systems; they do not specify particular emotions but can serve a large set of emotion-related goals. Effortful control, based on the executive attention system of the brain (Posner & Rothbart, 2007a), allows flexible response in the service of values, and it is a major focus of later chapters.

Temperament describes an individual's tendencies, dispositions, or capacities. These tendencies are not continually expressed; they depend on the appropriate eliciting conditions, that is, the content of situations. A fearful child is not continually distressed or inhibited. When experiencing novelty, sudden or intense stimulation, or signals of punishment, more fearful children are especially prone to a fearful reaction, experiencing it more rapidly and in response to lower intensities of stimulation. The child is also likely to show higher intensities of fear expression. Easily frustrated children are not continually irritable or angry, but when their intentions are blocked, or there is a failure of their expectations, or they are in pain, they are more prone to anger and frustration reactions than other children.

The Emotions

Human emotions and attention have been shaped over centuries of evolution. The emotions and attention are biological systems ordering feeling, thought, and action so as to deal with environmental challenges and opportunities (LeDoux, 1989). We share our emotions and orienting of attention with other animals. These reactions have been adaptive to our ancestors, signaling the meaning or significance of events to us and others of our species, and preparing us for action. Thus although temperament is individualized in our specific genetic makeup and through the experiences of our lives, it is also inherited by all of us.

Emotion networks have been conserved through evolution to allow species and individuals to deal with environmental and internally generated threat and opportunity. Tooby, Cosmides, and Barrett (2005) argue that emotions and their related motivations serve the purpose of *valuation*, discriminating situations from each other based on their positive or negative significance to us, and these valuations have been preprogrammed via our genes. With experience, valuation processes are applied to specific events in specific situations, providing meaning for our world. With this introductory description of some of the concepts of temperament, we are in a position to examine the history of these ideas.

A BRIEF HISTORY OF TEMPERAMENT

I now offer a brief history of temperament. This history is by no means complete, but it touches on some basic ideas from the past that are related to our current thinking. Although temperament can be traced back to the Indian Rig Vedas and the Chinese concept of ch'i (Needham, 1973), I begin this section with the Western approach of the ancient Greeks and Romans. Greco–Roman physicians, including Vindician, who in the fourth century C.E., identified temperamental types of persons as reflected in their patterns of emotion and behavior (Diamond, 1974).

Ancient Roots of Temperament

The term "temperament" is derived from the Latin *temperamentum*, or mixture, which came from *temperare* meaning to "mingle in due proportion." In Vindician's fourfold typology, the melancholic person is moody, with a tendency to fear and sadness, and seen as having a predominance of black bile. The choleric person is touchy, aggressive, and active, with a predominance of yellow bile. The sanguine person, sociable and easygoing, is seen as having a predominance of blood; the phlegmatic individual, calm, even tempered, and slow to emotion, is seen to have a predominance of phlegm. In our modern usage, a "temperamental" person is thought to be emotionally extreme, but the ancient view suggested that we *all* are prone to all of the temperaments; we differ in the strength and balance of these components.

Although Galen (second century C.E.) is usually given credit for the fourfold typology (Carey, 1994; Kagan, 1994), temperament ideas were actually well in place before his time and the full typology did not emerge in its complete form until later (Diamond, 1974). Nevertheless, Galen made an important observation about temperament in the young child: "The starting point of my entire discourse is the knowledge of the differences which can be seen in little children, and which reveal to us the faculties of the soul. Some are very sluggish, others violent; some are insatiable gourmands, others quite the contrary; they may be shameless, or shy; and they exhibit many other analogous differences" (as cited in Diamond, 1974, p. 604). Galen argued that if souls, that is, the essential nature of the young, were interchangeable, then children would be expected to act similarly from early in life, but they do not. Observing consistent differences in infants' and young children's behavior led Galen to argue that children differ from one other from the earliest days.

The fourfold typology of the Greco–Roman period put forward a number of ideas that remain important to our current thinking. First, the typology resulted from consistently observed patterns in the person's emotions and behavior; second, it was linked to human physiology as it was understood at the time—the bodily humors; and third, it was related to psychopathology, as in the relation between melancholia and depression and the relation between the choleric temperament and aggression. Temperament's meaning as a proportionate mixture also foreshadows Valentine's (1951) definition of temperament as involving a balance among tendencies.

Finally, the classic temperament types can be seen as prototypes for several of the basic emotions and motivations I discuss in this book. Positive emotion and stimulation seeking are linked to the sanguine type; fear and sadness to the melancholic; anger and irritability to the choleric; and general slowness in alerting and generating emotion and action to the phlegmatic type. When we consider recent work on temperament, we will see that three of the four types also correspond to three of the six temperament factors identified in childhood (Victor, Rothbart, & Baker, 2006) and in adulthood (Evans & Rothbart, 2007): aggressive negative affect (similar to the choleric type), nonaggressive negative affect (similar to the melancholic), and surgency (similar to the sanguine type). We do not identify the phlegmatic person, except perhaps by low scores on all the emotions, but phlegmatic tendencies are sometimes reported in temperament research involving children (e.g., Bates, Freeland, & Lounsbury, 1979).

The fourfold typology of temperament persisted through the Middle Ages and into the Renaissance (e.g., Burton, 1921; Culpeper, 1657), and was later found in the writings of Kant. Beginning with Wilhelm Wundt (1903), however, temperament typologies were abandoned; instead the basic dimensions on which people varied were identified. More recently, Kagan (1994), Robins (Robins, John, Caspi, Moffitt, & Stouthamer-Loeber, 1996), and others have reintroduced the idea of types, and some authors have mapped temperament dimensions onto the fourfold typology (e.g., Burt, 1937; Cattell, 1933; Eysenck, 1947; Wundt, 1903). The typology approach provides a simplified way of thinking about temperament, but it does not allow study of the conflict or balance between temperament tendencies as is possible in studying multiple temperament dimensions. I discuss some of the recent typologies in Chapter 3.

Temperament in the 20th Century

Two major approaches to the study of temperament were begun early in the 20th century. In Russia, Ivan Pavlov's (1935) laboratory carried out temperament research with dogs. Pavlov's approach was continued in the laboratories of Eastern Europe and in questionnaire studies of human temperament carried out in Russia and Eastern Europe (Strelau, 1983, 2008). The second approach, begun in Britain, used early versions of the statistical method of factor analysis on data from questionnaires; this method was later taken up by researchers in the United States. Both the Eastern European and the British approaches involved research on neurophysiology, and provided early frameworks for links between temperament and biology.

During most of the 20th century, however, these two approaches to adult temperament remained isolated from research and thinking about temperament in children. Most of the connections between the adult and child approaches have been relatively recent (e.g., Bates & Wachs, 1994; Halverson, Kohnstamm, & Martin, 1994; Rothbart & Derryberry, 1981). I now describe the Eastern European and British traditions in more detail, beginning with Pavlov.

Pavlov and the Eastern European Tradition

Almost all of us have a mental image of Pavlov's dogs from his research on the conditioning of salivation to sound, but few are aware of Pavlov's contributions to the study of temperament. In fact, a strong tradition in temperament study originated in Pavlov's laboratory and continues in Eastern European countries and Canada today (Rusalov & Trofimova, 2007; Strelau, 1983, 2008). Gray (1980) described in detail Pavlov's contributions to the study of temperament. Pavlov and his colleagues used as their subjects mongrel dogs that had grown up outside the laboratory (Gray). These animals were studied over a period of years and in a variety of experimental tasks, and researchers in Pavlov's laboratory came to know the individual animals well.

Classical conditioning responses of the dogs to a tone that preceded the presentation of meat powder were also analyzed subject by subject, and conditioning findings were seen as reliable only when they had been repeated from one dog to another. Thus, Pavlov and his collaborators became familiar with each dog's behavior across situations and over time (Gray, 1980). The dogs in Pavlov's laboratory were also known by name, not by number. Gray notes that the names given the dogs themselves sometimes indicated the individuality of the animals. For example, the dog "Gunshot" was described as a "lively" animal; "Milord" as a "calm, inactive" one; "Joy's" name speaks for itself.

Thus, Pavlov's laboratory created the necessary conditions for observing consistent and stable individual characteristics among the dogs, and after the first observations of dog temperament made by his student Nikiforovsky in 1910, Pavlov decided to study temperament himself. He also began to link the differences among the dogs to variability in the properties of the nervous system as he understood them (Pavlov, 1935; Strelau, 1983). To account for his findings on classical conditioning, for example, Pavlov had proposed the existence of excitatory and inhibitory brain processes. These processes were seen to underlie both conditioned learning and other aspects of behavior. Pavlov now proposed that both his laboratory animals and humans share these brain processes, with individual differences in temperament based on them.

If all the animals shared the same basic processes, how did Pavlov account for individual differences in the animals' behavior? Here is Gray's (1980) exposition of Pavlov's thinking:

> So we cannot account for Milord's inactivity by saying that he *lacks* [my emphasis] an excitatory process. What Pavlov did was to suppose that the functional parameters of these basic processes vary from animal to animal. Thus one dog may have an excitatory process which is particularly easily set into motion, or particularly intense . . . another may have an inhibitory process which is particularly difficult to set into motion . . . and so on. In this way, while preserving a unified theory of conditioning, one can nonetheless account for the peculiarities of the behavior of individuals. There is nothing surprising about this move. It is what we all do when we say that such a one is "quick to anger" or such another "hard to frighten"; anger and fear are common to us all, but we vary in our readiness to display them. (p. 106)

These ideas serve to elaborate the concept of temperamental reactivity introduced at the beginning of this chapter. By *functional parameters*, Gray refers to individual differences in the latency, intensity, and duration of activation of the psychological processes, similar to the reactivity differences described in our definition of temperament (Rothbart & Derryberry, 1981). This is a fundamental point about temperament and I will return to it again and again—the processes that underlie temperament are shared by all of us, but variation in the functioning of these processes is what I mean by temperament. Thus, from the very start, the study of temperament stresses ways in which we are alike as well as the ways in which we differ.

Pavlov (1935) was also interested in mental illness, and observed what he called *experimental neurosis* in the laboratory. This condition developed when a dog was required to make a very difficult conditioned discrimination. For example, a dog would be trained to salivate to the presentation of a circle (positive conditioning), but not to the presentation of an ellipse (inhibitory conditioning). The experimenter would then gradually change the circle to become more and more like an ellipse. When animals were required to make these discriminations over a period of weeks, their performance often drastically deteriorated. Dogs started performing incorrectly, not only to the difficult discriminations, but also to simple circles and ellipses. Some of these animals also became disturbed the moment they were put into the laboratory harness, howling and struggling to get away (Gray, 1980). Pavlov called this *experimental neurosis*, and he noted that some dogs were more prone to this condition than others (Strelau, 1983).

Pavlov also described distinctive categories of temperament, and related them to the dogs' conditioning ability and to how easily they succumbed to experimental neurosis (Pavlov, 1935; Strelau, 1983). The four categories of dogs described here include only the simplest of Pavlov's distinctions; later, his list grew to include over 30 different categories. The first of the four categories included dogs that were lively and active when stimulated, but became drowsy when they were not, for example, when they were required to wait quietly in harnesses with no stimuli presented. These dogs developed conditioned responses easily, and were unlikely to develop neurosis, even under the most difficult conditions of conflict. Pavlov saw this to be the ideal type of animal, and he linked it to the ancient *sanguine* temperament type.

The second group of animals established strong and stable conditioned responses but showed difficulty in adapting when conditions changed. This group also was unlikely to develop neurosis. Pavlov linked this group to the ancient *phlegmatic* type. The third category included dogs that formed positive conditioned responses easily, but formed inhibitory responses only with great difficulty, and their inhibition was easily lost. These animals were disturbed when an activity was interrupted, and often fell asleep or became aggressive when difficult discriminations were required. Pavlov linked this group to the *choleric* type.

Finally, dogs linked to the *melancholic* type developed conditioned responses only with difficulty, and were easily disturbed by distracting stimuli. These animals were also the most likely to develop experimental neurosis. Pavlov (1935) wrote least favorably about this fourth group, indicating that "They never fully adapt themselves to the conditions of life, are easily broken, [and] often and quickly become ill or neurotic" (1935, p. 338).

Pavlov felt that similarities between these categories of animals and the ancient temperament typology justified making strong links between temperament in dogs and humans, and to connecting the melancholic category to introversion and the lively and active sanguine category to extraversion.

Pavlov made value judgments about the temperamental characteristics he studied, and indeed, value judgments of temperament characteristics can be seen in the views of researchers up to the present day. The group of dogs Pavlov most valued, the sanguine dogs, was also the group that adapted best to his laboratory, and we might wonder whether Pavlov's need for cooperative subjects may have influenced his judgments. Pavlov's melancholic group of animals, for example, described as ill adapted to the conditions of life, might have adapted well to other circumstances, for example, as loving companion animals in a quiet home. Choleric dogs that had problems in the laboratory might also have adapted well to dominance contests within a wild dog pack. Pavlov's value judgments about dog temperament raised for the first, but not the last time, a question about the need to add evaluations to temperament characteristics. While the basic building blocks of temperament appear to vary little across cultures, for example, children's family, school, and culture often value some aspects of temperament more than others, and terms like "difficult children," to be discussed later, can also raise the question "Difficult for whom?"

Pavlov's (1935) temperament approach inspired much research in the Soviet Union and Eastern Europe. To get a brief glimpse of this work, we can look at two of the nervous system properties he proposed: strength and weakness of excitation. A general "law of strength" discovered in Pavlov's laboratory found that the higher the intensity of the conditioned stimulus (e.g., the louder the bell presented before the food powder), the greater the intensity of the response (e.g., the amount of salivation). Different dogs were also differently susceptible to the law of strength. Pavlov proposed that individuals who could continue to increase the strength of their response under high intensity or prolonged exposure to stimulation possessed "strong" nervous systems; those who easily lost the conditioned response had "weak" nervous systems. Pavlov associated the weak nervous system with the melancholic group of dogs. Later research by Nebylitsyn (1972a), using laboratory measures and drug studies of humans, indicated that individuals with weak nervous systems also showed lower sensory thresholds than those with strong nervous systems.

Serious problems developed for the Soviet tradition, however, when the nervous system properties they thought were general proved to be highly dependent on the specific stimuli used and the specific responses measured in the laboratory (Strelau, 1983). These results did not support the existence of the general nervous system properties that Pavlov (1935) had posited. Research on individual differences in threshold in the United States also indicated that sensitivity varied from one sensory system to another, for example, from vision to audition. Eventually, workers in Pavlov's tradition abandoned the notion of nervous system properties, and turned instead to the study of behavioral temperament traits (Nebylitsyn, 1972b; Teplov, 1964). With this change, researchers moved out of the laboratory and into the development of questionnaire measures (Rusalov, 1987; Rusalov & Trofimova, 2007; Strelau, 1972, 2008).

The British Tradition

Whereas temperament research in the Soviet Union originated in the laboratory and only later moved into the administration of self-report questionnaires, in Britain these events were reversed, with questionnaire research coming first and laboratory research later. In the Soviet Union, observations of behavior were also linked to properties of the nervous system from the beginning. In Britain, temperament dimensions were identified first, and theoretical links to the nervous system were made later, chiefly in work by Eysenck (1957, 1967) and Gray (1978).

Some of the first factor-analytic methods applied to temperament were used in British questionnaire research. These methods had been originally applied to the study of intelligence, and were then used to study the structure of temperament and character. Factor analysis reduces a large numbers of characteristic or trait measures to a smaller number of broad interrelated traits that are believed to underlie the more specific traits. In factor analysis, relations (and nonrelations) among variables are taken into account to identify a relatively small number of related variables, called latent dimensions or factors. When two measures are strongly related, either positively or negatively, they are likely to share the same factors; when correlations are low between measures, they are likely to be linked to different factors. These broad factors can themselves be factored, yielding still broader and hierarchically arranged dimensions.

In intelligence testing, for example, factor analyses by Cattell (1963), and Horn and Cattell (1966) identified hierarchical structures of individual differences in intelligence. At the top, there is general intelligence; at the next level, the broad factors of *crystallized* (facts and skills) and *fluid* (the capacities used to attain facts and skills) intelligence are found. At the next level are more specific factors of visualization, perceptual speed, and fluency. Although today, computers perform factor analyses quickly and easily, the pioneers of factor analysis labored for weeks over their data to identify shared commonalities across measures of traits. Webb (1915) and Burt (1937, 1938) published separate reports on the factor structure of temperament early in the 20th century, and their work, along with that of Heymans and Wiersma in the Netherlands (1906, discussed below), served as the beginning of a questionnaire tradition in research on temperament and personality.

Webb (1915) and Burt (1937, 1938) each used early forms of factor analysis on large groups of items written to measure the individual's emotionality, self-qualities, and intellect. Webb then had 20 judges observe and rate 194 college students on 39 qualities. He removed the variability in scores related to intelligence, and then asked what other general factors remained. He identified the factor w, which he defined as "consistency of action resulting from deliberate volition or will" (p. 34). It included items like "tendency not to abandon tasks in the face of obstacles," "trustworthiness," and "conscientiousness" versus items like "eagerness for admiration" and "readiness to become angry" (Deary, 1996, p. 994). Later reanalyses of Webb's data also yielded a factor labeled Extraversion–Introversion (Burt, 1937, 1938; Cattell, 1933; Garnet, 1918; Studman, 1935), assessing positive and outgoing behavior versus reserve and shyness.

Eighty years after Webb's (1915) original work, Deary (1996) reanalyzed Webb's data once again, and identified six factors resembling those later found by personality and temperament researchers: (1) Willfulness; (2) Extraversion; (3) Conscientiousness; (4) Affiliation; (5) Intelligence, Humor, Originality; and (6) Negative Mood. Deary saw these factors as similar to the "Big Five" or five-factor model (FFM) currently used to describe the structure of personality traits (Digman, 1990; Digman & Inouye, 1986; Goldberg, 1993; McCrae & Costa, 1987), although the match was not complete. The Big Five and FFM, to be discussed at greater length in Chapter 8, include the broad factors of Extraversion, Agreeableness, Conscientiousness, Neuroticism, and Openness.

Two decades after Webb's (1915) research, Burt (1937, 1938) identified another broad factor, labeled Emotionality or Emotional Instability versus Stability. The emotions in this factor were all negative ones. A similar factor was later identified by Eysenck (1947) and labeled Neuroticism. In a study of neurotic and delinquent children, Burt (1937) also discovered a more specific factor that was obscured by the general negative emotionality factor. One pole of negative emotion was oriented toward "submissiveness, sorrow, tenderness, and disgust, in a word, towards repressive or inhibitive emotions" (p. 182). The other pole "predisposes people towards assertive, angry, sociable, and inquisitive behavior, in short, towards active or aggressive conduct" (Burt, p. 182). Burt's analysis foreshadowed the later distinction between internalizing and externalizing behavior problems and emotions as described in Chapter 9 and findings on temperament that distinguish less assertive (fear, sadness, discomfort) from more assertive (aggressive) negative emotion (Evans & Rothbart, 2007; Victor et al., 2006).

By 1938, Burt had identified the factor of Extraversion–Introversion in addition to Neuroticism. By combining Extraversion and Neuroticism factors, he was able to derive the ancient typology. In this model, the melancholic person is the neurotic introvert, the choleric person is the neurotic extravert, the phlegmatic person is the emotionally stable (non-neurotic) introvert, and the sanguine person is the emotionally stable extravert. Eysenck (1947) would later put forward the same model.

What Eysenck (1947) added to Burt's (1937, 1938) model was a proposed physiological basis for these temperament dimensions. In an early model, he related extraversion–introversion to cortical excitation and inhibition, and neuroticism to limbic system functioning (Eysenck, 1957). In 1967, Eysenck offered a revised model based on the ascending reticular activating system and individual differences in arousability. Later, Gray (1978) proposed an alternative to Eysenck's model, using the dimensions of behavioral activation and inhibition, as well as a fight-and-flight dimension. Behavioral activation was seen as underlying an approach dimension and behavioral inhibition an anxiety dimension. Gray's initial work was mainly based on research with rats, but it continues to be one of the major current psychobiological models of temperament, along with models put forward by Cloninger (1986), Depue and Iacono (1989), Panksepp (1998), and Zuckerman (1991). I take up these models in more detail in Chapter 3. Before leaving Eysenck's work, however, I note that Eysenck too made value judgments about his temperament dimensions, just as Pavlov (1935) had done. Whereas Pavlov more highly valued the "strong," and more extraverted dog, Eysenck appeared to value the introverted person, whom he described as more reliable than the extravert.

Western Europe

Other research on temperament came out of Western Europe, where early Dutch research was influential, although it did not appear to affect Soviet or British work at the time. Heymans and Wiersma (1906) asked 3,000 physicians to each observe a family, including both parents and children, and to fill out a questionnaire on each person. An early form of factor analysis was then applied to over 2,500 questionnaires, extracting three broad factors: (1) *Activity*, the tendency to express or act out what is thought or desired; (2) *Emotivity*, the tendency to show body symptoms and to be fearful and shy; and (3) *Primary–Secondary Function*, the tendency to react immediately versus in a postponed and more organized way. These dimensions foreshadowed three of the broad factors of temperament we study today: Surgency, Negative Affectivity, and Effortful Control. I discuss these temperament factors in Chapter 2.

Heymans and Wiersma (1906) also crossed the extremes of each of these three factors, forming eight types. These were labeled passionate, choleric, phlegmatic, apathetic, sentimental, nervous, sanguine, and amorphous. Heyman and Weirsma's work also inspired longitudinal research on infants in Western Europe. Wallon (1925, 1934) in France, and later Meili and Meili-Dworetzki (1972) in Switzerland, studied individual differences in muscle tension and emotionality in infants, using video recordings of children's behavior, and finding stability over time in infants' distress to intense stimuli. The infant's distress reaction also predicted later behavioral inhibition or shyness at 5 and 7 years. The Swiss work showed a number of similarities to the more recent work of Kagan (1994) and his colleagues (see Zentner, 2008), as well as to work in our laboratory.

At about the same time as Wallon (1925), Carl Jung (1923) developed his theory of extraversion–introversion. Jung saw extraversion as related to a person's outgoing orientation, with rapid approach to external objects and greater physical activity. He described introversion as a disposition toward pulling away from external objects, with a greater preoccupation with internal states. Jung argued that both introverted and extraverted tendencies are present in everyone, but that for a given person, one of the tendencies will be more elaborated and conscious, the other more primitive and unconscious. Jung beautifully described differences in extraversion and introversion in young children:

> The earliest mark of extraversion in a child is his quick adaptation to the environment, and the extraordinary attention he gives to objects, especially to his effect upon them. Shyness in regard to objects is very slight; the child moves and lives among them with trust. He makes quick perceptions, but in a haphazard way. Apparently, he develops more quickly than an introverted child, since he is less cautious, and as a rule, has no fear. Apparently, too, he feels no barrier between himself and objects, and hence he can play with them freely and learn through them. He gladly pushes his undertakings to an extreme, and risks himself in the attempt. Everything unknown seems alluring. (1928, p. 303)

When psychoanalysts like Jung (1928) refer to a person's orientation toward objects, they include social objects (persons) as well as physical objects. Thus, the introverted child is also more wary in new social situations, approaching strangers with fear or caution; the introverted adult tends to react negatively to new situations or social gatherings, showing hesitation and reserve. The extraverted person more readily accepts, approaches, and acts directly upon both social and physical objects. An important idea here is that for extraverted persons, attention is more outwardly focused; introverted persons tend to focus attention more inwardly and are more introspective. Jung (1928) also suggested that the introverted attitude is inclined toward pessimism about future events; the extraverted attitude toward optimism.

Jung was also interested in the relation between temperament and mental illness, suggesting that introverts were prone to *psychasthenia*, "a malady which is characterized on the one hand by an extreme sensitiveness, on the other by a great liability to exhaustion and chronic fatigue" (1923, p. 479). Extraversion, on the other hand, was seen as predisposing the person to *hysteria*, "characterized by an exaggerated rapport with the members of his circle, and a frankly imitatory accommodation to surrounding conditions" (p. 421).

Early Research on Temperament in the United States

In the United States, Gordon Allport (1937, 1961) made major contributions to our understanding of temperament. He identified temperament as a subdomain of his trait-based theory of personality (1961). Like Valentine (1951) at the beginning of this chapter, Allport identified temperament with emotion, and defined temperament as "The characteristic phenomena of an individual's emotional nature, including his susceptibility to emotional stimulation, his customary strength and speed of response, the quality of his prevailing mood, these phenomena being regarded as dependent upon constitutional make-up and, therefore, largely hereditary in origin" (1961, p. 34). Allport, like Valentine, stressed individual differences in emotion in his definition and did not include attention (Thomas & Chess, 1977) and self-regulation, as others have done (Rothbart & Derryberry, 1981).

Cattell (1933a) also carried out research on temperament, asking college students to rate others known to them. He identified four factors of temperament: a Will factor like that of Webb (1915), with characteristics like persistent versus changeable, a Surgency factor; a Maturity factor, including qualities like good-natured versus malicious, a Kind on principle factor, versus absence of kindness; and a Well-adjusted factor, including qualities like emotional versus unemotional and balanced versus extreme.

Cattell (1957) later argued that what a person will do in a given situation depends on his or her traits, abilities, and motivations, and also on the extent to which the environment creates a *press* upon (that is, tends to elicit) those characteristics. If there is no press for fear, the trait of fearfulness will not be relevant to the situation. As the press for a given reaction increases, the trait will more strongly influence a child's behavior. Individuals high on a trait will be more sensitive to the environment's press on that trait than those low on the trait. This is another way of saying that you will not see evidence of a temperament disposition if the situation does not evoke it or press for it, but if the situation tends to elicit it, individual differences in reactivity will appear. This point also stresses the importance of environmental contributions to the child's experiences.

Thus, a young child may be fearful, but his or her parents may attempt to limit his or her exposure to threatening events. When parents avoid exposing the child to fear-provoking situations, or adapt situations so they will not press for the trait, the trait will be less evident, even though its potential for expression will continue. When the child enters school, for example, this new situation will exert a stronger press on the trait of fearfulness. The school setting is also likely to be less flexible and adaptable than the home environment, and teachers may be less (or more) likely than parents to use the child's temperament to inform their actions.

Temperament in Childhood

I now consider some of the early observations of temperament in childhood. The great normative studies of the 1930s in the United States followed infants' development on repeated occasions, searching for the "normal" or normative time at which children developed skills such as crawling or walking. The normative studies also led researchers to discover individual differences in temperament in young children (Gesell, 1928, cited by Kessen, 1965; Shirley, 1933). Researchers like Gesell observed large numbers of children; researchers like Shirley studied a small number of children intensively over time. The goal in both approaches was to establish a timeline for normal sequences of development, known as the "norms" of child development.

Following the small-sample approach, Mary Shirley (1933) intensively observed 25 infants over the first 2 years of their lives. Although she had originally planned to study only motor and intellectual development, she was struck by the differences among the infants that she called the "personality nucleus." Thus, in addition to the volumes on motor and intellectual development she had planned to write, Shirley added a third volume on the infants' core personality or temperament during the first 2 years. Shirley concluded her book by writing personality/temperament sketches of each of the children.

The frontispiece of Shirley's (1933) third volume, a picture of "serene Winnie and expansive Fred" (Figure 1.1), deserves our close attention. First, using Jung's (1928) terms, the photo suggests a distinctively extraverted attitude in Fred, and possibly an introverted attitude in Winnie. Second, the children's facial expressions suggest that they are having quite different emotional experiences in the situation. The twins are also engaging in, and thereby practicing, different behaviors, with a distinctly social bid from Fred and greater social reserve from Winnie.

As a thought experiment, imagine yourself as the photographer.

Would Fred and Winnie bring out the same or different reactions from you?
Would you be likely to pay more attention to Fred because you respond with delight to his joy and desire to be close to you?
Or would you attend more to Winnie, because you feel it is important to respond to the child who does not come forward?
Which child would you be likely to pick up and hold?

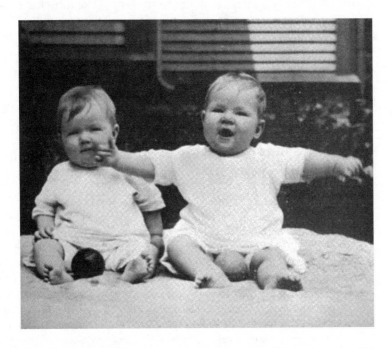

FIGURE 1.1. Winnie and Fred at 35 weeks. From Shirley (1933). Copyright 1933 by the University of Minnesota Press. Reprinted by permission.

The social interchanges of these two children with other people will influence others' expectations and behavior toward them now and in the future.

At the same time, the children's experiences in social interchanges will shape their own views of other people and themselves, and influence their future responses to others. Children's temperament reactions are thus likely to influence their mental models of people (as approachable or dangerous), and of the self (as lovable or unlovable). The influence of temperament on these views of the self and others will be automatic and reflected chiefly in the infant's behavior, but later it can be represented in statements about the self and other people, moving us more clearly into the domain of personality. I revisit these ideas in Chapter 5.

In her research, Shirley (1933) found both general changes in infants' temperament-related behavior over the first 2 years, and stability of differences in children's temperament over time. Based on her observations, Shirley developed at least seven principles of individual differences in infancy:

1. Differences can be seen as early as birth, in "irritability, in tone and timbre of the cry, in activity, and in tonicity of the muscles, as well as in the quality of reactions to the test situations" (p. 216).
2. The personality nucleus "may be observed in a variety of situations with consistent results" (p. 217). In Shirley's research, these included laboratory test situations and interactions of children with their families.
3. Age trends are consistent across the whole group of children, such as showing declines in irritability and distress proneness with age.
4. Each infant exhibits a pattern of traits that changes little with age, even when developmental change is occurring. For example:

> Virginia Ruth and James Dalton both decreased in irritability with age, in accordance with the trend of the group; but the former was consistently the most irritable and the latter the least irritable of the group. A behavior item, moreover, sometimes waned and lapsed, only to be supplanted by another that apparently was its consistent outgrowth. The baby who manifested the first characteristic in a high degree was high in the new trait also. When Virginia Ruth, Maurice, and Matthew gave up screaming, they became the most strongly addicted of the children to escaping from the examination. Similarly, Quentin's timorous crying gave way to apprehensive watching and that in turn to hiding temporarily behind his mother and being reluctant to play and talk in the examiners' presence. (pp. 218–219)

5. Similarities in traits are observed within families. Some families were characterized by shyness, or by high activity level, sociability, or proneness to distress. Shirley suggested that assortative mating, where like marries like, may have influenced these similarities.

6. She also notes that "in some instances specific training by the mother seemed to have little effect in counteracting a strongly established trait or developing one in which the child was weak" (p. 220). This is a critical issue in child development: How do the child's temperament and the parents' socialization attempts affect each other? I return to this question later in the book.

7. Finally, Shirley concludes that

> the evidence marshaled in this study is strongly on the side of innate differences in personality. The early appearance, pervasive nature, and relative stability and permanence of personality traits, their consistent pattern and their harmony with familial traits, all point to a hereditary basis. Developmental change in the frequency with which each trait is manifested supports the maturation hypothesis. To be sure, these results cannot be interpreted as conclusive evidence that personality potentials are laid down in the genes. But they do indicate that personality has its origin and physiological basis in the structure and organization of the nervous system and of the physio-chemical constitution of the body as a whole. Environment, it goes without saying, (also) has its influence on the physiological organism. (p. 220)

When the infants Shirley (1933) had observed were 15 years older, Patricia Neilon (1948) followed up on the sketches Shirley had written about the infants. She obtained independent personality descriptions of the children, who were now adolescents. A group of clinical psychologists then attempted to match the teenagers with their infant personality sketches. These judges performed considerably better than would have been expected by chance. Neilon's results suggested that at least some of the individual differences observed by Shirley in infancy showed considerable developmental stability.

Arnold Gesell (1928, cited in Kessen, 1965), another great normative developmental psychologist, filmed and studied hundreds of children in his Yale laboratory, and was similarly struck by the individual differences he observed. He also noted different developmental pathways among children, and suggested that while some characteristics of the children would be relatively stable, others would be more strongly influenced by socialization. An example of his thinking about developmental outcomes was presented in Gesell's description of CD in the Preface.

Gesell (1928, cited in Kessen, 1965) and Shirley's (1933) observations point to three fundamental concepts in our understanding of temperament and development. First, temperament traits form the nucleus or core of the developing personality and influence the directions or trajectories followed in development. Second, although relative stability of temperament traits across children is expected, outcomes will also depend strongly on developmental changes and on the child's socialization and experience. And finally, as Gesell's discussion of CD indicates, temperamental characteristics allow multiple pathways to developmental outcomes, so that a more surgent child like CD may become a delinquent or a good citizen, empathic or aggressive, depending on training and experience.

Clinical Studies of Temperament

After the work of the normative psychologists, temperament concepts generally disappeared from psychologists' discussions of social and personality development. During this period, social learning theories were in ascendancy. At least one influential theorist at the time argued that personality traits were merely social constructions, not true phenomena (Mischel, 1968), although he created measures of children's self-regulation that later showed the stability that would be expected from temperament or personality traits (Eigsti et al., 2006). During the heyday of social learning theories, environmental influences were seen as almost entirely responsible for personality differences, especially the child's history of rewards or punishments. Freudian or psychoanalytic theory was also influential during this period. It, like the social learning theories, emphasized effects of the environment rather than temperamental individual differences.

Theories of cognitive development views gained ascendancy from the 1960s onward, especially following publication of Flavell's (1963) important introduction to Piaget's theory, and these ideas came to be discussed in my later years in graduate school. As early as the 1940s and 1950s, however, a biologically oriented group of child physicians and clinicians were carrying out significant studies of temperament. Bergman and Escalona (1949), for example, identified children who were strongly reactive to low intensities of stimulation in one or more sensory modalities, especially sight, hearing, and touch. In the 1960s, Sybil Escalona (1968) proposed the fundamentally important concept of the child's *effective experience* on development. Her idea was that events in children's lives are experienced only as they are filtered through the individual child's nervous system, so that an environmental event is not the same for all.

Escalona (1968) noted, for example, that an adult's vigorous play with an infant may lead to pleasure in one child, yet to distress in another. By simply describing environmental events, she argued, we fail to capture essential information about the child's *reaction* to them, that is, the child's effective experience. Thus, we may observe parent–child interaction and note a parent's vigorous stimulation, such as bouncing or tickling the child. Coding the stimulation alone, however, does not capture the child's reaction as influenced by temperament, nor does it tell us anything about the child's experience in the situation. To study experience, we need to observe the child's behavior and physiological or self-reported reactions to the situation. One child may respond with animation and laughter; another may cry and attempt to get away. The heart rate, respiration, and/or cortisol response of two children may differ. One child may tell us he or she had a good time; another that he or she did not.

Murphy and Moriarty (1976) followed up a group of infants who had originally been studied by Escalona (1968). They studied preschool-age children's vulnerability, resiliency, and coping, and I discuss some of their important observations in Chapter 7. During the 1950s and 1960s, Fries and Woolf (1953; Fries, 1954) studied what they called congenital activity type. Korner (1964) studied neonatal individuality and developed an extensive observation schedule for the newborn, and Birns (1965) and her associates (Birns, Barten, & Bridger, 1969) developed some of the earliest laboratory assessments of temperament.

THE NEW YORK LONGITUDINAL STUDY

The most well known clinical studies of temperament in children, however, and indeed of all recent temperament research, was reported by Thomas and Chess and their colleagues in the early 1960s. Thomas, Chess, Birch, Hertzig, and Korn published the first of their volumes on children's reaction patterns in the New York Longitudinal Study (NYLS) in 1963. Later, Michael Rutter suggested they use the term "temperament" to describe their area of study, and this term was adopted for their future publications (Chess & Thomas, personal communication, 1992).

The NYLS findings arrived at a time when researchers in social development were also becoming aware of children's own contributions to their development, laying the groundwork for the study of temperament. These psychologists argued that social influence flows from the child to the parent as well as from the parent to the child. Robert Sears and his associates (e.g., Sears, Maccoby, & Levin, 1957) and others (Bell, 1968; Schaffer & Emerson, 1964) argued that influences in socialization are bidirectional; children are not born as homogeneous lumps of clay to be shaped into their differences by society. Instead, they show variability in behavior that can, in turn, elicit differences in the behavior and attitudes of their parents and teachers. The view that social influence works in both directions seems obvious to us now, but it was major news when it first appeared. At that time, behaviorism held sway in psychology and social learning theories attempted to account for individual differences almost entirely through parental reward and punishment.

Others who stressed children's contributions to their own development were cognitive developmental theorists like Piaget and Kohlberg. Piaget's (1954) observations of how children "construct" their views of the world, based on their experiences with it, emphasized how children influence their own development through their mental representations of events (see also Kohlberg, 1969). As children develop notions of their own self-identity, their thinking becomes an important determinant of the child's personality, and helps to shape concepts of self and others. Later, I consider models of the self and ideas about how cognition influences social development.

A fourth group of researchers were also actively studying the period of infancy (see Osofsky, 1979). One of the goals of their research was to describe the initial state of the infant and to study its relation to later development. Because the initial state of the newborn infant clearly varied from one infant to another (Escalona, 1968; Korner, 1964), early differences in emotions, activity, and attention were seen as providing the raw material for development. This work set the stage for the major contributions of Thomas and Chess (1977) and the NYLS, to be addressed in Chapter 2.

SUMMARY

In this chapter, I have offered a definition for temperament and distinguished temperament from personality. A brief account of adult models of temperament from ancient times was also offered. In Britain and Europe, early factor-analytic research yielded broad traits of introversion and extraversion, negative emotionality, and traits having to do with self-regulation. These dimensions of temperament are examined in more detail in Chapter 2. In that chapter, I also continue the historical review by describing Thomas and Chess's (1977) NYLS and some of its many insights. I then describe a more recent search for the structure of temperament in infancy and childhood, and the temperament dimensions that I and others have identified. In Chapter 3, I consider animal models of temperament and the brain architecture that may underlie these temperament dimensions.

CHAPTER 2

The Structure of Temperament

In the study of temperament, it is not enough to say *that* children differ from one another; we also wish to describe *the ways* in which they
differ. I now ask the question: What are the basic dimensions of temperament? Alexander Thomas and Stella Chess (1977) analyzed parent interviews and identified nine temperament dimensions. More recent research,
however, has revisited and revised their list of temperament dimensions. In
this chapter, I describe some of the measures we have used to discover the
structure of temperament. I then propose that basic temperament characteristics can be used as building blocks for personality, social development,
adjustment, and psychopathology. We begin, however, by continuing our
history of temperament and temperament research with an overview of
results from Thomas and Chess's pioneering study.

THE NYLS

In 1963, Thomas et al. published the first of their volumes on what they
called children's "primary reaction patterns." The term "temperament" was
used in all their subsequent books and papers (Chess & Thomas, personal
communication, 1992). With book titles such as *Your Child Is a Person* (Chess,
Thomas, & Birch, 1985), NYLS researchers argued that children's qualities
were not the simple result of their parents' treatment. Instead, children differ from each other from infancy onward, and are active agents in their

own development. Thomas and Chess (1977) also argued that sometimes a child's temperament makes being a parent difficult, and described a set of temperament traits they saw as "difficult" ones.

Thomas and Chess's Temperament Dimensions

Inspired by differences they had observed among their own adopted children, and reacting against the idea that individual differences were solely the result of parental influence, Chess and Thomas set out to study infants' reaction patterns in the NYLS (Thomas et al., 1963; Thomas, Chess, & Birch, 1968). First, they collected extensive interviews from 22 parents of 3- to 6-month-old infants. Parents were asked about their infants' reactions in a wide range of everyday situations including feeding, diaper changing, playing, and bathing. Here is an example of questions and answers from Thomas et al. (1963):

> INTERVIEWER: "What did the baby do the first time he was given cereal?"
>
> PARENT: "He couldn't stand it. . . . "
>
> INTERVIEWER: "What makes you think he disliked it? What did he do?"
>
> PARENT: "He spit it out and when another spoonful was offered he turned his head to the side."

As we have done in later temperament questionnaires, Thomas, Chess, and their NYLS colleagues were looking beyond parents' general judgments about their children to the concrete behaviors of the child that supported them.

From these interviews, large amounts of information were gathered about each child, and the researchers' next step was to decide how to analyze and summarize it. Chess and Thomas asked colleague Herbert Birch to help them organize the information they had gathered (Chess & Thomas, personal communication, 1992). To begin this task, Birch asked that each infant reaction, along with the setting in which it had occurred, be typed on a slip of paper (e.g., the infant's spitting out a new food, or kicking, splashing, or sitting quietly in the bath). Birch then sorted these slips according to the kinds of infant reactions that seemed to go together conceptually. Answers to the question about babies' movement in the bath, for example, were sorted into a category that also included activity in other situations, and later this dimension was called activity level. Answers to questions about how loudly and long a baby cried, or how vigorously he or she laughed, were sorted into an intensity category.

The nine categories that emerged from Birch's content analysis of infants' reactions came to represent the nine NYLS temperament dimensions (Chess & Thomas, personal communication, 1992; Thomas et al., 1963). These were labeled (1) *activity level*, defined as the level, tempo, and frequency of motor activity; (2) *rhythmicity*, the regularity and predictability of sleep, hunger, feeding, and elimination; (3) *approach versus withdrawal*, the child's first response, positive or negative, to novel objects, persons, or situations; (4) *adaptability*, the ease of modifying the child's response to new or altered situations in the direction desired by the caregiver; (5) *threshold*, the intensity of stimulation required for the child to respond; (6) *intensity*, the energy level of the child's reaction, irrespective of the kind of reaction or stimulation; (7) *mood*, "the amount of pleasant, joyful, friendly behavior as contrasted with unpleasant, crying, unfriendly behavior" (Thomas et al., 1968, p. 23); (8) *distractibility*, the interference with or changes in direction of the child's behavior in response to external stimulation; and (9) *attention span/persistence*, the duration of the child's activities and their continuation even when the child has become frustrated.

Over 100 families were later added to the NYLS, and all interviews were scored on each of these dimensions. In addition, the NYLS researchers used five of the nine temperament dimensions to categorize infants as "difficult" or "easy" (Thomas et al., 1963, 1968). Difficult children were described as withdrawing, having mostly negative mood, unadaptability to change, intense, and irregular. Infants who were located at the opposite pole of these five dimensions—high in approach, positive mood, adaptability, low intensity, and high regularity—were described as "easy." A "slow-to-warm-up" child was also identified, including infants who were withdrawing at first but low in the intensity of their reactions. Over time, they showed adaptability to change. When clinical psychologists and physicians used the NYLS labels of difficult, easy, and slow to warm up, they were able to argue that the parents were doing their best with a child, but their child was simply difficult to parent. Perhaps because the difficult, easy, and slow-to-warm-up categories were similar to ones parents were already using to describe their children, they have had tremendous staying power in the temperament literature, despite problems they have posed for research. I discuss some of these problems below. However, I begin by considering Chess and Thomas's (1986) contribution of the "goodness of fit" idea.

Goodness of Fit

Chess and Thomas developed the important idea of "goodness of fit" for thinking about temperament and development. Goodness of fit was said to occur "when the child's capacities, motivations, and temperament are adequate to master the demands, expectations, and opportunities of the environment" (1986, p. 380). Their idea was that a given situation will be a better fit for some children than for others, depending on the child's temperament. Thus, an active, athletic family may welcome an active and fearless infant, but the same child will be less appreciated in a family where quiet, sedate, and well-controlled behavior is valued. If parents welcome or adapt to the child's temperamental characteristics, there will be a "good fit"; if the child's behaviors meet with disapproval, there will be a "poor fit."

Sometimes, a "good fit" has been interpreted as being a direct match between the temperament of the child and the parent or teacher. It is important to remember, however, that there can be a good fit between caregiver demands and expectations and the child's temperament even when the child's and adult's temperaments are quite different. A family may actually value temperament characteristics that are dissimilar from the parents' temperament. An extraverted child, for example, may be valued in a shy family, given the positive value our society places on being outgoing (see Chapter 6), even though the parents themselves are shy.

Chess and Thomas (1984) gave as an example of a "poor fit" the case of Roy, a highly distractible child. As an infant, Roy's distractibility allowed his parents to soothe him quickly when he was upset; he was thus seen as a good baby and not at all difficult. As Roy grew older, however, his distractibility led his parents to see him as unreliable and forgetful. By the time he entered school, his mother often nagged him to get things done, and Roy coped with his mother's nagging by tuning out her messages. As seen by his parents, Roy's behavior did not improve over time, and his mother was unable to recognize that what had made Roy a "good" baby was now linked to his "difficult" and unreliable behavior at home and at school. One of the goals of Stella Chess's clinical work (Chess et al., 1985) was to point out to parents the continuities in their child's behavior over time, helping them realize that a temperament trait may be seen positively in one situation or period of development, but as a problem at another. Chess also helped them come to see their child as a separate person, independent from the parent's notions of what their child should ideally be, and to take the child's temperament into account in social interaction (Chess et al.).

Difficult Temperament

Thomas and Chess's longitudinal study followed their sample of infants over time, and a number of the children were followed into adulthood (Chess & Thomas, 1990). Meanwhile, the NYLS findings were greatly influencing developmental psychology, providing the basis for many studies of temperament in childhood. These included studies of children's difficultness. Recall that NLYS difficultness was based on high scores for children on intensity and negative mood, and low scores on approach–withdrawal, adaptability, and rhythmicity. This difficult temperament measure was based on an early NYLS factor analysis. Some researchers, however, have criticized both the concept and the way it is measured (Kohnstamm, 1989; Plomin, 1982; Rothbart, 1982).

There are several bases for criticism of the difficult child concept. One is that a given behavior may create difficulty for one adult, but not for another. In addition, a behavior that creates problems in one situation may not be a problem in another, and indeed may even be an asset. A long attention span, for example, may be helpful when children are busy amusing themselves, leaving their parents free to make dinner, but may become difficult when the child is called to dinner, and isn't ready to leave his or her activity. The case of Roy from the NYLS also illustrates that what is seen as easy and helpful at one age may be seen as difficult at another: distractibility thus may help in soothing the infant, but be related to the older child's being late for school and not completing homework assignments. Calling a child difficult also attaches a negative label to the child, even when most children's behavior is in fact sometimes "difficult," yet often "easy." Parents' perceptions of *what* behaviors are "easy" or "difficult" also vary from one culture to another, as I further discuss in Chapter 6.

Indeed, components of the Thomas and Chess difficultness category have been linked to positive characteristics. Withdrawal or fear, part of the "difficult infant" construct, predicts higher levels of conscience in preschool children and lower aggression later in childhood (Kochanska, 1991, 1995; Rothbart & Bates, 2006), although it also predicts later anxiety. Negative emotionality in adults is related to their ability to detect errors when they are solving problems (Luu, Collins, & Tucker, 2000). Cultural values also influence adults' views of whether a child is "easy" or "difficult" (Korn & Gannon, 1983; Super et al., 2008). Although industrialized Western societies usually associate difficulty with a child's proneness to negative emotion, for example, difficulty in Taiwan and Brazil is not associated with negative emotion, but instead with a weak and unhealthy infant (Mull, 1991, as cited by Wachs, 2000).

Finally, there is the problem that difficulty is often measured differently from one study to another. The five dimensions of difficulty: withdrawal, negative mood, unadaptability, high intensity, and irregularity that emerged from the NYLS factor analysis have not been replicated in later analyses. Rhythmicity typically does not cluster with the other measures, and thus is sometimes included in difficulty measures, and sometimes not. Distractibility and Resistance to Control are also sometimes included in the measure of difficulty because parents find these behaviors difficult, even though they were not part of the original construct. This wide range of definitions for difficulty causes confusion for those who read the research, and we need to be very careful in understanding how difficulty is measured in a given study.

At the same time, there *is* agreement that some aspects of a child's temperament create challenges for parents, and several studies have found that children who are high in negative emotionality and socially demanding are more likely to develop behavior problems later in life (Bates, 1989a, 1989b). Thus, difficulty could be defined as negative emotionality as proposed by Bates, Freeland, and Lounsberry (1979), or as resistance to control in older infants and children. In my own view, "difficulty" is a value judgment on specific temperament tendencies that has caused confusion in the field, although it is real in the mind of observers. I take up this issue in later chapters, but now consider measurement approaches to studying temperament by the psychologists who have followed Thomas and Chess's pioneering temperament research on children.

APPROACHES TO THE STUDY OF TEMPERAMENT

The most widely used approaches to measuring temperament in children have been questionnaires filled out by caregivers who know the child well, self-report questionnaires, naturalistic observations of children's behavior in the home or school, mechanical measures such as actometers that assess children's movement and activity, structured observations and cognitive tasks in the laboratory, and, when children have developed the necessary language and cognitive skills, the child's own reports about his or her reactions and behavior. Each approach offers advantages to the researcher, and in our laboratory at Oregon we have used all of them except actometers.

Questionnaires make use of the repeated observations caregivers have made of their children in many different situations. This satisfies the need for demonstrating that a trait is consistent across situations and stable over time, and allows a large number of temperament characteristics to be measured at the same time. With measurement of multiple temperament characteristics, we can also perform factor analyses to see which of the temperament dimensions are related to each other, letting us better determine the overall structure of temperament. Questionnaires are also relatively inexpensive to develop, administer, and analyze, and large numbers of families are available to take part in questionnaire research (Bates, 1989b, 1994). Overall, they have formed an essential element in large-scale studies of normal development and the development of psychopathology, as I discuss in Chapters 8, 9, and 10.

Other approaches to measuring temperament offer different advantages and disadvantages. In the laboratory, the child is exposed to a number of situations chosen to elicit a range of reactions. In the Laboratory Temperament Assessment Battery (LAB-TAB; Goldsmith & Rothbart, 1990), for example, children are exposed to a novel mechanical toy that moves in unpredictable ways, an approaching stranger, and masks that tend to elicit fear. Children's reactions to the events are coded from videotapes, and scores from each of the episodes are combined to give an overall fear score. Laboratory observations of temperament allow researchers careful control of the stimuli used to elicit children's behavior and fairly precise observations of the infant's or child's responses. In addition, observations and live coding of children's behavior in the home or school, or videotaping and later coding the child's reactions, give us information about children in their usual settings.

Because direct observations of temperament are more objective on the face of it than parents' reports, Jerome Kagan (1998) has argued that parent-report questionnaires should not be used in child development research. However, we (Rothbart & Bates, 1998, 2006) have reviewed evidence for agreement between parent-reported measures and other measures of temperament, and as the reader will see, many of the most exciting discoveries in the temperament area have come from parent-reported data, just as many of the most exciting discoveries in the personality area have come from self-report questionnaires.

Temperament researchers have been very aware of potential problems with parent and caregiver reports, but also know that laboratory and home observations have their own measurement problems and sources of error, as described below. In parent and teacher questionnaires, caregivers may not notice, or may fail to remember, the behaviors of their children. If caregivers are trying to describe their child in the best possible light or as having problems, they may also give biased reports. It may seem odd that parents would ever show a negative bias, but when parents are seeking clinical treatment for their children, they may exaggerate the child's negative qualities in order to get help.

Naturalistic home observations can avoid parent biases, but they bring with them different problems. Home observations are expensive and limited in what they can measure. Many temperament-related behaviors occur only rarely in the home, and the limited time we are able to spend in the home may not include them. Even if temperament-related behaviors do occur, repeated visits of the observer may be required to get enough information for a reliable measure (Epstein, 1984). In on-the-spot live coding of reactions, there are also limits as to how many different behaviors can be observed and recorded within a short period of time. Videotaping of the child's behavior is an improvement, but multiple cameras may be needed to capture both the child's behavior and the events that have led to the child's reaction. In our early pilot testing with multiple cameras (Rothbart, 1986), we found that cameras and their operators created a kind of circus in the child's home, calling the attention of the child and possibly influencing the behaviors we had set out to measure. With the recent miniaturization of cameras, however, this would presumably be less of a problem.

Although laboratory measurements offer considerable objectivity, other problems are likely to arise. When children are brought to a new and strange place, with strange objects and adults present, some children will become quite fearful or apprehensive, and their fearfulness can affect their other temperament-related reactions. The fear reaction may, for example, shut down or inhibit children's smiling and laughter or their expressions of anger. Other children will become more positively excited in the laboratory than in their usual settings, and may act more impulsively than usual.

Laboratory situations can also put artificial limits on children's responses. For example, in our laboratory observations (Rothbart, Derryberry, & Hershey, 2000), the infant was seated in a high chair while mechanical toys were presented; this situation prevents the child from leaving the situation or directly contacting the mother. If crawling away or clinging to the mother is the child's usual coping strategy for strangeness, this setting prevents their occurrence. The laboratory situation may also increase the child's distress because he or she is frustrated in his or her usual response. An additional problem is carryover effects from one laboratory episode to the next, especially if the child has become distressed in one episode (e.g., a mechanical toy) and is not completely soothed before the next one (e.g., a stranger approach). As in the home, the number of observations possible in a single visit is also very limited, and repeated visits to the laboratory may be necessary to measure any one temperament trait reliably.

More detailed discussions of the advantages and problems of each of these methods can be found in Bates (1987, 1989b, 1994), Goldsmith and Rothbart (1991), Rothbart and Bates (1998, 2006), and Slabach, Morrow, and Wachs (1991). In temperament research, we try to be aware of potential problems for each of the methods we use and to deal with them as best we can. We also use multiple methods in coming to conclusions about temperament. When similar findings are obtained from different methods, each with its own quite different strengths and weaknesses, we can feel a good deal more confident about what we have learned (Stanovitch, 1997).

Questionnaire Research

In measuring temperament traits, we wish to identify those responses of children that show consistency across situations and stability over time. A single measurement of a behavior does not allow us to determine consistency of reaction; multiple items or repeated measures are needed. To date, questionnaires have allowed the most extensive and fine-grained measures of temperament, and I describe these in some detail. Results from laboratory and home observations are added to elaborate on questionnaire findings. Laboratory studies in infancy are also described that have been used to predict parent-reported temperament in middle childhood (e.g., Rothbart et al., 2000).

In designing questionnaires, we create sets of items that will allow us to measure temperament across a range of situations. To minimize possible problems with the respondents' memory, we ask parents about recent behaviors of their children (e.g., during the past 2 weeks). To avoid asking parents to compare their child with other children (parents of first children, for example, may have very little experience with other infants), we ask about the frequency of occurrence of concrete behaviors (like spitting out food, turning away, splashing the bath water) rather than the presence of general traits. Because humans are able to make good judgments of the frequency of events (Hasher & Zachs, 1979), we ask how often a child performed a given action in a particular setting.

In the Infant Behavior Questionnaire (IBQ; IBQ-R; Gartstein & Rothbart, 2003; Rothbart, 1981), for example, parents are asked about children's distress when a toy is taken away, when they lose an object, or when they are restrained from an action (see sample items in Table 2.1). If parents who report high levels of the child's distress to limitations (anger/frustration) in one situation also tend to report high levels of distress to limitations in other situations, and parents who report little distress to limitations in one situation also tend to report little or no distress in other situations, we will find a positive relation or correlation between the items. Shared relations within a set of similar items are interpreted as measuring a shared underlying tendency, in this case, anger/frustration. Correlations could also result from a third influence, such as the parents' sensitivity to, or memory for, distress. Because of this, we seek support for our findings by using other methods as well.

TABLE 2.1. Scale Definitions and Sample Items for the Infant Behavior Questionnaire—Revised

Scale	Definition (sample item)
Factor 1—Surgency	
Approach	Rapid approach, excitement, and positive anticipation of pleasurable activities. ("When given a new toy, how often did the baby get very excited about getting it?")
Vocal reactivity	Amount of vocalization exhibited by the baby in daily activities. ("When being dressed or undressed, how often did the baby coo or vocalize?")
High-intensity pleasure	Pleasure or enjoyment related to high stimulus intensity, rate, complexity, novelty, and incongruity. ("During a peek-a-boo game, how often did the baby smile?")
Smiling and laughter	Smiling or laughter during general caretaking and play. ("How often did the baby smile or laugh when given a toy?")
Activity level	Gross motor activity, including movement of arms and legs, squirming and locomotor activity. ("When put into the bath water, how often did the baby splash or kick?")
Perceptual sensitivity	Detection of slight, low-intensity stimuli from the external environment. ("How often did the baby notice fabrics with scratchy texture – e.g., wool?")
Factor 2—Negative Reactivity	
Sadness	Lowered mood and activity related to personal suffering, physical state, object loss, or inability to perform a desired action; general low mood. ("Did the baby seem sad when the caregiver was gone for an unusually long period of time?")
Distress to limitations; anger/frustration	Fussing, crying, or showing distress while (1) in a confining place or position, (2) in caretaking activities, or (3) unable to perform a desired action. ("When placed on his or her back, how often did the baby fuss or protest?")
Fear	Startle or distress to sudden changes in stimulation, novel physical objects, or social stimuli; inhibited approach to novelty. ("How often did the baby startle to a sudden or loud noise?")
Falling reactivity/rate of recovery (negative loading)	Rate of recovery from peak distress, excitement, or general arousal; ease of falling asleep. ("When frustrated with something, how often did the baby calm down within 5 minutes?")

(cont.)

TABLE 2.1. *(cont.)*

Scale	Definition (sample item)
Factor 3—Orienting/regulation	
Low-intensity pleasure	Amount of pleasure or enjoyment related to low stimulus intensity, rate, pleasure complexity, novelty, and incongruity. ("When playing quietly with one of his/her favorite toys, how often did the baby show pleasure?")
Cuddliness	Expression of enjoyment and molding of the body to being held by a caregiver. ("When rocked or hugged, how often did the baby seem to enjoy him/herself?")
Duration of orienting	Attention to and/or interaction with a single object for extended periods of time. ("How often did the baby stare at a mobile, crib bumper, or picture for 5 minutes or longer?")
Soothability	Reduction of fussing, crying, or distress when soothing techniques are used by the caregiver. ("When patting or gently rubbing some part of the baby's body, how often did s/he soothe immediately?")

The Empirical Approach to Questionnaire Development

Two major approaches to designing questionnaires have been followed. One starts with a broad set of questionnaire items, collects responses to these items, and then uses statistical techniques like factor analysis to identify the items that are or are not related to each other. In factor analysis, if items in one group are more related to each other than they are to items in other groups of items, they are identified as contributing to a factor. The number of factors arising from this analysis gives the researcher an idea of the smallest number of organized groups of items present in the questionnaire. In turn, these groupings may represent shared underlying processes, giving us information about the possible biological structure of temperament.

Interpreting factor analysis is not wholly straightforward, and there is no single correct way to decide how many factors are present in a set of data (Gorsuch, 1983). However, even when different rules are used for deciding the number of factors, there is often considerable agreement in our findings. When agreement is found, and the factors also appear to be psychologically and physiologically meaningful, they give us an idea about how individual differences in temperament are organized.

THE EXAMPLE OF INTELLIGENCE

The first area in which the structure of individual differences was studied was in the measurement of intelligence. Thurstone and Thurstone (1941), for example, extracted intelligence factors from a large number of tests. The broad factors they found included *numerical quickness* (speed of calculation), *verbal understanding* (comprehension of words' meanings), *word fluency* (generating words), *perceptual speed* (noticing details), *spatial visualization* (of objects rotated in space), *memory* (for words, letters, or numbers), and *induction* (the ability to identify a rule describing a diverse set of information). Scores on a number of these factors are also related to an overall intelligence factor, called *g* for general intelligence.

A neural basis for the *g* factor has more recently been identified. John Duncan and his associates (2000) used positron emission tomography (PET) to identify the brain areas activated in adults when intelligence test items measuring *g* are presented. Adults' brain images were measured as they performed a wide variety of verbal, perceptual, motor, and spatial tasks that were highly correlated with *g,* and these were compared with images made during tasks that showed low correlations with *g.* Brain activations to the high-*g* tasks were found in the anterior cingulate and lateral prefrontal cortex, areas related to the control of thought across a broad range of tasks (executive attention) that we discuss in Chapter 3. It was exciting to see that an organization that had originally emerged from factor analysis of intelligence items was reflected in a specific brain organization. We are now finding this to be the case in temperament as well, as is also discussed in Chapter 3.

The Rational Approach to Questionnaire Development

A second approach to questionnaire building, called the *rational* approach, is more theoretical in its early stages, and this is the approach we have used in the development of temperament questionnaires. First, the temperament dimensions we wish to measure are identified. This is done through a thorough search of previous theories and studies of individual differences in temperament for possible dimensions of temperament (e.g., fear, anger, and positive emotion). We then create a definition for each dimension and write scale items based on that definition. In our initial questionnaire, we created scales for all nine of the Thomas and Chess (1977) dimensions, and added scales for fear and anger because of their presence in animal research (Diamond, 1957).

Items are written to fit the definition of each proposed dimension (see Table 2.1). For example, in developing the Infant Behavior Questionnaire

(IBQ; Rothbart, 1981), we defined activity level as a child's gross motor activity, including movement of arms and legs, squirming, and locomotor activity. Items were generated to fit the definition, and these items formed a test scale. I then sat down individually with parents who read and commented aloud on each item to make sure that the item was easy to understand. A large group of parents then filled out the test questionnaires on their babies, and statistical tests were performed to determine whether the items we expected to be related were in fact related to each other. Based on these data, we learned that infants who kicked and splashed in the bath also moved about in the crib, one of many correlations indicating a tendency of children to be more or less active. In some of our proposed dimensions, however, answers to the items we had expected to be related were not, raising questions about use of the dimension as an aspect of temperament.

Once a group of scales is constructed and administered to a large group of parents, factor analysis is performed to see relations among scale scores. In one broad factor, for example, children's scores on activity level were related to their level of smiling and laughter and to their preferences for seeking high-intensity stimulation (Gartstein & Rothbart, 2003). In addition to using this kind of exploratory factor analysis, confirmatory factor analysis can also be used to test whether a predicted organization of temperament is found. In confirmatory factor analysis, the researcher predicts that certain items or scales will contribute to one factor, while other items or scales will be related to other factors. The fit of different theoretical predictions to the data is then tested.

Averaging across Items

Whether we use questionnaires, home observations, or laboratory measures of temperament, multiple items are used to measure each trait or dimension. This is done because no single item or measure can give us a general measure of a given temperament trait or dimension. Because the definition of a trait requires that it show consistency across situations and stability over time, multiple items must be used. Another reason for averaging is that although an item or observation is expected to reflect temperament, temperament will be only one of many influences on any given reaction. Consider, for example, an infant's fearful reaction to a stranger. In addition to temperamental fearfulness, other contributions to distress may come from a passing negative mood, pain from getting a new tooth, discomfort from coming down with a cold, or the fact that this stranger was highly intrusive and disturbing, and would have frightened almost any child.

In some cases, these influences extraneous to temperament will increase the child's fear score; in other cases, they will lower it. We assume that these other influences occur at random, so that some of them will tend to give the child a higher score on an item, and some a lower score. The child's temporary state, mood, individual history, or other sources of extraneous influence will thus tend to cancel each other out when a number of items are averaged. By creating an overall score on a scale by averaging items, we expect that we will capture a consistent individual difference, and the quality of our measure of temperament will be improved. In parent-report questionnaires, we take advantage of the many observations a parent makes of an infant or a young child by writing multiple items. In self-report questionnaires, we take advantage of the many observations we make of our own thoughts, actions, and feelings, many of which are not available to outside observers.

Averaging is also used in laboratory measures. Thus, we repeatedly evoke a heart-rate reaction or an electroencephalographic (EEG) reaction through many presentations of a given stimulus. We then average over many measurements to remove effects of extraneous influences present in any single observation. In laboratory observations, multiple episodes measure the child's response to a stranger, a novel object, or a physically threatening situation, and episode measures are combined for the overall measure of the dimension. Because a large number of repeated observations are necessary to obtain good measurement in the laboratory, it is often difficult to measure more than one dimension on a single occasion. Perhaps because of this difficulty, researchers who limit themselves to laboratory studies have often measured only one or two temperament constructs at a time (see Kagan & Fox, 2006). They have most often concentrated on children's fearfulness, shyness, or behavioral inhibition, or on children's outgoing or impulsive tendencies. This is an important contribution, but it cannot capture the full range of temperamental variability.

THE STRUCTURE OF TEMPERAMENT IN INFANCY

We now consider the structure of temperament that has emerged in studies of infancy and childhood. Recall that Thomas and Chess (1977) and their colleagues identified nine dimensions of temperament in their parent interviews: activity level, rhythmicity, approach versus withdrawal, adaptability, threshold, intensity, mood, distractibility, and attention span/persistence. Thomas and Chess (1977; Thomas et al., 1963, 1968) also defined temperament as the *style*, but not the *content* of behavior, the "how," but not the "what" or "why" of behavior. Although Thomas and Chess said that they were not interested in the "what" of the child's reaction, several of their temperament dimensions do seem to measure what the child does rather than how he or she does it. Thus, in mood, positive versus negative emotion is measured. In approach–withdrawal, specific tendencies of the child toward or away from new objects or situations are measured.

Nevertheless, some of Thomas and Chess's (1977) dimensions do appear to deal with style. In the dimension of threshold, the child's sensitivity to different forms of low-intensity stimulation is measured across situations, and in the dimension of intensity, the strength of the child's reaction is also measured across many kinds of responses. If style were the essence of temperament, we would expect scores across a wide variety of stimulation situations (for threshold) and child responses (for intensity) to be interrelated. Two other style dimensions are rhythmicity and adaptability. Following Thomas and Chess's definitions, consistency of children's rhythmicity would be expected across sleep, feeding, and elimination; for adaptability, consistency of children's adaptability to what their parents desired would be expected, irrespective of what the behavior was or the situation in which it was measured. Although threshold, rhythmicity, adaptability, and intensity could easily be called "style," these were in fact the sets of temperament items that proved *not* to be related to each other; they did not yield reliable measures of temperament (Rothbart, 1981).

Revising the NYLS Dimensions

In the late 1970s, Doug Derryberry and I began our theoretical review of temperament models. The results of that review when combined with the results of our infant questionnaire work would influence how we saw the temperament dimensions identified by Thomas and Chess (1977) and how we thought about temperament generally (Rothbart, 1981; Rothbart & Derryberry, 1981). Because we wished to develop strong and reliable measures for the temperament dimensions Thomas and Chess had identified, and because we had found additional dimensions to explore from the behavior genetics and animal temperament areas, we set out to develop 11 scales for parent-reported temperament. These included the nine dimensions identified by Thomas and Chess, as well as scales for fear and frustration/distress to limitations.

The results of our research were a surprise at the time (Rothbart, 1981). We had expected the NYLS dimensions to yield internally consistent scales. In several cases, however, the items did not have strong enough correlations with each other to create consistent or homogeneous scales: infants, for example, did not tend to be intense across all temperamental dispositions. Some were intense in fear, but not intense in positive mood; some were intense in activity but not in fear. This meant that the intensity dimension was not represented as one of our final scales. Similarly, thresholds for reaction differed across situations and temperamental dispositions, and some infants responded to low intensities of fear stimuli, whereas others responded to low intensities of positive or anger producing stimuli. This meant we could not develop a homogeneous threshold scale. Adaptability in Thomas and Chess's (1979) model had to do with infants' general tendencies to adapt in the direction wished by the parents. This dimension was also not internally consistent. Some of the adaptability items had to do with how soothable the child was, however, and these items were related to each other, allowing us to develop a soothability scale. Rhythmicity was another scale that did not hold together: children who were regular in their bowel habits were not necessarily rhythmic in their sleeping and eating habits.

These results questioned Thomas and Chess's (1977) definition of temperament as "style," in that the style variables of intensity, threshold, adaptability, and rhythmicity showed little consistency across situations and responses. The reader may recall the findings by researchers in the Soviet Union that their temperament variables such as strength of nervous system did not hold up over different stimulus situations and different responses. This led them to move toward temperament questionnaires, where they could study the temperament dimensions that appeared more reliably across situations and over time (Strelau, 1983).

So if temperament isn't style, what is it? The results of our studies led us to take a much more biological view of temperament (Rothbart & Derryberry, 1981). Recall that Thomas and Chess had a dimension for mood, which was supposed to extend from positive mood at one pole to negative mood at the other pole. Using their model, it would not be possible for a child to be high on both positive and negative emotion. A similar dimension was approach–withdrawal, measuring a child's tendency to either approach or withdraw from novel stimuli and situations. Once again, however, we could not create homogeneous scales following Thomas and Chess's (1977) model. Instead, the mood scale fell apart into its positive emotion and negative emotion components, with its positive items linked to approach and its negative items to withdrawal groups of items from approach–withdrawal scale. Positive emotion items were related to approach and activity level, in a broad dimension of positive emotionality that we labeled Surgency. We took this name from Raymond Cattell's (1973) dimension of positive emotion and approach. This meant we could develop separate measures, allowing a given child to be high on *both* positive and negative emotionality, low on both, or high on one and low on the other. Our final scales measured fear, frustration, positive affect, activity level, duration of orienting, and soothability. See Table 2.1 for scale definitions.

Jenny Mauro and I (Rothbart & Mauro, 1990) later reviewed a large number of studies on the structure of temperament, finding considerable agreement in studies across laboratories. In these studies, when a style scale such as threshold was reliable, it was usually limited to a single kind of response, for example, sensitivity to dirty diapers. The revised list of temperament scales for infancy based on this review included fearful distress, irritable distress/frustration, positive affect and approach (surgency), attention span/persistence, and rhythmicity. Rhythmicity items were very limited, and usually related to only one response system, such as sleeping.

Mauro and I also found that researchers often used different names for measures that in fact were very similar, and similar names for measures that were in fact quite different (Rothbart & Mauro, 1990). For this reason, we have advised researchers who wish to use a temperament measure to look at both the scale definition and the items in the scale to make sure of what they are measuring. Studies of infant temperament scales with different names have also been found to measure quite similar dimensions. Goldsmith and Rieser-Danner (1986) asked mothers and day care teachers of infants ages 4–8 months to fill out three different infant questionnaires, the Revised Infant Temperament Questionnaire (RITQ; Carey & McDevitt, 1978), the Infant Characteristics Questionnaire (ICQ; Bates et al., 1979), and the Infant Behavior Questionnaire (IBQ; Rothbart, 1981). Several scales had been given different names in these instruments, but in all cases, the correlations among measures of similar dimensions were high.

The temperament dimensions emerging from our research with infants and young children also yielded dimensions very similar to dimensions of temperament identified in nonhuman animals. In animals, reactions to danger (fear), obstacles (frustration), or reward seeking (approach) have been called *emotional operating systems* by Panksepp (1998). Emotional operating systems have developed in animals over the course of evolution, allowing the organism to act in adaptive ways to environmental threats and opportunities. Applying this idea, temperament dimensions go beyond style definitions to include both the "what" (emotional operating systems) and the "why" (evolution) of behavior. They describe the sensitivity of emotional systems and related motivations, along with the efficiency of attentional systems, as discussed later in this chapter. Temperament dimensions that have emerged from other animal species are discussed in Chapter 3.

Over the years, we have identified additional temperament dimensions, and have also developed a broader and more fine-grained measure of infant temperament in the Infant Behavior Questionnaire—Revised (IBQ-R; Gartstein & Rothbart, 2003, see Table 2.1). In addition to the six scales from the original IBQ (activity level, fear, smiling and laughter, anger/frustration, soothability, and duration of orienting), new scales assess infants' approach, vocal reactivity, sadness, perceptual sensitivity, high- and low-intensity pleasure, and falling reactivity. Because advances in neuroscience have also led to increased interest in affiliative temperament systems (e.g., Panksepp, 1998), our revised questionnaire also included a scale for cuddliness, as a measure of affiliation toward others in infancy (Gartstein & Rothbart).

Factor analyses of scale scores in the IBQ-R yielded three broad factors of temperament in infants 3–12 months of age (Gartstein & Rothbart, 2003; see Table 2.1). The first we called Surgency, including scales of approach, smiling and laughter, activity level, and vocal activity. The second is a general factor of Negative Affectivity, with loadings from sadness, frustration, falling reactivity (contributing negatively), and fear. Fear, however, has very low loadings on this factor, and when we analyzed the data separately for older infants, fear formed a separate factor from the other negative emotions. We also extracted a third broad factor called Orienting/Regulation, including cuddliness, soothability, duration of orienting, and low-intensity pleasure. Higher Regulation was related to higher Surgency and lower Negative Affectivity. Factors, scales, and sample items from the IBQ-R are listed in Table 2.1.

THE STRUCTURE OF TEMPERAMENT IN CHILDHOOD

When we compare the structure of temperament in infancy with its structure in the preschool and primary school years, there are only a few differences, but they are important ones. When we developed the Children's Behavior Questionnaire (CBQ; Rothbart, Ahadi, & Hershey, 1994; Rothbart, Ahadi, Hershey, & Fisher, 2001) for 3- to 7-year-olds, we added a number of scales to broaden the content of the questionnaire. These had emerged from the IBQ (Rothbart, 1981) and from an adult temperament measure we had developed (Derryberry & Rothbart, 1988; see also Evans & Rothbart, 2007). The scales, with sample items, are given in Table 2.2. All of these scales proved to be homogeneous and appropriate for research.

Factor analyses of the CBQ scale scores also yielded three broad factors, shown in Table 2.2. These have emerged in studies performed in the United States, China, and Japan (Ahadi, Rothbart, & Ye, 1993; Kochanska, DeVet, Goldman, Murray, & Putnam, 1993). The first factor, called Surgency, includes scales measuring approach, impulsivity, high-intensity pleasure (sensation seeking), and activity level, with a negative contribution from shyness. The second, called Negative Affectivity, includes scales of discomfort, fear, anger/frustration, sadness, and soothability (contributing negatively). The third factor, labeled Effortful Control, includes inhibitory control, attentional focusing, low-intensity pleasure, and perceptual sensi-

TABLE 2.2. Scale Definitions and Sample Items for the Children's Behavior Questionnaire

Scale	Definition (sample item)
Factor 1—Surgency	
Activity level	Level of gross motor activity including rate and extent of locomotion. ("Tends to run, rather then walk, from room to room.")
Approach; positive anticipation	Amount of excitement and positive anticipation for expected pleasurable activities. ("Shows great excitement when opening a present.")
High-intensity pleasure	Amount of pleasure or enjoyment related to situations involving high stimulus intensity, rate, complexity, novelty, and incongruity. ("Likes to go high and fast when pushed on a swing.")
Impulsivity	Speed of response initiation. ("Often rushes into new situations.")
Shyness (negative loading)	Slow or inhibited approach in situations involving novelty or uncertainty. ("Sometimes prefers to watch rather than join other children playing.")
Smiling and laughter	Amount of positive affect in response to changes in stimulus intensity, rate, complexity, and incongruity. ("Smiles when looking at a picture book.")
Factor 2—Negative affectivity	
Anger/frustration	Amount of negative affect related to interruption of ongoing tasks or goal blocking. ("Gets angry when told she has to go to bed.")
Discomfort	Amount of negative affect related to sensory qualities of stimulation, including intensity, rate, or complexity of light, movement, sound, and texture. ("Is bothered by light or color that is too bright.")
Falling reactivity and soothability (negative loading)	Rate of recovery from peak distress, excitement, or general arousal. ("Rarely cries for more than a couple minutes at a time.")
Fear	Amount of negative affect including unease, worry, or nervousness related to anticipated pain or distress and/or potentially threatening situations. ("Is afraid of the dark.")
Sadness	Amount of negative affect and lowered mood and energy related to exposure to suffering, disappointment, and object loss. ("Cries sadly when a favorite toy gets lost or broken.")

(cont.)

TABLE 2.2. *(cont.)*

Scale	Definition (sample item)
Factor 3—Effortful control	
Attentional focusing	Tendency to maintain attentional focus upon task-related channels. ("When drawing or coloring in a book, shows strong concentration.")
Inhibitory control	The ability to plan and to suppress approach responses under instructions or in uncertain situations. ("Can easily stop an activity when s/he is told 'no.'")
Low-intensity pleasure	Amount of pleasure or enjoyment related to situations involving low stimulus intensity, rate, complexity, novelty, and incongruity. ("Enjoys sitting on parent's lap.")
Perceptual sensitivity	Amount of detection of slight, low-intensity stimuli from the external environment. ("Notices even little specks of dirt on objects.")

tivity. In Japan and the United States, but not in China, smiling and laughter also loads on this factor. These three factors are similar to higher-order factors identified by Sanson, Smart, Prior, Oberklaid, and Pedlow (1994) in 3- to 8-year-old Australian children, as well as to scales developed by Hegvik, McDevitt, and Carey (1982) for 8- to 12-year-olds, and by McClowry, Hegvik, and Teglasi (1993).

With this revised view of the structure of temperament in mind, we can now briefly review what we have learned about the early development of temperament. In Chapter 3, I relate the broad dimensions of temperament to animal and neuroscience research, and then move on to discuss how they may function in the development of personality and psychopathology (Chapters 4–9). I now consider the early development of major dimensions of temperament. These dimensions are surgency, negative emotionality (with the subconstructs of fear and anger/frustration), and effortful control. I begin with the broad temperament factor of surgency.

Surgency

The broad dimension of surgency has emerged from factor analysis of temperament scale scores in infants, children, and adults (Putnam, Ellis, & Rothbart, 2001). Surgency combines a disposition toward the positive emotions, rapid approach to potential rewards, and high activity level in a construct very similar to, and in adults, positively related to the personality factor of extraversion (Evans & Rothbart, 2007). Surgency/extraversion is a venerable temperament dimension, as can be seen in Kagan's (1994) book *Galen's Prophecy*. Surgency is also related to biological models that emphasize "approach" or "behavioral facilitation" (Depue & Collins, 1999; Gray & McNaughton, 1996; see Chapter 3 in this book). Individual differences in surgency-related behavior can be observed by the age of 2–3 months in smiling and laughter, vocal reactivity, and activity (Rothbart, 1989b). In infants whose surgent tendencies are strong, mothers talk about their children becoming "revved up" just at the sight of something interesting. When surgent infants are able to crawl and move about, they are also likely to set out quickly after exciting objects. Children low in surgency, on the other hand, are described by their parents as mostly sitting, moving only when they really want something.

Considerable stability of surgency and its components has been reported from early in development (Rothbart & Bates, 2006). Stability of a temperament trait means that infants with scores that are high or low on a measure tend to remain high or low in comparison with other children as they grow older. In our laboratory, we have found stability for positive emotion across the first year of life using two different methods: parent report (the IBQ) and home observation (Rothbart, 1986). Lemery, Goldsmith, Klinnert, and Mrazek (1999) measured parent-reported smiling and laughter, pleasure, and sociability, and found stability between 3 and 18 months of age. Infants' responses to laboratory episodes designed to elicit positive emotion, such as brief puppet shows, are also modestly stable in children between 9 and 33 months of age (Kochanska, Murray, & Harlan, 2000).

We used laboratory measures with infants who were seen at 3, 6, 10, and 13 months of age (Rothbart et al., 2000). The babies were videotaped while nonsocial events (e.g., small squeeze toys, a mechanical dog, a rapidly opening parasol) and social stimuli (e.g., an experimenter's speech to the infant, a peek-a-boo game) were presented. We coded smiling and laughter to these episodes, including the time to the infant's first positive reaction (latency), the intensity of the child's reaction, and its duration, and averaged these measures within each episode. Measures from different episodes were then averaged to yield overall measures of positive emotion. Approach was assessed in infants' latency to grasp small toys, and activity level was measured by the number of lines that 13-month-olds crossed as they moved among toys distributed across a grid-lined floor. Children who smiled and laughed more also showed more rapid approach and higher activity in the laboratory (Rothbart, 1988).

Later, when the infants were 7 years old, parents filled out the CBQ described previously (Rothbart et al., 2001). Smiling and laughter measured in the laboratory during infancy predicted the children's surgency as 7-year-olds, as reported by their mothers. Children who had rapidly approached objects at 6, 10, and 13 months were later described by their mothers as showing high positive anticipation, impulsivity, and activity at age 7 (Rothbart et al., 2000).

Other studies have also reported stability in children's activity and approach tendencies. Korner et al. (1985) found that motor activity in newborn infants when they were not distressed predicted later high activity level and approach at 4–8 years. In another study, stability of both approach and activity level was found between 2 and 12 years (Guerin & Gottfried, 1994). Finally, Caspi and Silva (1995) found that children who were high on approach or confidence at ages 3–4 tended to be rated as high on social potency and low on self-control at age 18.

In our longitudinal study (Rothbart et al., 2000), children who quickly grasped toys in the laboratory tended at age 7 to be lower in their attention control and inhibitory control, as reported by their mothers. These findings and those of Caspi and Silva (1995) suggest that when children have strong surgent tendencies, self-control may be difficult. If surgent tendencies are viewed as an "accelerator" toward action in the child, and inhibitory tendencies such as fear or effortful control as "brakes," then stronger accelerative tendencies may weaken the braking influence (Rothbart & Derryberry, 2002). To more completely understand the development of surgency, we thus need to study fear and effortful control.

Negative Emotionality: Fear and Anger/Frustration

The newborn infant shows relatively undifferentiated distress, but later it is possible to differentiate anger/frustration from fear. To measure these two negative emotions, we coded infants' distress to elicitors of fear (presentations of novel, intense, and unpredictable stimuli such as a mechanical duck and a monkey; a stranger's approach) and of frustration (placing attractive toys out of reach or behind a plexiglas barrier) (Rothbart et al., 2000). Infants expressed frustration by banging on the table or barrier and showing distress. They expressed fear by showing distress along with motor inhibition or withdrawal from a threatening object.

Fear

In our laboratory study, infants at 6 months readily approached and grasped the toys we placed before them (Rothbart, 1988; Rothbart et al., 2000). Some infants grasped the toys more quickly than others, but in general we observed rapid approach in what might be called "compulsive reaching" in the children. Some of the infants would rapidly grasp the novel and unpredictable toy object and then cry as they held it. By the time the infants were 10 months old, however, some of the infants who had grasped the novel and unpredictable objects quickly now showed greatly slowed approach, inhibition, or actual withdrawal from the objects, accompanied by distress (Rothbart). Infants' latency to approach and grasp low-intensity toys like little squeeze toys showed stability from 6 to 10 months, but their approach to novel and high-intensity toys did not show stability from 6 to 10 months, suggesting development of a fear system. These observations also indicated that children's surgent approach tendencies can be measured early in infancy, before their fear responses have fully developed, but that once fearful inhibition is demonstrated, many of the children will be less impulsive in fear-inducing situations.

After its appearance late in the first year, fear-related inhibition shows considerable stability over childhood and into adolescence (Kagan, 1998). Stability of fearful inhibition has been reported from 2 to 4 years (Lemery et al., 1999), 2 to 8 years (Kagan, Reznick, & Snidman, 1988), and from the preschool period to age 18 (Caspi & Silva, 1995). Guerin, Gottfried, Oliver, and Thomas (2003) have also reported stability of approach–withdrawal from infancy to adolescence. In our laboratory study (Rothbart et al., 2000), infant fear to mechanical toys, masks, and a stranger predicted later fear and shyness when the children were 7 years old. Infant fear also predicted later sadness, guilt/shame, and low-intensity (non-risk-taking) pleasure, as well as lower aggression. Fear in infancy did not predict later frustration/anger, and infant frustration/anger in infancy did not predict later fear or shyness.

Other long-term findings suggest that fear regulates approach. Infants who showed more fear in our laboratory at 13 months were later described by their mothers as showing lower positive anticipation and lower impulsivity, activity, and aggression (Rothbart et al., 2000). Fear thus appears to inhibit approach and aggression, resulting in greater control of action, and indeed temperament fearfulness is related to early development of conscience (Kochanska, 1997). These findings may seem surprising in that fear in our culture is often evaluated negatively, but in evolution, fearful inhibition is seen to protect the animal from approaching potentially harmful objects or situations. Psychological problems for humans can develop when fearful inhibition leads to rigid and overcontrolled patterns of behavior, limiting the child's positive experience (Block & Block, 1980; Kremen & Block, 1998). Fortunately, however, the development of temperamental effortful control during the preschool years will allow greater efficiency and flexibility in children's control of thought, emotion, and action.

There are also early precursors to later infant fear. Infant crying and motor reactivity to stimulation at 4 months of age predicts fearful inhibition at 14 months of age, whereas infant positive emotion and motor reactivity predicts infants' later exuberance or surgency (Calkins, Fox, & Marshall,

1996; Kagan, 1997). Once fearful inhibition is established, individual differences in the relative strength of approach versus inhibition under novel or intense conditions also appear to be relatively stable aspects of temperament (Rothbart & Bates, 2006). These stabilities in surgency versus fear and extraversion versus introversion are further discussed in Chapter 8.

Anger/Frustration

Anger and frustration occur when the child's aims or expectations have been blocked or limited. We measured anger/frustration by observing how infants reacted when a toy was placed out of reach or behind a plexiglas barrier (Rothbart et al., 2000). Some of the infants looked like angry older children as they pushed against the barrier and pounded on the table. Infants' frustration at 6 and 10 months also predicted 7-year anger/frustration, as well as other aspects of later negative emotion, including aggression, discomfort, guilt/shame, and low soothability. Greater infant frustration in infancy was also related at 7 years to higher activity level, positive anticipation, impulsivity, and high-intensity pleasure. While infant fear was thus related to later sadness, shyness and *weak* approach, as well as low aggression, infant frustration was related to later *strong* approach and higher aggression. Panksepp (1998) has proposed that when reward-related activities are unsuccessful, the anger/frustration functions of a "rage" system are activated. Strong approach tendencies are related to expectations of positive outcomes, but they are also related to frustration when positive expectations are not met. In our questionnaire findings for infancy and childhood, children with higher activity level have been consistently seen as more prone to anger/frustration.

The two forms of negative emotion, fear and frustration, differ in the extent to which they involve assertive action that is directed toward the outside environment, with assertive action linked to anger but not to fear. Anger and fear can thus be seen as the relatively assertive (anger) and nonassertive (fear) forms of negative reactivity to threat. Later in this book, I explore the possibility that nonassertive fear may form the roots of later *internalizing* problems (involving fear, anxiety, and sadness) and assertive anger/frustration the root of *externalizing* problems (involving anger, antisocial behavior, and aggression). I discuss these temperament reactions and their relation to the development of behavior problems in Chapter 9.

Although we have found evidence of differentiation between fear and frustration, a broad factor of negative emotionality is also often found (e.g., Gartstein & Rothbart, 2003; Rothbart et al., 2001). Children who show one negative emotion tend to show the others, so that there seems to be a general disposition of proneness to distress. This tendency is also seen in the broad personality factor of neuroticism. I consider possible neural under-pinnings of this general disposition to negative emotion in Chapter 3.

Effortful Control

Our factor analyses of the CBQ identified a general factor of effortful con-trol, composed of children's voluntary attentional focusing, inhibitory con-trol, perceptual sensitivity, and low-intensity pleasure (Ahadi et al., 1993). Although inhibitory control is not seen in early infancy, we have found a broad factor involving attentional focusing, attentional shifting, and inhibi-tory and activational control of behavior in adults as well as preschool-age, primary school-age, and early adolescent children (Derryberry & Rothbart, 1988; Evans & Rothbart, 2007). Children, adolescents, and adults who are high in effortful control also tend to be low in negative emotionality, in agreement with the idea that attention can be used to regulate emotion (Rothbart & Sheese, 2007).

We have defined effortful control as the ability to inhibit a dominant response (inhibitory control) in order to perform a subdominant response (activation control), to detect errors, and to engage in planning (Rothbart & Bates, 2006; Rothbart & Rueda, 2005). However, effortful control can also be seen as the ability to control one's actions (inhibiting and activating action), one's emotions, and one's attention (more efficient performance in conflict situations, higher persistence, and nondistractibility); can be more generally thought of as self-control. Effortful control has been found to undergo rapid development in children between the ages of 2 and 7 years, especially in the preschool years (Gerardi-Caulton, 2000; Kochanska et al., 2000; Roth-bart, Ellis, Rueda, & Posner, 2003). We have proposed that development of the executive attention system of the brain underlies children's develop-ing effortful control (Posner & Rothbart, 1998; Rothbart et al., 2007a). To assess executive attention, we have adapted tasks related to brain function in adults (Posner & Rothbart, 1998; Rothbart & Rueda, 2005) to use with young children, and these methods are described in Chapter 3.

Kochanska and her colleagues studied the development of effortful control in two large studies that followed children from 2 to 5 years and from 9 to 45 months of age (Kochanska et al., 2000; Kochanska, Murray, & Coy, 1997; Kochanska, Murray, Jacques, Koenig, & Vandegeest, 1996). They measured five skills involving the ability to suppress a dominant response in order to perform a subdominant response, including both delay and con-flict tasks. Beginning at age 2½ years (30 months), children's performance became highly consistent across these tasks, suggesting that an underlying quality of effortful control was developing. Children were also remarkably stable across age in their performance on effortful control tasks, and stability correlations were consistently high, as high as those for the stability of intelligence (Kochanska et al., 2000). Guerin et al. (2003) have also reported that toddler persistence predicts adolescent task orientation in parent reports.

The construct of effortful control brings powerful theoretical implications for temperament and development. Early theoretical models of temperament as reviewed in Chapter 1 stressed how our actions are driven by our level of arousal or by our positive and negative emotions. The control of approach by fear and the control of fear by strong approach tendencies fit with this kind of model. The trait of effortful control, however, means we are neither always at the mercy of emotion, nor of one emotional system's dominance over another. With effortful control, we can *choose* to approach situations we fear and inhibit actions we desire, giving a strong self-regulatory basis for action, conscience, and self-control. Effortful control also brings with it the possibility of self-regulated change. With the development of executive attention and effortful control we can observe our own actions, and select other actions based on our values and goals. Although the effectiveness of effortful control will depend on the strength of the emotional and motivational processes against which it is exerted, it provides the possibility for true flexibility of thought, emotion, and action.

Affiliation

Finally, let us consider a temperament dimension that we have studied only recently. This dimension of temperament has been inspired by research on the biology of behavior (e.g., Depue & Lenzenweger, 2006; Panskepp, 1998). We know that humans are social creatures, and that we share systems of affiliation with other social animals, including mammals, birds, and fish. These systems support bonds between mating pairs and care of the young (Insel, 2003). Depue and his colleague have distinguished the positive approach (surgency) dimension of temperament from positive enjoyment of closeness with others (Depue & Lenzenweger). This affiliative tendency further supports feelings of connection, care, and love. The affiliation system is thus related to affectionate and gratifying states of closeness to others. We have now measured affiliativeness in early adolescence and adulthood by self-report (Ellis, Rothbart, & Posner, 2004; Evans & Rothbart, 2007), and have developed an affiliative measure for our revised temperament measure in infancy and the toddler period (Putnam, Rothbart, & Gartstein, 2008). In infancy we use cuddliness as an indicator of social closeness.

Affiliativeness is not the same as security of attachment, because it does not chiefly involve the child's use of the parent as a secure base for exploration of the world, but additional research will be needed to explore the relation between affiliation and attachment. Because scales measuring affiliativeness have only recently been developed, little exploration of the stability of affiliation has been done. In a study that followed infants (3–12 months) to toddlerhood (18–32 months), however, we found significant stability for mothers' reports of their infants' cuddliness to toddlerhood (Putnam et al., 2008). Cuddliness in toddlerhood further predicted children's enjoyment of low-intensity pleasures in childhood (3–5 years), suggesting, in agreement with Depue and Morrone-Stupisky (2005), that affiliation is a general disposition to experiencing pleasure. We currently do not have an affiliativeness measure for childhood, but one may be developed in the future. I address the psychobiology of affiliation in Chapter 3.

A MODEL FOR THE EARLY DEVELOPMENT OF TEMPERAMENT

This brief introduction to the structure of temperament and its early development suggests a model like the one depicted in Figure 2.1. Here, reactivity and especially self-regulation develop over the early years of life, and self-regulatory temperament modulates early reactivity. The time of emergence is indicated from the top (earliest) to bottom (latest). There is a balance between temperament dispositions so that some traits can inhibit or activate other traits. Fear and surgency, for example, can inhibit each other, and fear can inhibit anger/aggression. Affiliation can inhibit anger/aggression, and effortful control serves as a general self-regulation mechanism, inhibiting or activating the negative emotions, surgency, and affiliation. Effortful control is an emotion-neutral process in itself, but it can serve many motivational purposes, including those of fear and anger as well as positive approach.

TEMPERAMENT TYPES

Our understanding of temperament traits and their relation to other each other allows us to better understand some of the recent typologies of temperament. Based on judges' ratings of individual characteristics, Block (1971) identified three personality types. The first of these, called *Resilient*, included traits of self-confidence, the ability to concentrate on tasks, adaptability to change, and verbal fluency. *Overcontrolled* individuals were shy, introverted, and lacked many social skills. *Undercontrolled* individuals showed little con-

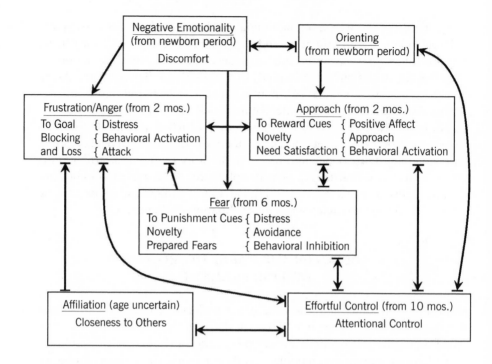

FIGURE 2.1. The development of temperament systems. Arrows and lines indicate relations of one system to another. Arrows = faciliation (positive influence); lines = inhibition.

cern for others and were impulsive, willful, and disagreeable. Three types of children have been identified in several studies of children and adolescents (see review in Caspi & Shiner, 2006). The studies have been carried out in different countries and with different ages of children (e.g., Asendorpf, Borkenau, Ostendorf, & van Aken, 2001; Caspi & Silva, 1995; Komsi et al., 2006). Methods for determining the types have also differed, with similar results, suggesting they may reflect reliable temperamental processes.

It is possible to relate these types to the temperament dimensions discussed in this chapter, and with the exception of affiliation, Komsi et al. (2006) studied 231 Finnish children at 6 months and again at 5.5 years, using the IBQ and CBQ. *Resilient* children were surgent, not very fearful (self-confident), and showed high effortful control (the ability to concentrate on tasks). *Overcontrolled* children were fearful (shy), less surgent (more introverted), and higher in effortful control. Finally, *undercontrolled* children were expected to be high in surgency and in negative emotion and also low in the three potential inhibitors of disagreeable behavior: the fear and effortful control that inhibit approach and impulsivity (surgency), and the affiliativeness inhibiting aggression that might hurt another person. In Komsi's study, undercontrolled children were high in negative emotion (including fear) and high in surgency and low in effortful control. In the future, we may be able to test whether, if the child is lacking in one kind of control (e.g. affiliativeness), his or her behavior may still be regulated by fear and/or effortful control, so that several other combinations of reactivity and self-regulation would be possible.

A CONCLUDING NOTE ON PARENTS AS INFORMANTS

In this chapter, the value of parents' observations to our understanding of the structure of children's temperament should be clear, even though there have been strong concerns about their use (e.g., Kagan, 1994, 1998). In our research and reviews, we have found consistent relations between parents' questionnaire reports and other measures of temperament, including laboratory and home observations (Rothbart & Bates, 1998, 2006). It is also clear that the understanding of the structure of temperament that we have gained from caregivers' reports provides rich connections to animal behavior, human personality, adjustment, and psychopathology, as is discussed in later chapters of this book.

SUMMARY

Research on the structure of temperament in infancy and in childhood indicates that a revision of the original NYLS nine dimensions is in order. During infancy, traits of fear, anger/frustration, surgency, and orienting regulation have been identified. At older ages, a broad trait of negative emotionality is frequently found, but the negative emotions of fear and anger are also frequently differentiated. Early childhood brings with it the important temperament characteristic of effortful control. In childhood, there is thus evidence for broad dimensions of surgency, effortful control, fearful distress, irritable distress, and general negative emotionality. Having briefly introduced the dimensions of temperament in childhood, I now turn to links between temperament and biology. For each of these dimensions, I briefly review animal studies and models for the neurological substrate of temperament.

CHAPTER 3

The Biology of Temperament

This chapter gives a brief introduction to the biology of temperament. This is a vast area of research, one that will require many more specific reviews as contributions continue to grow. I first consider how temperament concepts apply to other animals, and how we humans differ in the expression of temperament and personality from those animals. I also briefly review some of the biological models of temperament, and introduce the exciting new genetic methods now available for studying temperament. I begin, however, by considering temperament in my second favorite companion animal (the first is human), the dog.

Those of you who have a dog in the family may be familiar with how temperament concepts are applied to choosing and training a puppy. A wide range of puppy temperament tests are available, and books on raising dogs include methods for assessing the dog's temperament (e.g., Monks of New Skete, 1991; Volhard & Volhard, 2001; see also Lindsay, 2005). In choosing a puppy, you first observe the puppy's behavior. This includes watching the puppy interact with littermates, and noticing whether the puppy is the one who initiates activities with other dogs or remains indifferent, the puppy's tendency to dominate other animals (who wins in tug-of-war?), the puppy's tendency to be submissive or picked on by other animals, and the puppy's tendency to bite. You are also asked to observe whether the puppy is the first dog coming out of the group to greet you, whether it seems interested but hangs back, or simply doesn't pay much attention to you at all. What happens when you are alone with the dog? Is the puppy's tail up and wagging, or is it down? Does the puppy look away from you? Does the puppy come to you? Follow you? Ignore you?

The next tests assess the puppy's reactivity. What happens when you roll the dog on its back? Does the puppy struggle fiercely and bite, completely submit, or something in between? What happens when you gently pat the puppy's body from top to tail? Is there growling, quieting, cuddling, or attempts at escape? Rattling a set of keys lets you see the dog's alertness and curiosity. You can observe the puppy's reactivity to touch, loud sound, movement, or the presence of a strange object (e.g., an open umbrella). Does the puppy approach and bite the object, approach without attacking, run away, cower, or show no interest? Based on puppy temperament tests, Volhard and Volhard (2001) have identified six kinds of dogs and suggested how to match them with human families:

1. A dog who is *aggressive and dominant*. This dog can easily be provoked to bite, and may resist the human as a leader. Although an aggressive and dominant puppy is not a good choice for a family, the puppy can become a strong working adult, like a police dog.
2. A dog who is *self-assured and dominant*. This dog can be provoked to bite, but will follow the leadership of a human who is informed and firm. An owner who is indecisive and uncomfortable with training is not the best person for this dog.
3. A dog who is *outgoing and friendly*. This dog can adapt well when given regular training and exercise. Still, the dog may not be recommended for families with young children (the dog's exuberance may be too much for a young child) or for families that cannot provide the dog with needed exercise.
4. A dog whose *submissive* qualities lead him to look to the owner for leadership. This dog may lack self-confidence, but his or her gentle and affectionate qualities will make him a good family pet.
5. A dog who is *extremely submissive* and lacks self-confidence. This dog can become very dependent on the owner, displaying strong needs for social companionship and direction. Without special training, this dog can grow up to be shy and fearful, and may engage in fear-motivated attack.
6. A dog who is *independent and not very interested in people*. This puppy may mature into a dog who seems not to need the companionship of humans and demonstrates little affection.

We can use the Volhards' (2001) list to infer a set of puppy temperament traits: dominant/aggressive, outgoing/friendly, submissive/timid, affiliative, and curious/reactive to sensory stimulation or novelty. These traits, especially aggressiveness (related to frustration), outgoingness (related to extraversion/surgency), timidity (related to fear), curiosity (related to perceptual sensitivity), and affiliativeness, are similar to temperament traits identified in humans and discussed in Chapter 2. Dominance, however, has been little studied as a feature of human temperament, and when it has been studied, it has been linked to extraversion. Recently, longitudinal studies have followed up adult dogs who had been given temperament tests as puppies (see review by Lindsay, 2000). Fear and aggressiveness in puppies predict fear and aggressiveness in older dogs, but puppy dominance does not appear to be stable. Instead, dominance fluctuates with the animal's experiences in a particular group. If you are interested in a more highly standardized puppy test, see Lindsay (2005).

It is interesting that the Volhards' (2001) descriptions of young dogs are linked to suggestions about the best matches with families that might adopt them, recalling Thomas and Chess's (1977) idea of "goodness of fit." As a family pet, a dog who is too aggressive and dominating, too timid, too rambunctious, or too unsocial is likely to create problems for the family. A somewhat timid dog, on the other hand, may prove to be a good match for a wide range of relatively unskilled and low-energy dog trainers, whereas a strong and experienced dog trainer would likely be a good match for dogs up and down the temperament list.

In Chapter 1 I described temperament as it was observed in Pavlov's (1935) dog studies. However, temperament (sometimes called personality) has also been studied in chimpanzees, monkeys, gorillas, pigs, donkeys, rats, fish, and octopi (Gosling & John, 1999), as well as in horses, cows, cats, birds, and mice. A number of dimensions of temperament are seen in many species; others are more specific. Thus, guppies show variability in fear/avoidance and approach (Budaev, 1997); donkeys vary in obstinacy and vivacity (vivacity is likely related to surgency; French, 1993). Pigs show individual differences in aggression, sociability, and exploration/curiosity (Forkman, Furuhaug, & Jensen, 1995). In mice, two styles of coping reactions have been described: active coping, which includes aggressive behavior, and passive, nonaggressive coping (Sluyter & van Oormerssen, 2000). The actively coping mice appeared to be well adapted to an unchanging environment that involves defending a territory, whereas the nonaggressive animals were more adapted to changing environments, where caution may be needed to keep the animal alive. These differences in mouse temperament point up the way in which variability among species members supports the adaptation of the species. Depending on the environmental challenges and opportunities, one coping reaction may be adaptive and another not; in any case at least a subset of mice will survive.

Mice have been the major subject of genetic studies in animals, and in recent years, transfers of mouse embryos have been made from one mouse mother's uterus to another mouse's uterus. It has also been possible to breed aggressive and nonaggressive lines of wild house mice, implanting them into the uterus of mothers from the same or a different line to investigate prenatal intrauterine influences. Mice can also be assigned to their own or different mothers to test for socialization influences (Sluyter et al., 1996). Sluyter et al. found no effect of varying prenatal environment or of fostering male mice to mothers that differed on aggression, suggesting that intermale aggression in the wild house mouse is chiefly influenced by genetic factors.

Nonhuman Primates

Many of the most important experiences of my life have been ones where I realized how similar I was to others. One had to do with getting to know my male colleagues and realizing that most of the differences I expected did not seem to exist. Another was in watching *Tales of the City* and realizing how similar I was to its gay characters. A third experience occurred at the Chicago Zoo, where human visitors were standing on one side of a large glass cage, looking at the chimpanzees. At the same time, several chimpanzees were on the other side looking at us. A human father was carrying his young son, and held him up to get a better look at the chimpanzees. In turn, a chimpanzee mother lifted up her baby to better see the human child. Here were two parents with their children, and very little to distinguish between them. It brought tears to many pairs of eyes, including mine.

We now turn to those animals that are closest to humans genetically, the nonhuman primates. Three methods of studying temperament have been used in primate studies, and they are very similar to methods used in the study of temperament in humans. In one, coded observations are made of animals interacting in a social environment (Chamove, Eysenck, & Harlow, 1972). In the second, questionnaires ask caretakers to check the adjectives that best describe each animal in their care. The adjectives are carefully defined; after reading the definitions, caretakers rate each animal on each adjective, and scores are averaged to form scales. As in human questionnaire research, factor analysis allows study of the structure of the animals' temperament (King & Figueredo, 1977; Stevenson-Hinde & Zunz, 1978).

A third method involves laboratory observations: Here, the animals' reactivity to stimulation is studied, sometimes by adapting assessments of human newborns (Schneider & Suomi, 1992). Using these methods allows comparisons between different species, as well as studies of variability within species. They also allow comparisons between animals within the same species whose ancestors have adapted to different ecological settings (see review by Clarke & Boinski, 1995).

Chamove et al. (1972) observed rhesus monkey behavior in groups of four and factor analyzed the resulting behavior records. Three broad factors were identified: *Hostile*, including biting or grabbing other animals; *Fearful*, including withdrawal from both hostile and nonthreatening animals, and fear of the environment; and *Social*, which included play with other animals and objects, and positive contact with them. Gold and Maple (1994) used caretaker questionnaires to study temperament in captive gorillas. Adjectives were rated on a five-point scale. Factor analysis of the gorilla data yielded four factors, labeled Extraverted (sociable, playful, active, popular, curious, with negative loadings for the adjectives solitary and slow), Dominant (aggressive, effective, irritable, strong, opportunistic, and excitable—this factor could appropriately have been labeled aggressive/irritable), Fearful (fearful, apprehensive, insecure, tense, eccentric, with a negative contribution from confidence), and Understanding (showing warmth and understanding of other gorillas, equable, and motherly to others—this factor could also be labeled affiliative or nurturant).

Probably the animals with the greatest interest for us are those genetically close to us: the chimpanzees, which share approximately 98% of our DNA. Do these animals show an organization of emotion and behavior similar to what we see in humans? Van Hooff (1970) recorded over 50 behaviors in a group of chimpanzees, and King and Figueredo (1997) studied zoo chimpanzees using caretaker questionnaires. Their temperament factors included Submissiveness (an aspect of fear) versus Dominance or Aggressiveness, Playfulness, Agreeableness, Negative Emotionality, and Openness. King and Figueredo also identified Dependability, related to low aggression, impulsivity, and low unpredictable behavior, and possibly related to effortful control. There is thus considerable overlap of human and chimpanzee temperament dimensions: surgency, fearfulness, irritable/aggressiveness, affiliativeness, general emotionality/distress proneness, and openness (perceptual sensitivity and orienting).

The genes we inherit reflect evolved expectations about the kinds of environmental challenges and opportunities we will face. Humans and other animals encounter dangers, and threatening cues elicit responses of flight, freezing, or attack. Fear and approach systems have an evolutionary history going back beyond the mammals and animals with backbones to the fruit flies and sea slugs (LeDoux, 1996). Through our genes, we inherit structures that prepare us for the opportunities and threats our evolutionary ancestors have adapted to. Humans and other animals are also sensitive to rewards, and pleasure and positive anticipation are also linked to evaluation, action, and memory in many species.

Genetically based processes in physical structure, including brain structure, thus reflect and mirror the challenges and opportunities the animal will face in its expectable environment (Oyama, 1985). Animals' built-in reactions of fear mirror environmental danger, their anger reflects the blocking of goals; surgency reflects environmental rewards. Affiliation reflects our adaptation to others as social animals, orienting or perceptual sensitivity mirrors our alertness and responsiveness to change, and effortful control reflects a flexibility of thinking that can be used to obtain numerous goals such as safety, rewards, closeness to others, alertness to important events, communication, the ability to construct mental models of our environment, to learn and to change. These adaptations are built in to the genetic structure. We can see them as fundamental coping mechanisms that will be further shaped by the animal's experiences in different situations.

Individual differences in conscientiousness (effortful control) have been reported in studies of chimpanzees, but not in other nonhuman animals (Gosling & John, 1999). Affiliation, defined as affection and feelings of closeness to others, is an important dimension that has emerged from animal studies. It is not the same as surgent sociability or gregariousness, because shy persons may also have strong feelings of closeness to others. Because affiliativeness appears in animals and can be seen in human neural structures, we have added affiliation to our model of temperament. We have also added affiliativeness scales to our infant, early adolescent, and adult temperament questionnaires (Ellis et al., 2004; Evans & Rothbart, 2007; Gartstein & Rothbart, 2003).

Recently, studies of species similarities and differences have identified a neuron that we share with the great apes (gorillas, chimpanzees, bonobos, and orangutangs), elephants, and whales, but not with other animals (Allman, Watson, Tetreault, & Hakeem, 2005). This large cell, called the von Economo neuron, is present in the executive attention system described below (Allman et al., 2001) and is also in the frontal insula, a structure sensitive to the social emotions, including empathy, guilt, love, and even humor (Watson, Matthews & Allman, 2007). Allman et al. (2005) have suggested that this adaptation is particularly important to both self-awareness and social awareness, features critically important to a highly social species. It is interesting that sociality and the self would be so closely linked.

If there are similarities in emotion and attention between humans and our close relatives, how do we differ from chimpanzees? The differences mainly reflect human differences between temperament and personality. Humans have highly developed language and specific concepts of self and other. These views of ourselves in a social world add a new level of complexity to personality in the developing human. Indeed, personality in the older child and adult differs from temperament in the infant, and personality in the human differs from temperament in nonhuman animals. This is an important point because although we share aspects of reactivity and self-regulation with other animals, we also develop highly cognitive aspects of personality that have powerful effects on who we are.

TEMPERAMENT AND THE BRAIN

When we say that temperament is constitutionally based, we mean that temperament dispositions are supported by the nervous system. This means we can study temperament at the neural, neurotransmitter, and genetic levels as well as at the psychological level (Posner & Rothbart, 2007b). In our work on attention, we have identified relations between effortful control and the executive attention of the brain, as well as specific genes that support these networks (Posner, Rothbart, & Sheese, 2007; Rothbart, Sheese, et al., 2007). This kind of analysis is also being applied to emotional dimensions of temperament by Hariri (2009) and others.

I now consider some of the neural models of temperament, many of which have been based on observations of nonhuman animals (see also reviews by Konner, 2002; Posner & Rothbart, 2007a; Rothbart, Derryberry, & Posner, 1994; and Zuckerman, 2005). Two areas of research on the biology of temperament, neuroimaging, and molecular genetics have led to an explosion of information on biologically based individual differences, and progress in this area is very rapid (Canli, 2006; Nigg, Martel, Nikolas, & Casey, 2010). I will not go into detail on the anatomy of the brain and different methods of brain imaging here; these can be obtained in textbooks in neurobiology and cognitive neuroscience as well as other sources. One textbook possibility is John Martin's (2010) *Neuroanatomy Text and Atlas*. Some readers will likely read this section chiefly for general meaning.

Brain Models of the Emotions

As we have seen above, the brain processes information that is evolutionarily important to the animal's adaptation. This processing occurs through networks of neurons in the brain, and recent brain-imaging research allows us to explore the locations (sites) involved in this processing and the connections between brain sites during thinking and emotion. Emotion networks are broad inherited systems that order feeling, thought, and action

(LeDoux, 1989; Posner & Petersen, 1990). While other processing networks address the questions "What is it?" and "Where is it?" emotion-processing networks of the brain evaluate the meaning or importance of events for the individual (LeDoux). These networks address the questions "Is it dangerous?" Is it good for me?"; "Is it bad for me?" Because the emotions also include built-in coping mechanisms, they address the questions "What shall I do about it?" "Shall I go after it? Run from it? Attack it? Hide from it?"

Emotion reactions occur rapidly, often preceding other information processing of objects and situations that address the questions "What is it?" and "Where is it?" (LeDoux, 1989). Emotional evaluations are also important in consolidating memories of events (McGaugh, 2003). When the meaning and valuation of events has been coded and stored, emotion will influence both immediate and future reactions in similar situations. The expression of the emotions in the face, voice, and body also communicate the state of the infant or child to the caregiver and the state of the older child or adult to others (Campos, Barrett, Lamb, Goldsmith, & Stenberg, 1983). Emotional expression thereby provides a fundamental basis for social communication. I now go back to the dimensions of temperament identified in Chapter 2, describing briefly some of the brain structures thought to underlie emotional and attentional information processing. I begin with the negative emotions that include fear, anger, and frustration.

Fear

Fear is activated in the presence of threat, novelty, or signals of upcoming punishment, and its function is to avoid the danger and defend the organism. When fear is activated, ongoing motor programs are inhibited and responses that support coping with threat, such as fleeing, fighting, and hiding, are prepared (see review by Rothbart, Derryberry, et al., 1994). Fear responses, which can signal life-or-death situations, generally take precedence over other activities and emotions, and fear can inhibit or shut down the positive emotion/approach systems (Gray, 1978).

In Gray's (1978) model of the Behavioral Inhibition System (BIS), brain circuits including the orbital frontal cortex, medial septal area, and hippocampus are responsive to learned fear. This network opposes the Behavioral Activation System (BAS), an approach system described later in this chapter. Other investigators such as LeDoux (1987, 1989), have identified the amygdala as the critical structure in processing conditioned fear and other emotions. Neuroimaging studies of humans support amygdala involvement in both acquiring and expressing fear (Calder, Lawrence, & Young, 2001). The amygdala is also involved in recognizing fear (Calder et al.), and responds more strongly to novel than to familiar stimuli (Nishijo, Ono, & Nishino, 1988). The amygdala is not involved in the voluntary production of facial expressions of fear. Neuroscientists can also go beyond brain networks to study other levels of influence on emotion processing and expression. Hariri (2009), for example, has linked fear/anxiety to the psychological, brain network, neurochemical, and gene levels, and we can expect that other emotional systems will be analyzed in this way in the future.

The amygdala is also connected to autonomic and motor reactions including startle, motor inhibition, fearful facial expressions, and cardiovascular and respiratory changes (Davis, Hitchcock, & Rosen, 1987). Each of these reactions is part of the overall fear response, and just as persons can differ in their general dispositions toward fear, they can also differ in the networks that are part of the fear reaction. The amygdala also influences processing of information about objects within the cortex, and is linked to the executive attention system (Posner & Petersen, 1990). Anxious individuals show increased attention to threatening sources of information, whereas extraverted individuals show increased attention to rewarding sources of information (e.g., Derryberry & Reed, 1994).

Fear offers a good example of how quickly emotion processing can occur. In processing fear, the thalamus relays information about the object qualities of a stimulus (size, shape, color, etc.) through sensory pathways (LeDoux, 1989). At the same time, emotion information is rapidly routed for evaluation to the amygdala, where memories of the meaning of the stimulus influence early emotional processing. When we learn more about the event we may change our evaluations, but in the meantime projections back from the amygdala will influence subsequent sensory and object processing, and preparation for action.

The ancient Hindu story of the rope and the snake offers a good example of these processes. In dim light, we see a coiled object and immediately freeze, preparing to run away. When we later realize the object is a rope and not a snake, we are relieved, and we may laugh, shaking off the body tension that has prepared us for action (Rothbart, 1973). The amygdala supports motor activation via the corpus striatum and supports autonomic reactions (e.g., heart rate, respiration changes) via the hypothalamus. The autonomic nervous system provides body support for the coping actions that may be quickly required in situations of danger. Our heart races, our palms perspire, and we breathe more rapidly. The endocrine system (e.g., cortisol reactions) provides longer-term energy support for emergency action. These reactions are all part of the organization of the emotions that prepare us for evaluating and coping with threat (LeDoux, 1989).

Anxiety

Recent advances in neuroscience have also identified an "anxiety" system that supports a dimension of generalized anxiety or a disposition toward distress that is not linked to the particular cues that directly elicit fear (Davis, 1998; Rosen & Schulkin, 1998). This system involves the extended amygdala or BNST (bed nucleus of the stria terminalis) and is related to symptoms of posttraumatic stress disorder (PTSD; Patrick & Bernat, 2006). Watson (2005) and Krueger (1999) have pointed out that symptoms of psychopathology may be factored into two fear-related dimensions: one of these is called anxious–misery and the other is called fear. The anxious–misery (generalized anxiety) factor is linked to disorders of dysthymia, major depression, general anxiety disorder, and PTSD; whereas the fear factor is linked to social phobia, simple phobia, agorophobia, and panic disorder. The combination of these two factors defines the "internalizing" psychopathology that I discuss in Chapter 10.

Rosen and Schulkin (1998) suggest that the generalized disposition to distress may develop out of a fear system that was initially centered in the central amygdala, but that through a traumatic event led to the development of more general sensitivity in the extended amygdala (BNST). This idea links constitutionally based fear reactivity and the experience of traumatic events to the development of more general distress proneness. Although until now, most temperament researchers have not distinguished between fear and generalized distress proneness, work in this area is of great interest and importance.

Anger/Irritability

In Gray's (1982) model, circuits connecting the amygdala, hypothalamus, midbrain, and motor networks of the lower brain stem are involved in directly processing punishment and the failure to achieve expected reward (frustration), leading to *fight-or-flight* reactions. When pain or frustrating input is processed, these circuits can produce aggressive or defensive behavior. Panksepp (1982) discusses a similar neural circuitry in terms of a "rage" system (see review by Rothbart, Derryberry, et al., 1994: Rothbart & Posner, 2006).

Two different neural systems appear to be involved in different kinds of aggression. Aggression in the service of self-defense seems to be based on the same amygdala circuits used in the processing of fear (Blanchard & Takahashi, 1988). When the animal is protecting its resources or competing for new ones, however, a different neural system is involved, one based on the neuromodulator dopamine (DA; Lawrence & Calder, 2004). This system is linked to the production of offensive aggression (Smeets & González, 2000), and to the recognition of anger in the human face (Lawrence, Calder, McGowan, & Grasby, 2002). It is also linked to approach/surgency and there is evidence that the DA system supports irritable aggression (Depue & Iacono, 1989).

Negative Emotionality

A broad factor of temperament in humans is Negative Emotionality, including fear, anxiety, sadness, frustration/anger, and discomfort (Ahadi et al., 1993). Negative Emotionality is generally found to be independent of Surgency or Positive Emotionality so that people high in surgency may also be high in negative affect (Watson & Clark, 1992b). When measured in the same situation, however, activation of fear is likely to oppose the expression of surgency, or vice versa. In our observation of infants presented with emotion-inducing situations, they sometimes rapidly alternated between positive and negative emotions, and between approach and avoidance (Rothbart & Sheese, 2007).

Neural models can also be found to support general negative emotionality. First, we consider those brain circuits that underlie both fear and defensive aggression. If fear and defensive aggression share an underlying neural system, then general negative emotionality (sometimes labeled neuroticism; e.g., Eysenck, 1947) may rely on these shared networks. We often view and talk about a person as being "defensive," suggesting that he or she is highly sensitive to threats to the self-concept. A defensive person responds, often angrily, to events sensed as threatening.

A second link supporting negative emotionality is to general stress reactivity (McEwen, 2007). Stress reactions involve responses to threat via the autonomic nervous system, the hypothalamic–pituitary–adrenal (HPA) endocrine axis, and behaviors of fight or flight. Studies of stress reactivity include research on the HPA axis and cortisol reactivity (Gunnar & Quevedo, 2007), sympathetic and parasympathetic reactivity (El-Sheikh et al., 2009), and cardiovascular reactivity (Kagan, 1994) including studies of vagal tone (Beauchaine, 2001; Porges, Doussard-Roosevelt, & Mati, 1994).

One exciting aspect of considering proneness to stress as temperamental is that it gives us access to recent advances in the neuroscience of stress (e.g., Gunnar & Quevedo, 2007; Gunnar & Vazquez, 2006; McEwen, 2007; Sapolsky, Romero, & Munck, 2000). McEwen has suggested that changes in the body to compensate for stress reactions create an "allostatic load" that can over time be injurious to physical and mental health. In McEwen's words, "The common experience of being 'stressed out' has [at] its core the elevation of some of the systems that lead to allostatic overload: cortisol, sympathetic activity and proinflammatory cytokines, with a decline in parasympathetic activity" (p. 881).

Negative emotion is also regulated by general neurochemical systems and by circulating gonadal and corticosteroid hormones (see review in Rothbart, Derryberry, et al., 1994), influencing a broad range of negative emotions. Serotonin projections, for example, appear to moderate circuits related to both anxiety and aggression (Spoont, 1992). Low serotonin levels may thus increase a person's vulnerability to both fear and frustration, and contribute to general negative emotionality, including sadness and depression (Kramer, 1993). Genes influencing the serotonin pathway have also been linked to antisocial, aggressive, and impulsive behavior (Lesch, 2003). Finally, gonadal hormones are related to both positive emotion and aggressiveness (Zuckerman, 1991). We now continue our discussion by considering neural models that support surgency. These models provide a basis for desiring and moving toward positive rewards.

Surgency/Approach

A broad factor of surgency was described in Chapter 2; it includes activity, approach, and positive emotion. Based on animal research, models of approach-related networks have been put forward by Cloninger (1986), Depue and Collins (1999), Gray (1978), Panksepp (1982, 1998), and Zuckerman (1984). These models involve dopaminergic (DA) neurons and brain structures including the ventral tegmental area and the nucleus accumbens. When animals are more reward sensitive and approaching, these networks are more easily activated and the animal is motivated to seek the desired objects. Autonomic supports for action are also activated. This activation of incentive and reward networks has been linked to (1) the initiation of activity toward the reward, (2) anticipatory excitement and eagerness, (3) the exploration of novel environments, and (4) irritable aggression and anger when goals are blocked.

Reward sensitivity is also linked to positive emotion. Tellegen's (1985) research on personality yielded a broad factor he called Positive Emotionality that included pleasure and positive anticipation, and Watson and Clark (1997) have argued that positive emotion is at the core of individual differences in extraversion. In our research on infants (Rothbart, 1988; Rothbart et al., 2000), we found that smiling and laughter was related to how rapidly the infants grasped toys in the laboratory.

In fMRI research, Canli et al. (2001) found that adults who were highly extraverted showed greater brain activation to positive stimuli than to negative stimuli, with the activation reflected in widespread frontal, temporal, and limbic activations of both hemispheres of the brain. Adults who were high in neuroticism (negative emotionality), on the other hand, reacted more to negative stimuli than to positive stimuli, and the activation was more circumscribed (frontotemporal on the left side and deactivation in a right frontal area).

Approach–Withdrawal and Optimal Levels of Stimulation

Other models have been proposed to account for the way approach and fear/withdrawal seem to oppose one another. When we first observed a standardized stranger approach of infants in our laboratory (the stranger knocks, enters the room, stops, walks half way to the infant, who is sitting in a high chair, stops, and then approaches all the way), we realized that most children do not simply either approach or avoid the stranger. Instead they alternate between approaching, freezing, and withdrawing from the stranger. They also alternate between looking toward and away from the stranger and alternate smiling, watching, and showing distress.

One model of approach–withdrawal rests on the idea of an "optimal level" of stimulation. More fearful, cautious introverts are seen as more arousable and sensitive to stimulation at low intensities than social and outgoing extraverts (Eysenck, 1967). Introverts experience first pleasure and then later discomfort at increasing levels of stimulus intensity, showing a lower optimal level of arousal, that is, the point when pleasure is at its highest, just before the situation becomes overstimulating, resulting in discomfort. Because of a lower optimal level, the introvert seeks lower stimulus levels that lead to pleasure and avoids higher levels of stimulation that lead to discomfort. In Strelau's (1983, 2008) temperament model, more strongly reactive individuals also carry out activities to maintain their optimal levels of stimulation by holding down exciting stimulation. Less reactive individuals will seek exciting stimulation. Thus the most commonly used coping strategies of individuals will differ, depending on their reactivity. The development of coping is further described in Chapter 6.

Berlyne (1971) proposed a model in which arousal resulting from the intensity, novelty, or surprise value of a stimulus activates two motivational systems. One is pleasure-related, involving approach. This system is activated at lower levels of intensity; the other system involves distress and withdrawal, and is activated at higher levels. The two systems oppose each other, and individual differences in the strength of these two systems create variability in the optimal level of arousal for the person. The optimal level is the point at which the person's approach and pleasure tendencies are at their highest, but withdrawal processes do not yet dominate. Schneirla (1959) put forward similar ideas, describing Approach and Withdrawal systems related to the intensity of stimulation across a broad range of species. Two system approaches are helpful in allowing for the very rapid alternations of approach and withdrawal that we have observed.

In humans, differences in the activation of the right and left cerebral hemispheres have also been related to approach and withdrawal. Higher frontal left-hemisphere EEG activation to stimulation is related to higher positive emotion and lower negative emotion; higher frontal right-hemisphere activation to higher negative emotion and lower positive emotion (see review by Davidson, 2003). Resting EEG balance is also related to individual differences in positive and negative emotional reactivity. Fox, Calkins, and Bell (1994) found that infants with stronger right-frontal EEG activation between 9 and 24 months of age showed more fearfulness and inhibition at 4 years of age than did other children. Shy children also showed right-frontal asymmetry. Other findings do not always agree with this model. Canli et al. (2001), for example, using brain imaging, found in adults that negative stimuli in comparison with positive stimuli activated greater *left* than right frontal and temporal cortex in persons higher in neuroticism. More research is needed to address this model.

Affiliation

Depue and his colleagues argue that there are two broad networks related to rewards (Depue & Collins, 1999; Depue & Morrone-Strupinsky, 2005). The first, the network for surgency discussed above, is strongly related to feelings of desiring, wanting, and positive excitement, and to the rapid activation of responses that will move the organism toward potential reward. The second, the affiliation system, is related to affectionate and gratifying states of closeness to others.

Panksepp (1986b) argues that affiliative and prosocial behaviors depend in part on opiate projections from higher limbic regions (e.g., the amygdala and cingulate cortex) to the hypothalamus. Brain opiates are linked to emotions of social comfort and bonding, and opiate withdrawal leads to irritability and aggressiveness. Because lesions of the hypothalamus can dramatically increase aggression, Panksepp (1986a) suggests that this region normally inhibits aggressive behaviors controlled by midbrain regions. When aggressive tendencies are suppressed, friendly, trusting, and helpful behaviors are possible. Depue and Morrone-Strupinsky (2005) further identify opiate-related systems of affiliation related to affectionate and gratifying states of closeness to others.

Panksepp (1993) reviewed research suggesting links between social bonding and the hypothalamic neuropeptide oxytocin (OXY) involved in maternal behavior, feelings of social acceptance, social bonding, and reduction of separation distress. OXY is also released during sexual activity in both females and males. In Cloninger's (1987) theory, reward dependence is a human temperament dimension that ranges from emotional dependence, sympathy, sentiment, persistence, and sensitivity to social cues at one pole to social detachment, coolness, tough-mindedness, and independent self-will at the other. Cloninger sees reward dependence as supporting social motivation.

Emotion and Attention

Emotion processing most often occurs at the same time as other information processing in the brain, including object recognition and location processing, language, vision, audition, and so on, each of which involves its own underlying neural networks (Posner & Petersen, 1990; Posner & Rothbart, 2007a). Each source of information can also be acted upon by attention. In a thought experiment, keep your eyes focused on a single location, while concentrating on what you see in your central focus of attention. Second, while maintaining your focus, turn your attention to what you see to the right or left; third, on sound; fourth, on how your stomach feels; fifth, on your emotional state; and so on. Connections between the executive attention system and the emotional-processing networks allow the person to select emotional or other information for conscious processing. In this way, at any given moment, we may or may not be aware of our emotional evaluations or preparation for action (Bush, Luu, & Posner, 2000; Posner & Rothbart, 1992), just as we may not be aware of sounds or sights that are available to us.

Attention and emotion systems influence each other, with attention selecting or avoiding information about emotion, and emotion affecting how easily we can shift or focus our attention (see review by Rothbart & Sheese, 2007). In anger, for example, we tend to focus on the agent or object we see as preventing us from attaining our goal. At the same time, motor systems and thoughts about how to remove the obstacle are activated. When we think about what is preventing us from getting what we want, we may also repeatedly rehearse the situation and what we can do about it. In states of fear, we may monitor the dangerous object, our own feelings, and possible routes of escape in the immediate situation, or we may relive the fearful situation in our thoughts. Attention is also used in thinking our way out of difficult situations, and after the event, in deciding what we are going to do the next time the situation occurs. When we are under severe threat or stress, however, we may find this kind of thought to be very difficult.

Attention is also essential to reading the state of other people and understanding and communicating with them (Goleman, 1995; Matthews, Zeidner, & Roberts, 2002). This use of attention influences our acceptance by others (Parker & Asher, 1987). Information about the state of others is important to our adaptive behavior, and failure to adequately process social information can also be involved in the development of disorders (Blair, Jones, Clark, & Smith, 1997). Attention, for example, is implicated in the neurotic process. When a person's attention is focused on threatening stimuli or on the precarious state of the self, information about others is less accessible. When we are afraid or angry, we may thus be cut off from information that would have helped us respond appropriately to others. On the other hand, our own empathic distress can be used to inform us about how others feel.

I now turn to models for attention networks, which have been studied at the psychological, neurochemical, and genetic levels, and can serve as a model for the investigation of other temperament systems.

Attention Networks

Three brain networks support different operations of attention: the alerting, orienting, and executive attention networks (Posner & Petersen, 1990; Posner & Rothbart, 2007a). Here I consider the orienting network and the executive attention network that supports effortful control. Orienting involves the selection of locations, aligning one's attention with important signals in the external or internal environment (Posner, 1980). Visual orienting may be *overt*, involving eye movements to the location, or *covert*, where eye movements are not involved. As seen in the thought experiment, we can attend to one location, while at the same time monitoring events that are peripheral to it. The visual orienting system has been associated with posterior brain areas, for example, the parietal lobe and frontal eye fields (Corbetta, Kincade, & Shulman, 2002). Orienting is often studied by presenting a signal indicating where the next event is likely to occur, thus directing attention to the cued location (Posner).

Orienting to novelty is an important reactive aspect of attention, and children differ in how quickly they orient to a novel event and how long they attend to it (see review by Ruff & Rothbart, 1996). In infants, individual differences in duration of orienting are related to smiling and laughter,

and vocal activity, suggesting that orienting may be part of an early positive reactivity or interest system. As the child develops reaching, crawling,
and walking (Gartstein & Rothbart, 2003; Rothbart, 1988; Rothbart, Derryberry, et al., 1994), orienting will be linked to motor approach. Early in
development, orienting plays a central role in the regulation of emotion. It
continues to maintain that role but to a lesser degree as the executive attention system develops (Rothbart, Sheese, Rueda, & Posner, in press; Sheese,
Voelker, Posner, & Rothbart, 2009). In adults, orienting to a novel object has
been shown to draw into play the executive attention system discussed in
the next section (Shulman et al., 2009).

Temperamental effortful control is supported in part by development
of the executive attention network of the brain (Posner & Rothbart, 2000,
2007a). Executive attention involves volitional or willed action (Posner &
Rothbart, 1991, 1994). Areas of the midfrontal lobe, including the anterior cingulate cortex (ACC) and dorsolateral, ventral, and orbital prefrontal
cortex, appear to support this network (Botvinick, Cohen, & Carter, 2004;
Casey et al., 2005; Vogt, Finch, & Olson, 1992). The ACC is also linked to
the limbic system, including the amygdala, and is very closely tied to the
control of emotion. It has close connections to the motor systems that are
located adjacent to it. The ACC connects widely different aspects of attention (e.g., attention to the content of words, environmental locations, or
internal feelings). Activity in the ACC is modified by DA input from the
underlying basal ganglia.

Executive attention is often studied in tasks involving conflict. One
conflict task is the Stroop task, where subjects are instructed to report on
the color of ink (e.g., red) of a word, while ignoring its color name (e.g.,
blue; Bush et al., 2000). Here, conflict is created between our strong tendency to read the color name rather than the ink color. Another task is
the flanker task, in which there is conflict between a central target (e.g.,
an arrow pointing right) and surrounding flanker stimuli (arrows pointing
in the opposite direction to the central arrow) that may conflict with the
target. Resolving conflict in the Stroop task and flanker tasks activates the
ACC and lateral prefrontal cortex, parts of the executive attention network
(Botvinick, Braver, Barch, Carter, & Cohen, 2001). Effortful control has been
linked to performance on conflict tasks, indicating a connection between
effortful control and executive attention (see Rothbart & Rueda, 2005; and
Posner & Rothbart, 2007a, 2007b).

There is evidence for the ACC as part of a network involved in regulation of action, cognition, and affect (Allman, Hakeem, Erwin, Nimchinsky,
& Hof, 2001; Bush et al., 2000; Rothbart & Sheese, 2007), and further divi-
sions within the ACC are also important. Dorsal areas of the cingulate have

been linked to the regulation of cognition, and more ventral areas to the regulation of emotion (Bush et al., 2000). The ventral portion of the ACC, related to emotion regulation, shows a high level of tonic activity even at rest (Fox et al., 2005). Activation of the dorsal area also inhibits activation of the ventral area and vice versa (Drevets & Raichle, 1998) suggesting a tradeoff between cognitive control and emotional control. Although additional areas of the cingulate have also been found (Rudebeck, Bannerman, & Rushworth, 2008), the general division into affective and cognitive areas remains supported. Activation of the executive attention network also leads to decreased activity of the amygdala when a person is asked to ignore negative information (Hariri, Mattay, Tessitore, Fera, & Weinberger, 2003).

Questionnaire measures of effortful control in adolescents and adults have also been linked to the activation of executive attention brain areas involved in self-regulation (Kanske, 2008; Whittle, 2007). Kanske found that questionnaire measures of effortful control (Evans & Rothbart, 2007) were related to performance on conflict tasks, whereas self-reported anxiety and depression were related to lower performance on conflict tasks. Low effortful control was also related to EEG measures of high activation in the ventral (emotion-related) ACC. Whittle related measures of the Early Adolescent Temperament Scale (Ellis et al., 2004) to the size of brain structures and their activity. She found that the size of the dorsal (cognition-related) ACC was related to mothers' reports of greater effortful control, whereas ventral (emotion-related) ACC activation was related to lower effortful control.

Emotion thus affects the direction and time course of attention, and attention can be used to control emotion just as emotion influences attention. These processes differ among individuals, reflecting each person's temperamental reactivity and self-regulation. In adults, negative emotionality, neuroticism, and trait anxiety are related to the speed and duration of orientation to threat (e.g., Mogg, Bradley, & Williams, 1995), as well as to altered patterns of attention toward detecting errors (Paulus, Feinstein, Simmons, & Stein, 2004). Neuroticism is also linked to the difficulty a person has in disengaging his or her attention from sources of threat (Derryberry & Reed, 1994, 2002). Extraversion, on the other hand, is related to difficulties in disengaging attention from rewarding stimuli (Derryberry & Reed, 1994).

Summary

Models from neuroscience have been frequently associated with temperament dimensions, following the ancient tradition of linking temperament to underlying physiology as it was understood at the time. Models have been described here for fear, anger/aggression, general negative emotionality, approach, and affiliation. The orienting and executive attention networks have also been described. This is a very active area of research, especially in human brain-imaging studies, and will continue to grow. Another area of intense activity is research on molecular genetics. I now turn to contributions of behavior genetics and molecular genetics research to the study of temperament.

TEMPERAMENT AND GENES

Behavior Genetics

Research in behavior genetics has addressed the question of a biological basis for temperament by estimating the amount of variation in a trait that can be attributed to genetic variation within a population of people. In twin studies, differences between identical (monozygotic, or MZ) twins and fraternal (dizygotic, or DZ) twins are compared. MZ twins, who share 100% of their inherited genes, are expected to be more alike than DZ twins, who share 50% of their genetic material. Estimates of genetic influence in twin studies have been substantial for most broad temperament and personality traits. In general, genes have been found to account for 40–50% of the variability in temperament and in the Big Five and FFM personality measures (Krueger & Johnson, 2008; also see discussion by Zuckerman, 2005). The Big Five and FFM measures are also highly correlated with measures of temperament in adults (Evans & Rothbart, 2007). The Big Five and FFM measures with the corresponding temperament factors are extraversion (surgency), agreeableness (affiliation vs. anger/frustration), neuroticism (negative emotionality), conscientiousness (effortful control), and openness (orienting sensitivity).

Adoption studies, where adoptive and biological siblings are compared, give generally lower heritability estimates than twin studies. Both twin and adoption studies provide support for both genetic and environmental influences on individual differences, although the effects of being raised in the same family appear to account for little of the environmental influence (Krueger & Johnson, 2008). Environmental influences tend not to be shared within the family, as might be expected for children who have quite different experiences with parents and siblings.

Tellegen et al. (1988) studied adult MZ and DZ twins who either had been raised together or had been separated early in life and raised apart. Overall correlations of traits for MZ twins raised away from each other were high and quite similar to those found for identical twins raised together, with heritability estimates of about 50%. Correlations for MZ twins raised apart were considerable for stress reaction (negative emotionality), sense of well-being, control, low risk taking, and aggression. For the broad traits of positive emotionality, negative emotionality, and constraint (a combination of effortful control and fearful inhibition), only positive emotionality showed evidence that MZ and DZ twins raised together were more similar than twins raised apart. These findings suggest shared family influences on positive reactivity, although most twin studies have found little evidence for the influence of being raised in the same family (Krueger & Johnson, 2008).

Goldsmith, Buss, and Lemery (1996) reviewed six studies of behavioral genetics in children that also found clear heritability of temperament. Questionnaire measures showed a shared family influence for positive emotionality and approach, supporting Tellegen et al.'s (1988) research with adults. Goldsmith et al. (1996) also found evidence for both genetic and shared family influences on CBQ effortful control, suggesting that effortful control is also influenced by family experience.

Although behavioral genetics research argues for strong heritability of individual differences in temperament, the findings are based on the usual environmental circumstances experienced by developing children within a given sample (Krueger, South, Johnson, & Iacono, 2008). The analysis thus does not tell us what the heritability *might* be if the environments were different. They also do not let us know *how* temperament and personality outcomes develop. Zuckerman (2005) raises a number of additional cautions in interpreting heritability studies. In 1995, Zuckerman addressed the question of "What is inherited?" in this way:

> We do not inherit personality traits or even behavior mechanisms as such. What is inherited are chemical templates that produce and regulate proteins involved in building the structure of nervous systems and the neurotransmitters, enzymes, and hormones that regulate them. . . . How do these differences in biological traits shape our choices in life from the manifold possibilities provided by environments . . . ? Only cross-disciplinary, developmental and comparative psychological research can provide the answers. (pp. 331–332)

Experience and environment build changes in brain structure and functioning (Posner & Raichle, 1994) both before and after birth (Black & Greenough, 1991). This view is very different from the idea that genes give us a hard wiring that will determine our future temperament and personality.

Recently methods of molecular genetics have allowed researchers to make more precise linkages of genes and temperament, and have found that environmental effects often depend on the temperament of the child. I now turn to some of the findings in this area.

Molecular Genetics

The mapping of the human genome has provided an exciting new direction for understanding the role of genes and environment in development. In research on individual differences in attention, for example, the variations in at least two genes have been related to the executive network as measured by the Attention Network Test (ANT) in adults. One is a variation in the dopamine D4 receptor (DRD4) gene; another is a variation in the monoamine oxidase (MAOA) gene, related to the synthesis of dopamine and norepinephrine. In a genetic imaging study, variations in these genes were also related to differences in brain activation within the ACC, a structure in the executive attention network (Fan, Fossella, Sommer, Wu, & Posner, 2003). Executive attention can also be influenced by other genes related to DA (Blassi et al., 2005) and serotonin (Reuter, Ott, Vaitl, & Hennig, 2007). Genes may interact in their influence on performance. For example, it was found that the DRD4 and the serotonin transporter gene interacted to influence the duration of orienting during infancy (Auerbach, Faroy, Ebstein, Kahana, & Levine, 2001). Specific genes have also been linked to aspects of emotional temperament, including fear and aggression (Panskepp, 1986b, 1998).

In attention studies, the presence of the 4-repeat variation of the DRD4 gene has been associated with greater difficulty in resolving conflict (Fossella, Posner, Fan, Swanson, & Pfaff, 2002). Children with the less common 7-repeat allele of this gene show behavioral aspects of attention-deficit/hyperactivity disorder, but do not show deficits in executive attention based on conflict tasks (Swanson et al., 2000). The 7-repeat variation appears to be more related to sensation seeking, a reward-related temperament trait, than to effortful control. This genetic variation of the DRD4 gene, which developed over the course of human evolution, may have conveyed an advantage for humans who were attracted to novelty, as groups of ancient humans migrated out of Africa (Ding et al., 2002).

Gene–Temperament Interactions

Molecular genetics studies also allow us to look for interactions between genes and environment in producing temperament and personality outcomes in children and adults. We examined the DRD4 7-repeat gene, related to sensation seeking, and parenting as they related to 2-year-old children's temperament (Sheese, Voelker, Rothbart, & Posner, 2007). Children with this variation showed temperamental characteristics that depended on the style of parenting. Children with the DRD4 7-repeat gene whose mothers gave the child high support and autonomy during a free-play interaction showed normal levels of activity and impulsivity. However, children with this variation whose parents did not provide support and autonomy showed high activity level, high risk taking, and impulsivity—all indicating risk for attention-deficit/hyperactivity disorder. Children with no 7-repeat allele showed relatively low levels of activity, risk taking, and impulsivity, regardless of parenting (Sheese et al., 2007).

Presence of the 7-repeat allele may also lead to greater influences of the environment, including parenting and culture, on the child. Greater sensitivity to the environment may also lend an evolutionary advantage as cultural learning gains in importance (Sheese et al., 2007). For example, it has been found that there is a stronger influence of parenting in the presence of the 7-repeat allele than for children without this allele (Bakermans-Kranenburg & van IJzendoorn, 2006; van IJzendoorn & Bakermans-Kranenburg, 2006). Bakersmans-Kranenberg, van IJzendoorn, Pijlman, Mesman, and Juffer (2008) also performed a parenting-training intervention. This training decreased externalizing behavior, but only for those children with the DRD4 7-repeat allele. This finding is important because assignment to the training group was random, thus ensuring that the result is not due to something about the parents other than the training.

In another study of gene–environment interaction, Caspi et al. (2002) investigated an MAOA genotype in relation to the experience of maltreatment in a large sample of children. Children who had been maltreated and who also possessed a variation of the gene that resulted in high levels of MAOA expression were found to be especially likely to develop antisocial behavior problems by adulthood. O'Connor, Caspi, De Fries. and Plomin (2003) studied a group of adopted children, identifying genetic risk by measuring the biological parents' questionnaire self-reports of negative emotionality. At age 12, 23 of the 171 adopted children had also experienced a significant separation from their parents. When there had been no separation, children's genetic risk had no effect on adjustment. If there had been a separation, however, the genetic risk predicted poor adjustment. In these studies, a combination of a genetic disposition and an environmental risk was particularly likely to lead to poor adjustment and antisocial outcomes.

Suomi and his colleagues (Champoux et al., 2002) have studied specific genes and environment in rhesus monkeys, testing for the serotonin-related 5-HTTLR gene. Monkeys with the 5-HTTLR short-repeat allele showed higher levels of distress in a temperament assessment than those without it. In human studies of infants, a similar association has been found, with the 5-HTTLR short-allele linked to higher distress and lower orientation scores (Auerbach et al., 1999; Ebstein et al., 1998). In monkeys, however, lower orientation scores were found *only* for monkeys who had been reared in nurseries with same-age peers, but not if they were raised by their mothers. Suomi and his colleagues suggest that mothers' care and control of their infant's experience may have buffered or protected against the effects of their genetic characteristic, and this has been found in studies of the development of attachment in human children (Barry, Kochanska, & Philibert, 2008). We interpreted our findings with 2-year-olds in a similar way: the DRD4 variation is related to high activity and sensation seeking, but good parenting may serve to moderate and regulate this tendency (Sheese et al., 2007).

Animal Studies of Environmental Influence on Temperament

Researchers studying laboratory animals have used inbred strains to control for heredity while studying the effects of early experience on later behavior. One surprising early finding was that when newborn rats had received some kind of handling by the caretaker, rather than being left alone, they showed less emotionality and stress reactivity later in life. Newborn rats who had been removed from the nest and handled, or even given shocks or been shaken, showed later lower fear and stress reactions than animals who had not (Levine, Haltmeyer, Karas, & Denenberg, 1967; see review by Konner, 2002). Recently, however, Meaney (2001) and his colleagues have found that the later lowered reactivity of the animal is linked not to the handling itself, but to the behavior of the mother rat after the pup is returned to the nest, having been taken out and handled (Diorio & Meaney, 2007). After its return, the mother licks and grooms the pup extensively, and the mother's behavior is linked to lower later fear. Even when handling did not occur, the mother rats who licked and groomed their offspring more raised bolder pups. "They explore more in the open field, indicating less fear, and they have more receptors in the amygdala for anxiety reducing drugs—that they probably use to calm themselves naturally. In addition, they are physiologically less stress-responsive" (Konner, 2002, p. 224).

More extreme stress, such as prolonged separation from the mother, has the opposite effect, increasing fearful reactivity (Spencer-Booth & Hinde, 1971). Nevertheless, animal research clearly indicates that emotional reactivity is influenced by experience. Meaney (2001) sees this as the programming of neural networks by the early environment. These animal studies offer support of human research on the effects of childhood trauma and neglect on patterns of behavior and reactivity to stress (Felitti et al., 1998).

"Knockout" Animals

By artificially introducing mutation in the cells of mice, it is possible to abolish (or knock out) the activity of a preselected gene. Interbreeding mice with mutations produces a generation of mice that have inherited the mutation from both parents, and carry two copies of the mutant gene. These are called "knockout mice." Characteristics of knockout mice have been used to provide clues about a gene's normal role in development. For example, by deleting a single gene, mice have shown a dramatic reduction in nurturance and affiliation (Brown, Ye, Bronson, Dikkes, & Greenberg, 1996). When genetic manipulation was used to increase the number of vasopressin receptors in the brain, a strain of unsocial field mice was transformed into animals with more outgoing and gregarious temperament (Young, Lopez, Murphy-Weinberg, Watson, & Akil, 1998). Single gene deletions have also produced heightened aggression (Nelson & Young, 1998) and anxiety (Parks, Robinson, Sibille, Shenk, & Toth, 1998; Pattij et al., 2002). An important concern in interpreting this research, however, is that when genes are missing from birth, there may be compensations in behavior during the animal's development that could be confused with the more direct effects of a missing gene. Nevertheless, these studies provide promising prospects for future understanding of the biology of temperament.

SUMMARY

In this chapter, I have considered some of the temperament characteristics that we share with nonhuman animals, and noted why the distinction between temperament and personality is important. I have also briefly touched upon some of the brain networks seen to underlie individual differences in temperament. Chemical templates inherited in the genes contribute to brain structures that are reflected in our temperament characteristics, and we can now trace links between our genes, brain structure, and behavior. We are also able to study links between genes, parenting, and behavior at different stages of development. Future research will increasingly link development of the nervous system to changes and continuities in temperament, and will consider periods of specific interest such as toddlerhood, adolescence, and aging. Beginning with Chapter 4, I look at children's temperament in interaction with experience during early development.

CHAPTER 4

Infancy

In this chapter, I begin our study of social and personality development, starting with the days just following birth. To do this, I rely heavily on our understanding of the early dimensions of temperament. Because infants are social organisms from the very start, I also recognize that it is necessary to consider development within the caregiver–infant relationship. Later in life, children will see themselves as separate objects, describe themselves, evaluate themselves, and even make decisions about who they wish to be, but in the beginning the infant lacks the elaborated thought and the language, effortful attention, and controlled action that allow those kinds of decisions. Temperament can be seen clearly during this period.

The temperamental core of personality in early infancy includes distress proneness, orienting, and soothability. By 2–3 months, we will also see positive affect, approach and surgency, frustration, cuddliness and affiliation. These dimensions affect the child's interactions with the social and physical world. The infant's reactions that are initially based on temperament will be adapted during repeated interchanges with others and the environment. The child's expectations about the world and significant figures in it will also be developing, and the child's adaptations and expectations will be built around what the environment offers: soothing; opportunities for food, play, and exploration; frustration when the child is removed from playing with objects or the objects are taken away; threats in the form of strange persons, objects and situations; and the expectable rhythms of eating, playing, and sleeping.

TEMPERAMENT IN THE NEWBORN

All healthy newborns show varying states of arousal and emotion (Korner, 1972; Wolff, 1987). These include states of sleep, distress, calmness, alertness, activity, quiet, and acceptance or rejection of stimulation. The quality of these states varies from child to child and early temperament differences will be reflected in the infant's states and state regulation. Distress proneness, self-soothing, and soothability are important aspects of temperament in the newborn infant. We begin by looking at two of the quite different newborn infants described by Brazelton and Cramer in 1990, Robert and Emily. Robert is a physically active newborn, yet he quiets when placed on his mother's stomach. He moves his hand easily to his mouth for self-soothing and can make well-organized crawling movements with his legs when placed on his stomach. When bathed, he cries loudly, but then quiets rapidly when wrapped in a swaddling blanket. Brazelton and Cramer judged that Robert would create few challenges for his caregivers in the early months.

The second child, Emily, is much more uneven in her states. She awakens suddenly, making jerky movements and crying. She appears to be unable to bring her hand to her mouth. When startled, her arms and legs are thrown out to the sides, she becomes distressed, and seems unable to soothe herself. Her mother finds her difficult to soothe, and worries because she seems so different from her first two children, who had been more like Robert. However, Emily's mother is open to observing her daughter and notices that

> Emily preferred gentle handling and subdued noises. Whereas she might turn away from a loud noise or an abrupt stimulus, she'd turn toward a gentler, softer one. If she [Emily's mother] spoke gently to her as she built up to crying, she could "bring Emily down" to a quiet, alert state. If she stroked her gently or gave her a finger to suck on, Emily used it to keep herself quiet. Even when she was awake and upset, her mother soon found that handling her, rocking her in a containing embrace, or standing her up to bounce gently on her legs became ways that organized Emily and calmed her upset, driven states. (Brazelton & Cramer, 1990, pp. 81–82)

Emily's mother is doing what parents can do when they are sensitive to the preferences of their babies. It is as clear to me as yesterday when the nurses swaddled our firstborn son in a receiving blanket, and we brought him home. After we loosened his blanket, he began to cry very loudly, and picking him up and walking with him did nothing to soothe him. After some scary moments, we remembered that he had been calm when he was swaddled. It took me several tries to develop a good blanket-wrapping technique, but over a period of hours, we saw that swaddling really did serve to "bring him down." Swaddling is used for soothing and infant-state regulation in many cultures, and Chisholm (1978) has suggested it may have a place in industrialized cultures as well. Later, we discovered that a pacifier and vigorous rocking were equally effective for soothing our son.

Assessing Temperament in Newborns

From the start, the child's reactive distress occurs in the context of the caregiver's soothing. In fact, the other-regulation provided by the caregiver in combination with the self-soothing and soothability of the infant provides an early example of infant reactivity, self-regulation, and caregiver regulation. We will see examples of this kind of interaction throughout development, but now we turn to ways of assessing the newborn's temperament.

Two major methods have been used to study newborn temperament: one is the Brazelton Neonatal Behavioral Assessment Scale (NBAS; Brazelton & Nugent, 1995; Brazelton, Nugent, & Lester, 1987); the second involves more standard observations of the infant in the hospital or laboratory (Birns, 1965; Riese, 1987). The NBAS developed out of the newborn neurological examination used to assess the infant's physiological well-being by observing the newborn's reflexes and changing states. The NBAS includes ratings of autonomic, attentional, and motor responsiveness (reactivity) of the newborn and the child's state changes during the exam. The NBAS is an interactional assessment, meaning that the tester tries to elicit the best possible performance in each infant. This means that the NBAS is not completely standardized, and there is variability in how it is done, depending on what the tester believes will create the best conditions for each child. This raises problems when we wish to use standard procedures for measuring temperament. Because it emphasizes the baby's competencies, the NBAS has also been used to demonstrate to parents the many adaptive skills of their newborn.

Strauss and Rourke (1978) carried out a factor analysis of 10 samples of newborn NBAS ratings, identifying four major factors, which can be taken as early temperamental differences among children: (1) *orienting*, chiefly to visual stimuli, when the child was quiet and in an alert state; (2) *irritability*, tension, and *activity*; (3) *soothability* and rapidity of build up of distress; and (4) overall susceptibility to *distress*. Newborns who showed greater orienting to the outside environment were also less susceptible to distress. This balance between orienting and negative emotion will be seen later in infancy (Harman, Rothbart, & Posner, 1997), and greater attentional control has been linked to lower negative emotionality up to adulthood in our temperament research (Derryberry & Rothbart, 1988; Evans & Rothbart, 2007; Rothbart & Sheese, 2007).

The link between activity and irritability is also very interesting. In an early study, Fries (1954) assessed newborn activity using a startle test (dropping a padded weight on the bed close to the infant's head). Infants were rated as quiet if their movement in reaction to the event lasted less than 10 seconds, active if it lasted more than 25 seconds, and moderately active if they were in between. Fries also observed the infant's frustration reaction when the breast or bottle was removed while the infant was sucking on it. Infants who were more active on the startle test also showed stronger motor reactions to this frustration. Quieter infants continued to make sucking movements and often fell asleep shortly after the nipple was removed. The relation between higher activity level and greater frustration reactivity has also been observed throughout the study of temperament in infancy and childhood (Rothbart, Derryberry, & Hershey, 2000; Rothbart & Derryberry, 2002), although connections between activity and positive enthusiasm (surgency) are also clear.

Birns (1965; Birns et al., 1969) observed newborn distress reactions to application of a cold disc to the infant's skin or to removing a pacifier. Infants were followed up at 1, 3, and 4 months of age, and their social responsiveness was observed at 3 and 4 months. Newborn distress proneness was related to higher irritability, and to lower smiling and vocal reactivity to social stimulation at 3 and 4 months. In the Louisville Twin Study (Matheny, Riese, & Wilson, 1985; Riese, 1987), newborn irritability predicted 2-year-old higher distress, lower attentiveness to stimuli, and responsiveness to observers, and more variability in motor movement, although the predictions from the newborn did not hold for the ages below 2. Newborn irritability in the NBAS also predicted 15-month-old irritability, unsociability, and unadaptability (Larson, DiPietro, & Porges, 1987) on the ICQ (Bates et al., 1979). Orienting in newborns with disabilities was also related to greater social participation and social competence when the children were 3 years old (Bakeman & Brown, 1980). Thus, newborn orienting, activity, distress proneness, and soothability differences can be seen early in life and show some continuity with later temperament.

CAREGIVERS' AND INFANTS' DEVELOPMENTAL ISSUES

The infant is social, and infant, child, and adult personality develops through social interchanges. During the first years of life, infant development is rapid. Each major change in the child can also create a new challenge for the parent, just as the parent's responses or lack of responsiveness can create adaptational challenges for the child. Sander (1962, 1969) observed 30 pairs of infants and their mothers in the hospital and then at their homes over the first months of life. Over the course of these observations, he identified a series of major *issues* or challenges faced by caregivers and infants early in life. Each of these issues can be related to the children's temperament, their developing self-regulation, and their relations to others. Sander described his approach in this way:

> After following ten or fifteen of the pairs we could begin to anticipate the time of appearance of some of the important concerns the mother would express, or, on the other hand, feel relieved about. This gave the impression that we were watching a sequence of adaptations common to all the different mother–infant pairs, although acted out somewhat differently by each. Each advancing level of activity which the child became capable of manifesting demanded a new adjustment in the mother–child relationship. (1969, p. 1)

An example of a change that requires adjustment from the caregiver is the infant's ability to get about by crawling or walking. When children can move from place to place and go after objects, and cannot be moved from one place to another without protesting, the parents face issues related to the child's growing autonomy and independence. One way the caregiver may cope with these issues is to baby proof the house so that infant and parent desires do not conflict too often. This minimizes the need for running after and correcting the child, and is less likely to contribute to the child's frustration.

How the early issues are dealt with is built into the history of infant and caregiver adaptations to each other, and each adaptation affects future interactions. This is what development is all about, and we cannot truly understand the child's temperament and personality without tracing this social history. The developmental issues identified by Sander (1969) with one added from Margaret Mahler (1967), are listed in Table 4.1. The first is the issue of initial regulation.

Initial Regulation

Newborns show more gradations between wake and deep sleep than at any point later in life, and these are organized into infant states (Korner, 1972). They also show rhythmic changes in sleep and wakefulness, hunger, and elimination. These range from the rhythms of sleeping and waking (circadian rhythms), through 4- to 6-hour rhythms of alertness (ultraradian

TABLE 4.1. Infant Developmental Issues

Issue	Span of months	Prominent infant behaviors (that became coordinated with maternal activities)
Initial regulation	1–3	Regulation of infant's eating, sleeping and states of emotion and attention, including needs for soothing and arousal.
Reciprocal exchange	3–4	Activities of infant care, such as feeding, dressing, and bathing, become reciprocally coordinated. Infant smiling is part of the infant-mother social exchange.
Hatching	4–5	The infant has more control over orienting his or her attention and may be directing it away from the caregiver.
Initiative	5–9	Activities are initiated by the infant to gain the mother's proximity and attention, and the infant sets out to actively manipulate the environment.
Focalization	9–15	The infant seeks proximity with and attends closely to the mother, focusing on her to meet his or her needs.
Self-assertion	14–20	The child develops a concept of self and engages in self-assertive activity that may come into conflict with the desires of the mother.

Note. Data from Sander (1969) and Mahler (1967).

rhythms), to more rapid rhythms of scanning, sucking, body movement, and respiration. Sleep–wake and other rhythmic states are easier to see in some infants than in others, and being able to "read" the signals of the infant is of great importance to the caregiver. For example, noticing the infant's reflex of rooting (moving the head and lips toward the caregiver's body in response to touch), the caregiver can see some of the earliest signs that the infant is hungry. In time, the infant will "read" the mother's preparations for feeding, bottle or breast, and will avidly prepare for a meal.

The first issues Sander (1977) observed involved *initial regulation*, that is, the regulation of the infant's eating, sleeping, and states of emotion and attention. The infant's temperamental irritability and soothability, as well as infant orienting, will both contribute to state regulation. Some infants can soothe themselves easily, sucking on a thumb or pacifier, rubbing the face, hair, or body. Self-soothing behaviors are shown in the womb, and some infants are born sucking their thumb. In contrast, some infants are more at the mercy of an extended period of distress than others, and a variety of soothing techniques are used by the caregiver to bring the baby to a calm, and often, sleeping state. The caregiver's goal is to assist the infant in moving from distress to a calm, alert state, and from distressed wakefulness to sleep. If there is a universal social issue in infant development, it is likely this one, although different cultures will vary in how it is handled.

The regularity of the environment makes a contribution to infants' sleep–wake rhythms from the very start. For the first 10 days of life, Sander, Julia, Stechler, and Burns (1972) assigned newborns randomly to either a single caregiver who was sensitive to their needs, or to the normal hospital routine where a rotating series of nurses followed a more strict schedule. Infants in the single caregiver group developed earlier differentiation of day–night sleep and greater stability of sleep cycles, and these persisted over the first 2 months of the infant's life. Infants in the single caregiver group were also more regular in feeding.

Many issues involving regulation of state can reoccur later in development. Soothing the young infant to a calm or sleep state is a challenge during the newborn period, but later in the first year, the issue of the child's sleeping through the night often occupies both infant and parent, and sleeping issues can continue into the preschool period (Bates, Viken, Alexander, Beyers, & Stockton, 2002). Sleep regulation issues also are seen in adolescence, when many young people sleep a great deal and do not function well early in the day (Carskadon, 2002). Still later, issues of sleep and waking develop in aging (Foley, Ancoli-Israel, Britz, & Walsh, 2004). In Chapter 9, I consider how disorders of regulation, including sleep problems, can develop.

Soothability

Like most parents preparing for a second baby, we thought we had learned how to soothe any infant from what had worked with our first child. Our first child required vigorous rocking and rhythmic stimulation, and the frequent use of a pacifier for soothing. When we used these techniques with our second child, however, not only did they not soothe him, but they appeared to make him more distressed. He preferred to soothe himself, lying quietly while self-calming, and he completely rejected the pacifier. Our second child preferred lower levels of stimulation than the first, a difference I discuss later in connection with optimal levels of stimulation.

Individual differences in proneness to distress and soothability create challenges for the caregiver who is trying to soothe the infant. Infants who are more distress prone are also more difficult to soothe (Crockenberg & Smith, 1982), creating a special challenge for the caregiver who is trying to regulate the infant's state. Leerkes and Crockenberg (2002) found that mothers of irritable infants who successfully soothed them showed greater feelings of effectiveness than other parents. On the other hand, parents can become discouraged when their children do not seem to respond to them. Escalona (1968) described how a mother felt when she "expended loving efforts without the immediate gratification of seeing the babies respond. Maternal feeling and behavior depend heavily on the mother's perception of herself as someone who know[s] what is best for the baby and who knows herself effective in tending and satisfying his needs" (p. 108). Parents who see their infants as more soothable also show greater sensitivity to their infants (Ghera, Hane, Malesa, & Fox, 2006), or perhaps the parent only *seems* to be more sensitive to the infant because the infant is easier to soothe. It is very difficult to disentangle each member's contribution to caregiver–child interaction.

Soothability also influences the child's expectations about others. Infants will be developing expectations about caregiver soothing as well as learning what they can do to soothe themselves. Their view of the other-regulation situation is also very different from that of the parent. For example, infants do not yet have a cognitive model of the self. Thus, while parents are making judgments about the soothability of the infant and about their own capacity to soothe the child, the infant is making no such judgments. The parent thinks about the situation using the words and categories he or she has picked up from others and the advice of experts; the infant uses no such words and categories. Looking at the larger family unit, we see that both mothers and fathers are affected by infant crying. Wilkie and Ames (1986), for example, found that infant crying was related to fathers' negative views about themselves and negative views about their partners as wives and mothers. Crockenberg and Leerkes (2003) found that mothers who reported that their infants showed greater distress to novelty also reported lower satisfaction with the support they received from their partner. They expressed greater satisfaction with the partner when the child was highly soothable.

A model for early soothing is depicted in Figure 4.1. One of the first things to notice about this figure is that in addition to regulation by the caregiver, infants come into the world with mechanisms for both self-soothing and enlisting the soothing of others. Newborns suck their thumb, finger, and hands, and they turn away from higher-intensity stimulation (Lewkowicz & Turkewitz, 1981). During the first months of life, developmental changes will lead to the infant's increasing control over orienting and greater control over self-soothing.

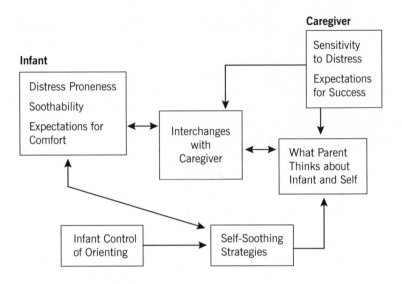

FIGURE 4.1. A model for infant soothing.

Orienting, Soothing, and Coping

The soothing techniques that are effective with infants change over the course of early development. Parents of newborns are more likely to use physical methods such as holding, walking, and rocking but by 3 months they will be distracting the child by presenting interesting sights or sounds (Jahromi, Putnam, & Stifter, 2004). Does distraction work in soothing infants? We studied orienting to distractors and soothing in 3- and 6-month-old infants (Harman et al., 1997). Infants were first shown a sound and light display that led to distress in about 50% of the infants. We then presented the infants with interesting visual and auditory distractors such as sound-making toys. As infants oriented to the distractors, their facial and vocal signs of distress disappeared. As soon as their orienting stopped, however (e.g., when the object was removed), the infants' distress returned to almost exactly the same level as they had shown prior to the presentation of the distractor. We experimentally determined that this distress was not a frustration effect due to the removal of the object. An internal system, which we called the *distress keeper*, appeared to keep track of the infant's initial level of distress, so that it returned when the infant's orienting to the novel event was lost. In later studies, we found that infants could be quieted by distraction for as long as 1 minute, without affecting their level of distress once the orienting was ended (Harman et al.).

For younger infants, the adult can present distractors that control the infant's orienting during soothing. By 4 months of age, however, infants have gained a good deal of control over their *own* orienting (Johnson, Posner, & Rothbart, 1991). They are now able to anticipate *where* the next visual event will be located in a repeated sequence of locations (Clohessy, Posner, & Rothbart, 2001; Haith, Hazan, & Goodman, 1988). They can disengage their gaze from one visual location and move it to another rather than being apparently stuck on the first position (Ruff & Rothbart, 1996). Infants' control over orienting is also linked to lower distress proneness and higher soothability as reported by their parents (Johnson et al., 1991).

How do infants come to use attention to control their own emotion? We observed a number of changes in the use of attention by infants who visited our laboratory four times between 3 and 13 months of age (Rothbart, Ziaie, & O'Boyle, 1992). As they grew older, infants increasingly looked away from distressing objects. Looking away appears to be an effective strategy for the infant to regulate his or her own arousal within a comfortable range. Field (1981) found that 4-month-old infants showed heightened heart rate in the period just before they looked away, and lowered heart rate while they were looking away.

Infants in our study also increasingly turned to their mothers when arousing stimuli such as masks and mechanical toys were presented. By 13 months, infants' disengagement (looking away) from the stimuli was related to lower levels of expressed distress in the laboratory. There was also some stability from 10 to 13 months in infants' patterns of looking away, mouthing, hand-to-mouth soothing (e.g., thumb or hand sucking), approach, and withdrawing the hand, suggesting that the infants' soothing strategies were becoming habitual by the last quarter of the first year of life.

Between the ages of 3 and 13 months, infants' use of passive methods of self-soothing such as thumb sucking decreased, and infants used more active methods, including attacking the mechanical toys by hitting them or throwing them off the table, and waving their arms. Infants who had shown the greatest distress in the laboratory at 3 months, however, tended to persist in self-soothing by self-touching or sucking. Once a mechanism for emotion regulation develops, it may persist because it has brought relief to the child, even though more sophisticated emotion regulation strategies can become available at a later time. This idea is very important as we think about the persistence of children's social and personality adjustments. What works in one time and at one place may be carried over to future situations, even when the methods may not be effective.

Other studies have found that infants who used disengagement of attention to soothe themselves were able to directly decrease their levels of distress (Stifter & Braungart, 1995), and we have proposed that early mechanisms for coping with negative emotion may later be transferred to the control of cognition (Posner & Rothbart, 1998). In support of this idea, infants' use of self-regulation in anger-inducing situations predicts their ability to delay reward when they are preschoolers (Calkins & Williford, 2003). Mischel and his colleagues (Sethi, Mischel, Aber, Shoda, & Rodriguez, 2000) observed children's ability to delay gratification, that is, to choose to wait for a larger reward when a smaller reward was immediately available. When toddlers diverted their attention away from a desired stimulus while waiting for it, they were better able to resist temptation. Toddlers' use of distraction strategies also predicted their later ability to delay gratification.

Culture affects how infants are soothed by their caretakers and whether they are soothed at all. When I was born, my mother was a young woman barely graduated from high school. She had married a school teacher and was living in Reedpoint, Montana. Her own mother lived in North Dakota, and she and my father were alone in their parenting. She searched for information on how to raise me, her firstborn, and looked to the experts for help. The U.S. Department of Agriculture published pamphlets (the Child Care Bulletins) on how to raise children, and at that time they were strongly influenced by the childrearing advice of the behaviorist John B. Watson. Watson's (1930) views on raising children were based on a rather Puritan interpretation of learning theory. He argued that children should be fed on a 4-hour schedule; no exceptions. Any love responses directed toward the child by the parent were discouraged. They would only create a child who was riddled by dependency and inadequacy; these responses were to be avoided. The parent was to treat the child objectively, avoiding any nurturant emotions or behavior.

I have asked my mother how I handled this situation. She said I didn't cry very much but engaged in a lot of self-soothing. I sucked my thumb and twirled my hair to bring myself down. I may have felt somewhat helpless, with the only predictable thing the orderliness of feedings, which occurred whether I was hungry or not. On the other hand, there were some positive consequences of my attempts to adjust to the Watson regime. I developed language early; it allowed me to communicate with my parents and also led to their approval. My sister was born when I was 14 months old, and my mother would leave me to watch her when she went outside to hang up clothes. My mother remembers me coming out, not much more than a baby myself, to tell her that the baby was crying. My early experience involved little soothing from others, but it may have set me on a road that would make words and the communication of ideas important to me for the rest of my life. And my sister? She cried so much that my mother couldn't bear to follow the 4-hour feeding schedule. She gave it up and fed Carol when she was hungry.

Reciprocal Exchange

The second issue described by Sander (1962, 1969) is called *reciprocal exchange*, defined as back-and-forth exchanges in smiling, spoon feeding, vocalizing, and other activities. Here, we observe the influence of temperamental differences in smiling and laughter, vocal reactivity, orienting, and possibly affiliation. At 3–4 months, the infant has become more oriented to the outside world, and smiles and coos to social stimulation (Emde, Gaensbauer, & Harmon, 1976; Ruff & Rothbart, 1996). Active positive interchanges between parent and infant are now possible, and the infant's smiles, coos, and extended gaze enchant us (Stern, 1985). Selma Fraiberg (1977) described the social interchanges shown by caregiver and infant in poetical language:

> During the first six months, the baby has the rudiments of love language available to him. There is the language of the embrace, the language of the eyes, the language of the smile, vocal communications of pleasure and distress. It is the essential vocabulary of love before we can speak of love. Eighteen years later, when this baby is full-grown and "falls in love" for the first time, he will woo his partner through the language of the eyes, the language of the smile, through the utterance of endearments, and the joy of the embrace. In his declarations of love he will use such phrases as "When I first looked into your eyes." "When you smiled at me." "When I held you in my arms." And naturally, in his exalted state, he will believe that he invented this love song. (p. 29)

This loving period between infant and caregiver developing at about 2–3 months is related to the infant's brain development. At 1–2 months of age, the infant's gaze tends to become strongly focused on a stimulus location in what has been called "obligatory attention" (Ruff & Rothbart, 1996; Stechler & Latz, 1966). Obligatory attention is in turn dependent on development of the cerebral cortex (Johnson et al., 1991; Johnson, Posner, & Rothbart, 1994). After the first month, the infant can focus visual attention strongly, but brain mechanisms allowing the child to switch attention from one focus to another are not yet available. If infants are looking at an inanimate object, such as a checkerboard, they may look so long that they become overstimulated and distressed. Expressions on a parent's face regularly change and the face bobs and moves about, so unless the parent over-stimulates the baby, or purposefully adopts a still face (described below), distress is unlikely. Instead, babies gaze into their parent's eyes for extended periods, smiling and cooing.

These infant responses have strong effects on the parents' feelings. Robson and Moss (1970) asked mothers when they first felt their child recognized them as a special person, when they first saw their child as an individual, and when their own feelings of love toward their babies developed. Many mothers reported that these feelings did not develop until the child's smiling, eye contact, and vocal responsiveness at 2–3 months. Infants differ in their tendencies to smile and laugh, and in their orienting, and these differences will affect the nature of the caregiver–infant relationship.

In contrast to their attempts to soothe and change the state of distressed infants, caregivers often try to stimulate their infant's smiles. Smiling and laughter from the child is read as "I like it," and the caregiver is likely to repeat the previous stimulus or a variant on it when the child has responded positively (Rothbart, 1973). The encouragement of positive emotion can also be influenced by culture. Caudill and Weinstein (1969) found that American mothers stimulate and arouse their infants to a much greater extent than Japanese mothers. In the United States, parents also often introduce toys into the interaction. For example, a stuffed bear is made to hop over the blanket and to nuzzle the infant's tummy, or a rattle is shaken before the infant's eyes and then placed in the infant's grasp. Japanese interactions more often occurred directly between infant and mother. Bornstein and his associates found that American mothers responded more to their infants when the infant oriented to physical objects; Japanese mothers responded more when the infants oriented to them (Bornstein, Tal, & Tamis-LeMonda, 1991; Bornstein, Toda, Azuma, Tamis-LeMonda, & Ogino, 1990). These differences were found even when infants from Tokyo and New York did not differ temperamentally.

Caregivers and infants show reciprocal interchanges in many cultures, and the language mothers and other caregivers direct toward their infants at this time is quite distinctive (Snow, 1972). Mothers tend to speak in higher frequencies, using shorter utterances and long pauses, and to exaggerate the range of their speech. This speech, called *motherese*, is likely to attract the child's attention (Fernald & Kuhl, 1987) and to lead to smiling and laughter, movement, and vocalization in the infant. Recent studies have looked for the effective ingredient of motherese, finding that the mother's expression of positive emotion is of primary importance (Singh, Morgan, & Best, 2002; Trainor, Austin, & Desjardins, 2000). Although infants usually prefer mothers' speech to infants when compared with mothers' speech to adults, they will prefer the mother's speech to an adult when it contains greater positive emotion in comparison with her speech to an infant.

Child–infant interchanges in reciprocal exchange provide good examples of Escalona's (1968) concept of *effective experience*. One child is active and prone to smiling and laughter, and engages in positive interactions with objects such as a mobile, even in the absence of other people. A second child is less active, and engages in positive interactions with objects only when the caregiver is there to present the mobile and add social stimulation. When the *active* child is being stimulated by the parent, on the other hand, he or she may be distracted away from the mobile and toward the caregiver. Thus the effective experience of the active child alone with the object appears to be similar to the less active child's experience while playing with the object *and* the caregiver, although the two situations are objectively quite different. The presence of particular toys in the home, then, will have different outcomes depending on the temperament of the child and when, how, and with whom the child interacts (Escalona, 1968; Wachs, 2000).

In temperament studies, some infants smile much more than do others, smiling more quickly, more intensely, and over a longer period (Rothbart et al., 2000). These children are also prone to vocalize. When these infants are old enough to reach or crawl, they tend to be more active, approach new objects more quickly, and move around more. Some infants, however, rarely smile, and some may be easily overstimulated when the parent tries to elicit smiling and laughter. When an infant is blind, for example, it may be difficult for the parent to get the child to smile (Fraiberg, 1977). Sensing this lack, the parent may increase the intensity of stimulation in trying to elicit a smile from the infant; this in turn may overstimulate the child.

Although mothers of blind infants often agreed that they were using high-intensity stimulation to elicit smiling, one mother suggested to Fraiberg (1977) that parents can look for cues other than smiling and laughter to know that the child is happy and engaged. These included movements of arms and hands toward sound-making objects. Following the mother's suggestion, Fraiberg was able to teach parents to use other cues, like the infant's body orientation and movement, to see how the child was feeling and what he or she wanted, that is, to "read" the infant without depending on smiling and laughter cues.

When we look at the lovely parent–infant interchanges in sighted infants more closely, we see a good deal of regulation by both the caregiver and the infant. There are repeated changes of focus of attention of both participants, looking toward and then away from the partner (Brazelton & Cramer, 1990). Caregivers adapt to the child's self-regulation in two ways: first, they read the infant's looking away to say that the child has had enough stimulation. The parent then lowers the intensity of the inter-action. Second, when the child is unsmiling and unreactive, they tend to increase the stimulation. In these examples, the caregiver's response is con-tingent on the infant's. Bigelow and Birch (1999) found that 4-month-olds preferred interacting with a woman who had previously interacted with them contingently than with a woman who had interacted with them in a noncontingent way.

These natural approaches of caregivers are reflected in a training pro-gram developed for parents interacting with their infants (Field, 1977). In this program, parents of easily overstimulated infants are instructed to imi-tate their baby. When the baby smiles, the mother smiles, when the infant looks away, the mother looks away, and so on. This simple rule effectively lowers the level of stimulation the child experiences, and leads to less over-stimulation and distress. With a slow-to-arouse infant, on the other hand, the mother is instructed to try to get and keep the infant's attention (Mal-phurs et al., 1996). Here the caregiver increases rather than decreases the intensity of the infant's stimulation. These two strategies serve to match the parent's behavior to the excitement requirements of the child's tempera-ment. When the infant's reactions are not easy to read—as in the case of blind infants—parents can also look for other signals that communicate the child's state (Fraiberg, 1977).

In Sander's (1969) view, what is important here is how each member of the interaction affects the behavior of the other and also changes when the other's behavior changes. This pattern is called *coregulation* by Fogel (1992). Coordination in timing between parent and infant is also important. Beebe and her colleagues (2000) have used a statistical technique called time-series analysis to look at the coordination of infants' and mothers' vocalizing to each other. It is interesting that the rhythms of mother–infant "conversation" are very similar to those of two adult speakers, and that mother–infant coordination predicts later positive outcomes (Jaffe, Beebe, Feldstein, Crown, & Jasnow, 2001).

Patterns of coordination will continue in interchanges throughout life, involving a number of social processes. One is emotional *contagion*, where pleasure, anger, or fear is displayed by first one, and then the other partner in the interchange. The second involves direct *imitation*, where one person's novel or interesting act is copied by the other. In caregiver–infant interac-tion, imitation goes in both directions, with caregivers often imitating the facial expression or movement of the infant, as when the parent opens his or her mouth wide during the infant's feeding. When the infant replies with a similar action, a simple reciprocal game is begun. A third process is seen after the development of *language*, when young children repeat variations on the words of others, and older children and adults relate stories on similar topics to each other in conversation. Finally, each person serves to arouse or sooth the other.

Are there potentials for problems in this interaction? Yes. Not only may parent and infant responses be uncoordinated and out of phase with one another, but the parent may not be able to read the infant's signals so that he or she either overstimulates or understimulates the child. I revisit disorders of regulation in Chapter 9. For now we return to caregiver–infant interactions, to see what happens when infants have gained greater control of their own orienting and may orient their attention away from the caregiver. This is the period Margaret Mahler (1967) has called *hatching*.

Hatching

By about 4–5 months, cortical brain development allows the infant to more easily disengage from one focus of visual attention and to shift to another location (Johnson, Posner, & Rothbart, 1991), and this advance in the infant's control of attention creates another issue for the parent. During reciprocal exchange, the caregiver–child couple are often closely synchronized. The two appear to have eyes only for each other. The mothers' behavior also to a great degree determines the nature of the interchange. As infants start to develop greater control of their own orienting, however, they can begin to look around for other possible sources of interest than the caregiver. When this happens, the parent is no longer the child's sole focus of attention.

Using Mahler's (1967) metaphor, the child now begins the "hatching" process, breaking out of the caregiver–infant shell into a larger world, first through orienting and later through locomotion. With this new increase in the infant's control of attention, parents may feel sorry to have lost their earlier closeness to the baby and may try to demand the infant's attention. Other parents adapt to the change by sitting the infant on their knees, with the child faced away from the parent. In studies done in the United States, facing the child outward was done more often with boys than with girls (Goldberg & Lewis, 1969). The period of hatching raises the more general issue of the child's autonomy versus connectedness with others, an issue that will reemerge repeatedly throughout life.

At 4 months, infants differ from each other in how long they orient or maintain interest (Ruff & Rothbart, 1996). Infants control the eyes first, with gaze control generally preceding control of other motor systems as the child physically moves out into the world. The hatching seen in the infant's orienting will soon be followed by the child's ability to crawl or walk during the period of initiative, in the next of Sander's (1969) issues. Issues of the child's orienting or interest will nevertheless continue with development, and they will come to be central to how the child learns (Posner & Rothbart, 2007a). I discuss the topic of interest and learning in Chapter 7.

Initiative

The next developmental issue emerges at about 5–9 months (Sander, 1962, 1969). At this age, infants become increasingly active in going after and getting what they want, with temperamental differences in activity and approach. Organized physical approach occurs as the infant gains control of the arms and hands for reaching and the torso and legs for crawling and later walking. Whereas in earlier periods the caregiver tended to control the interaction, the child's new goal-related activities lead the caregiver to realize that he or she may no longer be in charge. Sander notes that some parents who had very much enjoyed interacting with their infants when the parents were in apparent control of the interaction saw the child's intention and initiative as the first skirmish in what would be a continuing battle of wills. Parents may even take a position like the one taken by one of Sander's families: "Ned has to learn that he doesn't win, that we win" (1969, p. 208).

The period of initiative also marks the beginning of a set of interactions between the infant and the world that will continue for a lifetime. These interactions can result in the child's development of skills and can result in feelings of mastery, effectance, and competence—or of discouragement and feelings of helplessness (Harter, 1983, 2006). Individual differences in the strength of temperamental approach and fearful inhibition will be of central importance in these interchanges. Differences will also be seen in the child's persistence in pursuing a goal, his or her response when approach is blocked, and in the kind of negative emotion the child expresses when a goal is blocked or an object lost (anger/frustration or sadness). As we have noted, stronger frustration tends to occur with temperamentally more active children (Rothbart & Derryberry, 2002).

Temperament contributes considerably to infant action and thinking. Joseph Church (1961) wrote of infants' approach toward objects in this beautiful language:

> There are forms that ask to be grasped, textures that invite palpation, and holes and crevices that invite probing with a forefinger. It is the way the environment feeds back to his actions that forms the baby's schemata; the paper that crackles or tears, the plastic toy that skitters away from his awkward

fingers, the chair that refuses to budge, the toy car that rolls backward and forward but not sideways, the food that sticks to hands, the flavors and odors and sounds that come from everywhere, the pliancy and resiliency and heft and intractability of things. (p. 40)

The child is responding to and learning about the physical world, and developing actions for and expectations about it. He or she is also responding to and learning about the caregiver: the caregiver's hair, clothing, glasses, jewelry, and the features of the caregiver's face, the sounds and words and facial expressions that the caregiver offers in response to overtures from the child.

When Church (1961) speaks of feedback from the environment, he is talking about how the object's response to the infant's action influences the infant's expectation and behavior toward the object in the future. The child's ability to create effects also influences his or her general tendencies to approach change and newness. Taken in their extreme, these tendencies describe a child who most often says "yes" to new experiences, a child who says "no," and a child who says "Give me a little time, please." These orientations are also shaped by social interchanges, including the caregivers' responsiveness to the child's desires, their play and talk with the child, and the materials they provide for the child to explore. The extent of the child's approach will also be shaped by limits the caregiver sets on the child's actions, and sometimes these limits are severe. In our laboratory, one of the infants approached laboratory materials only after considerable encouragement by the experimenter. The parent told us that her 13-month-old infant had already learned not to touch things that were on the table.

More active children may conflict with their caregivers when the adult limits exploration, and the resulting frustration may then lead to anxiety or belligerence in the child. Children in institutions, on the other hand, may have so little experience with what objects and persons are "good for," that they become quiet and apathetic. In the child's early developing orientations, we see feelings of interest, competence, and mastery, and also feelings of discouragement, anger, helplessness, and lack of interest. Children who are more or less active will differ in the kinds of emotional patterns they are likely to develop, with anger more likely in active children, and fear and sadness in less active children. They will also differ in their styles of learning. Fries and Woolf (1953) suggest that less active children will often gain experience by watching and listening or quiet exploration rather than through the "active muscular interaction" and trial and error of more active children (p. 52).

Focalization

Sander's (1969) issue of focalization is seen at about 9–15 months. Children can now establish and maintain physical closeness to their parents through crawling or walking. Previously, they could bring their parents to them through distress cries, and their smiling and cooing encouraged the parents' engagement (Bowlby, 1969). Now, however, the children are able to seek out both social and nonsocial interests, following their own agendas. Seeking the parent can be heightened by the child's developing fear of strangers, although in some children, fear of strangers is observed a good deal earlier (Rheingold & Eckerman, 1973). Children differ in their dispositions toward fear. Individual differences in fearfulness have also been called behavioral inhibition to novelty, and have been extensively studied and reviewed by Kagan and Fox (2006) and their colleagues. Whereas some children become distressed to novel or challenging stimuli and are likely to freeze or move away, other children not only do not become distressed, but may make approaches toward exciting objects. In our laboratory, some of the infants would pick up a rapidly moving mechanical toy, smile, and kiss it.

The child's increased desires for the parent's comfort and soothing during the period of focalization may lead to ambivalent or even negative parental reactions. If the parent feels the child is demanding too much, he or she may refuse to provide what the child seeks. In turn, the child may still use stronger attempts to get close to the parent. Sander recorded these remarks of the mother of a 14-month-old: "She bothers me all day. I can't do anything. I can't sit down to read a paper or anything because she always tries to get up on me, and when I'm in the pantry, she's in the pantry; when I'm in the kitchen—if I'm sweeping, she's gotta sweep" (in Sander, 1964, reprinted in Sander, 2007, p. 19). Sander notes that the child is now actively vying for the mother's attention. During the period of hatching, the mother may have felt a lack of the infant's attention, but now the mother herself is the child's prize, including her attention. Children are here following their own (autonomous) desires, yet their actions are directed toward connectedness with others. True self-assertion will come later, as the cognitive self-construct develops. We discuss this development in Chapter 5. Issues of connectedness will be seen in full force in the intimate relationships of adulthood, when one member of a couple often appears to need a greater amount of attention and service from the other.

This would seem to be a period when individual differences in infants' affiliativeness are clearly seen. However, this temperament dimension has been little studied, and we have much to learn about affiliation and its relation to other temperament dimensions and to the child's social experience. In the next section, we see similarities between affiliation and Bowlby's (1969, 1973) model of attachment.

Attachment

Children's behavior during Sander's (1969) period of focalization is part of the process that John Bowlby (1969, 1973) called attachment. Bowlby defined attachment theory as "a way of conceptualizing the propensity of human beings to make strong affectional bonds to particular others and of explaining the many forms of emotional distress and personality disturbances, including anxiety, anger, depression and emotional detachment, to which unwilling separation and loss give rise" (1977, p. 201). Attachment is clearly linked to love and affiliation, and our attachments to others can also lead to anxiety at the threat of loss of the attachment figure, and to sadness or anger at loss or separation. Moreover, these reactions are often unexpectedly strong. What might account for the strength of the emotions when attachment is threatened? If we consider attachment in terms of evolution as Bowlby (1977) has done, we see how remaining close to familiar others can keep the child safe from possibly mortal danger. In an evolutionary view, threats to the child's attachment bonds can be equivalent to threats to the child's physical safety and integrity, requiring strong and immediate reaction.

Attachment issues continue throughout childhood, especially when the child's fears become heightened during periods of developmental vulnerability, and they persist into adulthood as we pursue our own security through our attachments to others. Bowlby argues that "Whilst attachment behavior is at its most obvious in early childhood, it can be observed throughout the life cycle, especially in emergencies" (1982, pp. 668–669). We know how losses of significant others through separation or death affect us, even when the attachment figures have not been seen for decades, and in later chapters, we will consider the power of perceived rejection in older children and adults.

The infant's attachment to a mothering figure and the mothering figure's attachment to the infant develop at first through the mother's reactions to the infant's crying, clinging, sucking, and orienting, and are affected by aspects of temperament. Cooing and smiling to the parent are then added, and later (in Sander's [1969] period of focalization), the child actively attempts to maintain closeness to the attachment figure by following and seeking. Over the first year of life the infant also becomes more selective in attachments, preferring familiar figures to strangers.

A period of heightened attachment seeking in the toddler and preschool years is often followed by a decrease in the child's seeking of support. "As the child gets older, and especially when he is past his third birthday, his demands tend to ease. Other interests and activities attract him and occupy his time, and there is less that alarms him" (Bowlby, 1969, p. 356). Bowlby notes that in the early years, children are developing "working models" of caregivers and others, determining who their attachment figures are, where they are located, and how they will respond to the child. Children are also developing working models of the self in relation to others even before the self-construct develops, including how acceptable or unacceptable the child feels in relation to the reactions of attachment figures.

If we view attachment through the lens of temperament, we see that some children will feel more vulnerable due to their more sensitive fear systems. Bowlby (1973) also observed individual differences in children's temperamental fearfulness: "It must be assumed that genetic differences play some part in accounting for variance between individuals with regard to susceptibility to fear. Very little is yet known about their role in humans, but it is well documented in the case of other mammals" (p. 187).

Many studies have been directed toward children's security of attachment. Ainsworth (1973) defined attachment as the organization of the child's thoughts, feelings, and behaviors in relation to a particular caregiver, including feelings of security, safety, and trust in the caregiver's dependability (Bretherton, 1985; Sroufe, 1979). Infants' attachment security is most often measured using the Strange Situation, a laboratory observation developed by Mary Ainsworth (1973), where infants and their caregivers come to a playroom equipped with toys. A series of separations from the mother, appearances of a stranger, and reunions with the mother are then acted out. The Strange Situation is often quite stressful for the child, and the child's soothability and positive emotion during reunions with the mother are taken as a measure of the child's attachment security.

Some children may become distressed during separation, but they greet the mother positively when she returns and are easily consoled. These are called "secure" or category "B" children. A second group, the "insecure avoidant" or "A" children, tend to be not very distressed during separation and are likely to avoid or ignore the mother when she returns. A third, the "C" or "insecure ambivalent" group, may cling to the mother even before she leaves. They are often seriously distressed by the separation, and when the mother returns, they stay close to her, but may also show anger when the mother directs her attention to them. Some of these children become so distressed that they are inconsolable. In Ainsworth's view, attachment security develops as a function of parents' sensitive responsiveness to their infants (Ainsworth, Blehar, Waters, & Wall, 1978), and research does indicate a modest relation between the two (Bakersmans-Kranenburg, van IJzendoorn, & Juffer, 2003). However, measures of the mother's sensitivity and ability to soothe are also likely to be influenced by the reactivity, soothability, and clarity of signals of the child.

A good deal of research has investigated how temperament is related to attachment. Bell (1989) was one of the first to suggest that newborn temperament predicts later attachment security. He cited four studies showing a direct link between newborn irritability and later attachment behavior. One measure that predicted later insecure attachment was the child's negative reaction to the withdrawal of a pacifier (Bell, Weller, & Waldrop, 1971). Newborn infants who were more distressed when a pacifier was removed also cried more in reunion episodes of a Strange Situation at 14 months, and were more likely to be categorized as insecurely attached (see also Calkins & Fox, 1992).

Unfortunately, some of the studies on temperament and attachment carried out after Bell's (1989) review used temperament questionnaires that were not very reliable. More recently, however, interesting relations between temperament and attachment have been found. The avoidant group appears to be paradoxically more approach oriented to the toys in the laboratory, and the ambivalent group appears to be more fearful than the children in the other categories (Burgess, Marshall, Rubin, & Fox, 2003). This suggests an interaction between the child's temperament and experience in the development of attachment. Although most children seek security with the parent when they are afraid, children who are more fearful are likely to have had a greater history of depending on the parent for comfort. If the parent then suddenly fails to respond (by soothing and making the child feel safe), the child's insecurity will be heightened (Bowlby, 1969). Other children may have experienced little soothing from others, and rely on their own self-soothing for relief.

van den Boom (1989, 1991, 1994) predicted later attachment from newborn infant temperament measures and measures of the mother's sensitivity in the home (with sensitivity thought to be the major contributor to the child's secure attachment). Infants in the study had been born to low socioeconomic status (SES) mothers. To assess newborn irritability, van den Boom averaged results of two administrations of the NBAS, at 10 and 15 days. She selected a distress-prone or irritable group that included 17% of the infants; these children scored highest on NBAS measures of peak of excitement, rapidity of build-up, and irritability. An equal number of infants who had scored below this level formed the nonirritable group (van den Boom &

Hoeksema, 1994). Infants in the irritable group of newborns were significantly more likely to appear in the insecurely attached categories (especially in the avoidant category) at 12 months. In this study, measures of mothers' sensitive responsiveness in the home using Ainsworth's coding method did not predict security of attachment.

Because van den Boom had also observed the infants and mothers in their homes, she found that mothers of children in the irritable group, especially the infants who would be later categorized as avoidant, tended to ignore their infant's crying for long periods, and to use soothing methods that were not very effective (van den Boom & Hoeksema, 1994). Over time, they also played with their infants less. Other mothers, especially those of infants who would later be classified as ambivalent, were more variable: sometimes they used effective soothing, at other times the soothing techniques led to increased infant distress. van den Boom (1989) suggested that the infant's irritability and difficulty in soothing may have made it hard for these mothers to be sensitive.

van den Boom (1989, 1994) then designed an intervention study with a larger sample of low-SES irritable infants. As before, infant temperament was measured at 10 and 15 days, and only irritable infants and their caregivers took part in this study. van den Boom made three visits to the home when the infants were between 6 and 9 months of age. She taught half of the mothers how to soothe and play with their babies. Mothers were also taught how to read the infant's cues and to offer prompt and effective soothing, and how to positively interact with their babies at times when the child was not upset. van den Boom's intervention resulted in greater responsiveness and stimulation by the mothers, greater infant sociability to the mother, better self-soothing, and higher levels of exploration in later infancy. It also produced more secure attachment when infants and mothers were tested in a Strange Situation at 12 months.

What does van den Boom's (1989, 1994) research mean for understanding the relation between temperament and attachment? She showed that highly irritable newborns in lower-SES homes had a higher likelihood of insecure attachments. She also observed that high irritability in the newborn and young infant may lead to lower levels of effective soothing and lower positive interactions with the mother. van den Boom's (1989, 1994) intervention study also indicated that *changes* in the caregiving environment can lead to greater attachment security in the irritable infant.

From a temperament point of view, security of attachment as measured in the Strange Situation is a result of a complex set of parent–child interchanges. These interchanges are related to the mother's responsiveness, the infant's stress response, approach, fear and frustration tendencies and their affiliativeness, and the history of the mother–child interaction (Rothbart & Derryberry, 1981). Over the course of these interactions, some children will have learned that the mother provides soothing. Others will not learn this connection, either because they chiefly soothe themselves, or because their mothers rarely offered soothing, or because the mother's soothing was not very effective. Although security of attachment is often thought of as a trait of the child, in fact, it describes the child in a relationship with a particular adult. This relationship is often measured on only one occasion in the Strange Situation. Children's security of attachment with the mother can also be quite different from their security with the father. Finally, children's experiences in soothing can differ from one culture to another, just as parents' attitudes toward and methods of soothing can differ historically, depending on changing values of the culture.

THE TEMPERAMENTAL CORE OF PERSONALITY

In this chapter we have seen the beginnings of the child's orientation toward people and objects, toward connection with and independence from significant others. Connection develops through regulation and soothing, reciprocal exchange in play, and security as the child comes to the parent for comforting. The infant's tendencies toward autonomy are especially seen during the periods of hatching and initiative, and the period of *self-assertion* is discussed in the next chapter. The two social orientations of connection and autonomy have been given many names, including expressiveness and instrumentality, communion and agency, and homonomy and autonomy. The balance between connection and autonomy in each of the child's relationships will provide a lifelong set of issues for development.

The child's temperament influences the nature of the child's first experiences and expectations. The child's strategies for self-soothing, seeking help and comfort from others, obtaining rewards, and avoiding harm during this time are also developing into consistent ways of coping. Crying may not lead directly to relief, but children can soothe themselves by sucking on their thumb, hands, fingers, shirt, or blanket. Caregivers may not be responsive to the infant's overtures for affiliation, but older children can seek out interchanges with others who are more favorable, or they may create them in fantasy. A more fearful child may stay as close as possible to the parent in strange places, whereas a more surgent child is likely to greet the social world with open arms and exploration.

SUMMARY

In this chapter we have looked at early individual differences and how they develop within the social and physical environment. We have seen that infants and their parents and caregivers face a number of issues during the first year of the child's life. As the infant develops, more adjustments will be required as the parent and child serve to regulate each other. During the first year, the parent typically makes more adjustments than the child, but as the child's capacities for self-regulation develop and as more demands are made on the child in the home, neighborhood, and school environments, the child will take on greater responsibilities for adjustment. I have also discussed how individual differences in the child's temperament are related to issues and adjustments. Even by the end of the first year, however, not all temperament systems are in place. Temperamental effortful control is developing slowly, and we will see its influence more clearly in the toddler and preschool years—and in the next chapter.

CHAPTER 5

The Self
and Structures of Meaning

In Katherine Nelson's (2007) book on the development of children's minds, she defines *meaning* as that which is perceived as relevant or significant to the person "on the basis of needs, interests, present context, or prior history" (p. 9). She notes that meaning "applies across the biological spectrum, as well as across development. . . . One part of meaning is dependent on biology, that is, on what is essential to the organism" (pp. 9–10). The "biologically determined sensitivities" of the infant are seen in the child's initial temperamental reactivity and self-regulation. Early in life, emotional reactions or sensitivities are automatic, but as the child responds to events, he or she develops expectations about the future. By studying these kinds of meaning we go beyond the study of concepts as definitions or units within theories to a more inclusive understanding of knowledge as it functions in our lives (Rosch, 1999). Through initial reactions and memories of events, temperament helps to shape the individual's understanding of the world, and the meanings he or she gives to it. Later, meanings will come from language and will be phrased in propositions and beliefs. At first, however, meaning structures stem directly from temperamental reactivity.

111

AUTOMATIC MEANINGS

As we have noted, the child is a part of the caregiver–infant unit, and from the start, caregivers will provide the "other-regulation" that infants may lack in self-regulation. In the caregiver–infant setting, the child's emotional expressions communicate how the child is feeling, and the child's self-regulatory behavior also provides information to the caregiver about the infant's state. This allows the caregiver to interpret the meaning of events to the child before the child has the language to describe their meaning. The caregiver can also react automatically to the intensity and frequency of the child's behavior. In 1974, Richard Bell proposed a *homeostatic* model to account for the kind of mutual regulation that develops between the child and the caregiver:

> Briefly, it is assumed that each participant in a social or caregiving interaction has upper and lower limits relative to the intensity, frequency, or situational appropriateness of behavior shown by the other. When the upper limit for one participant is reached, that participant is likely to react in such a way as to redirect or reduce the excessive or inappropriate behavior (upper-limit control reaction). When the lower limit is reached, the reaction is to stimulate, prime, or in other ways to increase the insufficient and nonexistent behavior (lower-limit control reaction). (p. 13)

Homeostatic models of temperament apply throughout the lifespan. An example given by my husband and me provided great delight to our two children. We would set out on a road trip, with the boys in the back-seat of the car, and my husband would choose some intense and, to my mind, highly repetitive music for our entertainment, for example, a Bruce Springsteen song, turned to a high volume. Immediately after he adjusted the volume up, I would adjust it down, and this exchange would continue for some time to the great amusement of our children. Another example concerned our infant children and their grandparents: one grandparent provided high-intensity soothing stimulation (e.g., vigorous rocking); this quieted the older child, but unsettled the second, increasing his distress. The other set of grandparents provided quiet cuddling, which left the second child satisfied, calmed, and content. The more active infant, however, was much more interested in the world beyond the lap, arching his body out of his grandparents' grasp to pursue excitement, and leading his grandparents to wonder whether he liked them.

The homeostatic model also applies to later sibling interactions. Two siblings, for example, can set the excitement level of their interchange so high (e.g., through loud argument, complaints, or physical fighting) that the more distress prone of their parents is likely to intervene. In this way, the children's interaction can affect the number of people taking part in the interchange. Older children and adults also "read" the other and attempt to adapt to the other's state. Thus, homeostatic models can be seen operating in adult couples. One partner becomes distressed easily; the other steps in to soothe or reassure the first. One partner worries and ruminates on negative possibilities; the other reassures, allowing for more flexibility in the couple's decisions and activities. Interchanges of this sort can become consolidated over time and consistently repeated. When a partner is later lost to death or divorce, the partner left behind may be confused about how to act, now that they are suddenly required to take on qualities of the lost partner.

Conscious control is not needed for these homeostatic adjustments, although we can observe ourselves engaging in them, shifting from automatic to conscious control. The infant's built-in system of signals, including signs of distress, contentment, or approach, lets the parent know about the child's levels of toleration and enjoyment. When the child appears displeased, the parent may automatically lower the intensity of the interchange or give the child more attention. When the child appears bored, the parent may increase the intensity of his or her contribution or add novelty to the interchange to make the situation more exciting.

When our children were infants, one of the things I most enjoyed was relying on this direct parent–infant communication and just "doing what came naturally." Here, the caregiver's own temperament and personality will also make a contribution. For some parents, reading and responding to the child's cues will be easier than for others, and this may be due in part to ambiguous and hard-to-read cues from the infant or to the nature of the caregiver's attention. Some infants are simply harder to "read" than others (Bell, 1974) so that a more conscious analysis of the child's cues may be needed, at least at first, and some caregivers may be unlikely to read the child's cues in detail.

This automatic approach can also prove to be harmful, however. In infancy, if a parent becomes too upset at the child's crying and does not exercise the needed self-control, he or she may become angry and injure the child (Bell, 1974). It is important for the adult to recognize that the parent and the child do not carry equal responsibility for their interchanges. Instead, the *adult* bears responsibility for care of the child and for building his or her self-regulative qualities. Knowing this, one knows that the parent is responsible for self-control. If the parent responds with anger to an older child's anger, for example, an escalation of negative interaction is likely to result.

A more conscious approach allows caregivers to realize that they need not react automatically, even if they have a strong urge to do so. Instead, they can pause, analyze the situation, and change their own behavior to produce a better outcome for their children. They can also recognize that what they have just done is not helpful, and choose to act differently in the future. This approach is also helpful in other situations where one wishes to change one's more or less automatic behavior, as I show in Chapter 9. Parent-support organizations can actively support this kind of awareness and responsibility in the parent, and clinical psychologists have recently focused on "mindfulness" as allowing for change. It is important for the adult to recognize that the parent and the child do not carry equal responsibility for their interchanges. Instead, the adult bears responsibility for care of the child and for building his or her self-regulative qualities.

EMOTIONS AS STRUCTURES OF MEANING

Recall that emotion addresses questions of evaluation: "Is it good for me? Is it bad for me?" New events attract the child's attention. If the event is not seen as meaningful or important, attention wanes and habituates over time (Ruff & Rothbart, 1996). If the event elicits an emotion, however, an organized set of reactions occur. These involve not only evaluations of events but also the enactment of strategies to deal with them. Emotion involves the perception of objects of desire, leading to positive emotions and approach; objects of threat, leading to withdrawal and attack; or the loss of valued objects, leading to anger or sadness. Both Guidano (1987) and Nelson (2007) have observed how the emotions represent meanings that operate before language, and I have adopted Nelson's term "meaning structure" to refer to emotional reactions as well as to the later cognitive meanings coded in language. Children will differ in the sensitivity of their meaning structures depending on temperament. What is a threat to one child can be nonthreatening to another; what is an exciting possibility to one child may be unappealing to another. Further structures of significance and meaning will develop according to the child's life history, that is, his or her experiences in specific situations with specific people, and parents may do all they can to make sure these experiences are manageable for the child.

IMPLICIT AND EXPLICIT KNOWLEDGE

For many years, psychologists resisted the idea of unconscious influences on one's feelings, cognition, and action. This may have resulted in part because social learning theorists rejected Freud's theory of the unconscious, but the unconscious processing of information is now an important topic for cognitive psychology. This research and thinking has given us a number of names for different kinds of knowledge: implicit and explicit, procedural and declarative, and automatic and effortful. Knowledge can be implicit and automatic, shown in actions and procedures, or explicit and declarative, shown in rules and stories about situations and people. A common example of implicit knowledge is the motor skill of riding a bicycle or driving a car. Language can be used to teach these skills, but the automatic skill that results is likely not to involve language. Explicit knowledge, on the other hand, is conscious, as when we recognize an object or person and put it into a category, or tell a story about ourselves. Explicit knowledge is available to us from our storehouse of facts, methods, principles, propositions, and beliefs. If a child is asked to describe a bicycle, the description will involve explicit knowledge. This is conscious knowledge that can be put into words; it is usually but not always expressed in language. Explicit knowledge is also called declarative knowledge.

Infants' temperament offers a set of automatic procedures for dealing with the environment, and these procedures are open to learning from the environment. Meaning structures in the child can be implicit or explicit (they are explicit when a word is put to describe a category), but early in life, they tend to be implicit and related to our automatic reactions to events. Let us consider a common example: At the beginning of what will prove to be a significant interaction, a temperamentally fearful child meets his uncle. The uncle, happy to see the child, moves up close, pinches the child's cheeks, and greets him loudly. For the more fearful child, this experience is a distressing one and the child pulls away. The next time the uncle appears, even though he doesn't come up quite so close, the child again becomes distressed and tries to escape. Now, the mere sight of the uncle leads to the child's anticipation of distress, so that the "meaning" of the uncle is threat. In addition, the uncle may come to think that the child does not like him, or that the child is disagreeable.

The child's temperament in this way is being made specific as a meaning structure applied to a particular interaction with a particular person. The child's reaction involves the autonomic nervous system and neuroendocrine preparation for energy and action. It includes tendencies toward flight, freezing, or attack as preparations for coping, and the child's attention may be particularly focused on the threat and on routes for escape from it. The child's fear reactions become further consolidated during each repeated interaction between the uncle and the child, as the child anticipates the uncle's approach by crying or pulling back.

The infant and his uncle have developed, in Robert Hinde's (1997) term, a "relationship." A relationship involves a repeated set of interactions between two people, so that the behavior of each person comes to take into

account the behavior of the other. There is continuity over time in a relationship. It is affected by past interactions, observations of others' reactions,
and expectations about upcoming interactions. Later in life, relationships
can also be affected by the things other people say about the partner. Each
older partner can then describe the relationship and tell stories about its
history. These descriptions and stories will be affected by the experiences of
each partner in the relationship.

Now imagine a temperamentally more surgent child with the same
uncle. The uncle pinches the child's cheeks and the child laughs, holding
out her arms to be picked up. Like the fear reaction, this positive reaction
may become consolidated over repeated interchanges between child and
uncle. The sight of the uncle now provokes smiling and excited vocalization
from the child, along with a "pick me up" posture. Later the child looks
forward to meetings with the uncle and assuming the reactions are mutual
and other adults do not interfere, a positive relationship will develop.

If the uncle were to have made a milder and less intense approach, the
more fearful child may also have had positive experiences to carry forward
to future interactions. A third situation is also possible: If the child is low in
both fear and surgency, he or she may show little reaction to the uncle, even
though when the uncle interacts with the other children, he is experienced
as either threatening or positively exciting. The less reactive child is unlikely
to carry strong emotional expectations or motivated actions forward to the
next meeting.

When fearful children are exposed to the approach of a stranger, they
are more disposed to become upset than less reactive children. After a number of such frightening experiences, the fearful child may show a stronger
general orientation away from new people. The less fear-reactive child is less
likely to experience distress and will be less likely to develop an avoidant
orientation. More negatively reactive children are also treated differently
by adults (Crockenberg & Acredolo, 1983; Linn & Horowitz, 1983). Highly
surgent infants, on the other hand, may lead adults to provide even higher
levels of stimulation, producing further positive excitement, smiling, and
laughter.

Over time, an implicit meaning structure based on temperament links
the child's emotional evaluation (fear or pleasure), the child's coping action
(approaching or moving away), and later, the child's and uncle's explicit
knowledge about the event and the other person (this person is dangerous,
a lot of fun, this child doesn't like me). This analysis brings us to a basic
question about the development of temperament and personality: Can a
child develop meaning structures that are specific to only one person or to
only some people, or need they apply to *many* people in order for them to be

part of a child's personality? In a temperament view, the child *can* develop meaning structures particular to a single person or group, and these specific relationships can be important components of the personality. Indeed, some of a person's most significant and life-influencing ideas and behaviors may *not* extend across multiple situations or to multiple people, but be quite specific.

Significant relationships can also exist with one's work, one's travel experiences, or one's possessions. In Gogol's (1965; original 1842) great story *The Overcoat*, the hero moves from a powerful attachment to his work as a clerk (bringing home extra work to do for pleasure in his spare time) to a possibly even greater involvement with his new overcoat, leading to a tragic outcome. Both the work and the overcoat are given elaborate structures of meaning, influencing and being influenced by, the social environment. It has been said that we all come out from under Gogol's overcoat; it describes how an object of meaning may become the most important thing in a person's life; it also acts as a cautionary tale.

If we are willing to allow that a single relationship with a person or attachment to an object or activity, can be a part of one's personality, if we accept that meaning structures and relationships need not qualify as "traits," we can take a much broader view of personality. Relationships and meaning structures add richness to the usual trait models of psychology and they are important components of the child's personality, along with the child's model of the self and identifications with others. Dweck (2008) calls meaning structures *beliefs*, and identifies them as significant components of personality. The fearful child in our example will later learn the name of his uncle and may account for his own distress by believing (wrongly) that the uncle is a bad or dangerous person. The uncle may also come to believe that the child doesn't like *him* or that the child himself (or the uncle himself) is unlikable. The more fearful child may cope with threatening events by withdrawing or becoming quiet, and interactions with others may follow a similar pattern to those shown with the uncle. Nevertheless, the child's coping responses will also be shaped by the situation: A child may usually withdraw from a threatening person or run to his or her parent, but when withdrawal is not possible and the caregiver is not present, strong distress may result. Adaptations are always selected from the possibilities present in the situation, and they change as the child's history changes.

We not only develop explicit constructs of ourselves, but constructs of others, and the judgments we make about others and about the self are strongly linked to our emotional reactions to them. Once we are able to make declarative judgments about others or ourselves, we are adding another dimension of meaning, and it is important to remember that the meanings carried implicitly in our emotions and action tendencies may be quite different from the meanings coded in our beliefs and language. Thus, it is possible for a person to say that he or she likes or even loves another person, while experiencing feelings of aversion in that person's presence and avoiding him or her whenever possible. These two different levels of meaning or knowledge may or may not agree. To the degree they are in agreement, we may call the personality more integrated or more authentic.

Different experiences would have been possible for the temperamentally fearful child and the uncle. Perhaps the uncle is at first intrusive and the child shows distress and pulls away. The mother then suggests that the uncle not directly approach the child, but instead talk quietly, directing attention toward the mother while waiting for the child to come to him. Following the mother's instructions, the uncle directs his attention away from the child and quietly talks to the mother. The child, less threatened, watches this interchange and, feeling safer, offers a toy to the visitor. The uncle accepts it and quietly thanks the child. The child then takes back the toy. This kind of interchange can set the stage for more positive future interactions between the child and the uncle, as long as the adult can keep his potential intrusiveness in check. There is the possibility of both the repair of a disrupted relationship, and the creation of different outcomes in the relationship. Our lives are lived in possibilities.

The more surgent child may also have been frightened by the interchange. Let us say that the child finds her uncle's approach exciting, and grabs his glasses. He pulls back, saying loudly, "Hey—don't do that!" which frightens the child. Although the child is temperamentally disposed to a positive reaction, her own fear reaction has now been activated. This response, similar to that of the first child, may be consolidated over time. For the more surgent child, however, most interchanges with new people or even later interchanges with the uncle are likely to be positive, so that this interchange will be an exception. Because situations generally lead to positive reactions, the child is still likely to be assessed as surgent on trait measures.

Some children will show a great deal of variability in their reactions from one situation to another. For the fearful child, for example, some situations (e.g., at home, with well-known adults in familiar places) will have been experienced as safe; other situations (e.g., strange people and situations, crowds) will be more threatening. This child is likely to behave differently in situations that vary in their potential for stress. For the surgent and outgoing child there is likely to be more consistency across these situations, because the child is rarely threatened and will be generally more approaching.

DEVELOPMENT OF SELF-REPRESENTATIONS

Up until now, we have chiefly discussed the more automatic responses of the child, and the implicit learning related to them. Now we turn to what is probably the most important explicit meaning structure, the representation of the self. With the development of representations of the self, we are clearly going beyond temperament to cognitive structures of personality, but temperament is likely to influence the content of these structures. During the second year of life and beyond the child is developing a cognitive model of the self, and children's goals and experiences can now become linked to the self as an object among other objects. Feelings of volition are also attached to the model of the self, creating what we can call the *ego-self*, and cognitions of "I am doing this" and "I am feeling that" are added to the child's more automatic and nonconscious actions.

New possibilities for meaning and control also arise as the child uses language to describe the self and others, and to place the self within a personal history or narrative. Because self-related thoughts are laid upon basic temperament and because they carry with them new strengths and vulnerabilities, I discuss the early development of the self in some detail. The model of the self, seen in relation to the meaning of others and of events, takes personality beyond temperament and into an explicit cognitive level of understanding and meaning.

Early Aspects of Self

Even though the cognitive model of self is not yet developed, several aspects of self will have already been experienced during the first year of life. During the early months, infants' experiences of distress, pleasure, sleepiness, and alertness have been described by Sander (2007) as constituting a *state self* (see Figure 5.1). It may also be seen as an experiential self, based on the feelings of the body. Emde (1983) similarly refers to an *affective core* of the person that is seen very early in life. This level of self, however, would be expected to change as the child's state changes.

Later, as the infant's expectations and intentions develop (4–8 months), the infant's approach and avoidance tendencies are experienced in what we can call an *agentic self* or *sensorimotor self* (Rothbart, 1989b). The infant can now initiate a "conversation" or play with the caregiver, with expectations that the partner will respond (Case, 1991). Social learning theorists like Bandura (1986) have stressed conscious judgments of self-efficacy, that is, the *belief* that one is able to master and control future issues and situations. However, sensorimotor experiences of mastery (as when the infant rolls

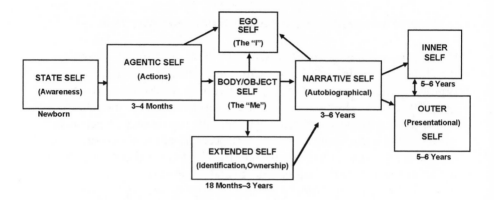

FIGURE 5.1. Early development of the self.

over for the first time) or uncertainty (as when the infant hesitates before beginning an action) appear to be present much earlier than verbally available cognitions.

The infant anticipates rewards as he or she pursues objects and acts on them. Frustration is also experienced when an expected event does not occur, a desired goal cannot be reached, or a valued object is lost. With the onset of fearful inhibition during the second half of the first year, feelings of uncertainty are also developing. Temperamental reactivity influences the child's approach, frustration, and avoidance, and thus contributes to the experiences of the agentic self. The agentic self is also seen as the child bases actions on past experiences and anticipates outcomes.

The Body or Object Self

Later, the identification of the *body self* develops. Between about 15 and 24 months, evidence for the body self is seen in the mirror test originally used in primate studies (Amsterdam, 1972; Lewis & Brookes, 1978). In mirror studies, a spot of red is surreptitiously placed on the child's face, and the child's reactions to seeing his or her image in a mirror are then observed. At younger ages, the infant tends to treat the mirror image as a playmate, not noticing the spot, but by 21–24 months, 75% of infants recognize themselves in the mirror by trying to rub off the spot from their faces (Lewis & Brookes). This is called mirror self-recognition, and it appears to be part of a cognitive model of the self. Mirror self-recognition, for example, is linked to children's use of personal pronouns such as *me* and *mine*. Self-recognition and the use of personal pronouns are also related to children's pretend play with a doll, where the child pretends to feed the self and then pretends to feed a doll (Lewis & Ramsay, 2004). In this play, the child appears to be treating the doll as another self.

Temperament is related to the age at which an infant shows recognition of the body self. Lewis and Ramsay (1997) found that infants with higher stress reactivity at 6 and 18 months showed earlier self-recognition. They suggest that the internal experience of negative emotion may lead to a greater focus on the inner self, and to earlier recognition of a self (Lewis & Ramsay). Negative emotions may also be linked through evolution to strong motives to protect and defend one's person, leading the negatively reactive child to an earlier cognition of the body self as something to be protected and defended. If more fearful children are more sensitive to threat, they may also develop a greater sensitivity to feelings of lack of personal control. Predicting and controlling events would be important to these children. In our unpublished longitudinal research, children who as infants were more fearful in the laboratory, were at age 2, more strongly concerned about being in control and in charge of games, events, and outcomes. Indeed, control may continue to be a major issue with the child who is more vulnerable to threat.

Two-year-olds are also able to identify pictures of themselves and to differentiate their own picture from pictures of other children. Embarrassment and shame are self-conscious emotions that begin to be shown at about this age, and the appearance of these emotions is related to the development of self-recognition (Lewis, Sullivan, Stanger, & Weiss, 1989). Embarrassment and shame are also related to a distress-prone temperament (DiBiase & Lewis, 1997). Children who are more fearful and easily frustrated in infancy are more likely to later show shame and guilt, two important self-related emotions that are part of the personality (Kochanska & Aksan, 2007; Kochanska, Gross, Lin, & Nichols, 2002; Rothbart, Ahadi, et al., 1994).

During the toddler period, the child's models of body self and ego self appear to become linked in self-willed action. Two-year-olds, for example, often insist on doing things themselves (Bronson, 2000). At this age, however, children's skills are not well developed, and children often become frustrated when they are unable to achieve what they want. When the child's goals are at odds with the caregiver, the caregiver may also intervene, removing an object or moving the child, creating further frustration. When the young child's frustration becomes severe, temper tantrums may result. Kopp (2009) reviews research indicating a peak of negative behavior at "about the time of heightened consciousness of self, while communication skills are still limited" (p. 41). The peak of temper tantrums is reported at 17–24 months (Kopp, 1992), the peak of physical aggression at 2½–3½ years (Nagin & Tremblay, 2005), and the peak of negativism at 2½–3 years (Tremblay & Nagin, 2005).

Sander's Issue of Self-Assertion

We now return to the last major issue of Sander as it emerges in toddlers. The issue of *self-assertion* was seen by Sander (1962, 1969) in children 14–20 months of age. At this time, children are developing constructs of the self and others as separate entities through the *body-self* construct. With the growing sense of self and self-related intentions come increases in the child's self-assertion, or *ego-self*, and power struggles between caregiver and toddler may result.

How do parents discourage or encourage children's self-assertion? Children's insistence on doing things for themselves and their powerful reactions to frustration often set the stage for battles for control with the parent. Other parents, however, may so frequently grant their child's demands and wishes that the child comes to expect that personal demands will be obeyed by others. Parents may also encourage self-development by asking the child to choose between options: "What would you like to eat? Which of these outfits would you like to wear?" It is always important to remember what a child is learning in a given situation: If the child is offered many choices, he or she may come to demand even more. Other parents are more ambivalent about controlling their children. They want their child to be assertive, but do not wish to give up their authority as parents. These parents may be inconsistent in their reactions.

Sander (2007) suggests that issues during this period involve the parent defining areas where the child may establish self-assertion, and areas where self-assertion is not allowed. This can be called *setting limits* for children. Issues of self-assertion, like other early issues, will be influenced by the child's temperament. Children who are highly surgent and goal oriented, for example, may be more likely to clash with their caregivers. If the child is also prone to distress, coercive exchanges between the child and parent may develop (Patterson, 1982).

In coercive interchanges, one participant performs an action or says something that the other finds painful and punishing. In response, the other participant behaves in ways to cause the first participant pain. For example, the child hits the parent or says, "I hate you," and the parent returns pain for pain by striking the child. The child then responds by screaming. The parent spanks the child, and so on. Each participant responds with actions resulting in pain to the other. The interaction continues in mutual escalation until one participant gives up and leaves the interaction, and this is frequently the parent. Patterson (1982) observes that coercive interchanges are reinforcing to both participants. The one who terminates the cycle is reinforced because the pain stops when the cycle is over; the other partner experiences both the stoppage of pain and also the feeling of "winning out" in the interchange. Coercive interactions can train higher levels of aggressive behavior in both the child and the parent.

Issues in 2-year-olds' self-assertiveness can also include children's negativism, with "no" becoming the child's favored response to requests or demands from the parent. In our research, children who were temperamentally more distress prone as infants were more likely to show negative reactions to suggested activities as late as 7 years of age (Rothbart, Ahadi, et al., 1994).

Parenting Styles and Self-Assertion across Cultures

In parent–child interactions during the period of self-assertion, we see the development of parenting styles that have been studied by Baumrind (1967). She identified three styles of parent control. The first is called *authoritarian*, where the parent consistently asserts control and may use physical punishment to achieve it; the second is *permissive*, where the parents generally let their children follow their own desires, and give the child what he or she wants (when the parent cannot put up with the child's demands any longer, however, he or she may angrily punish the child). The third is *authoritative*, where the parent attempts to encourage feelings of competence and self-assertion in the child, but at the same time attempts to set boundaries for the behavior. Here the parent lets the child know when an action is acceptable and when the behavior is not allowed. The authoritative parent is also more likely to explain to the child why a behavior is not allowed.

One temperament-related item that is left out of Baumrind's (1967) model is how the child's behavior may be shaping the parent's style of interaction. For example, the parent is unlikely to continue using a style that does not work. The parent may at first try an authoritative approach, but find that a child is not responsive to it. This may lead the parent to move in the direction of a more authoritarian or more permissive style. It is quite possible then for a parent to use chiefly one parenting style with one child, and a modified or quite different form of that style with another child in the family. The parent may also use a combination of styles depending on the child and the issue. Just as the relationship is shaped on the child's side by his or her experiences, so the parents' relationship with the child can shape the parents' experience (Bell, 1974).

One of the most exciting aspects of writing this book has been to learn more about how cultures can influence the child's and parent's experience. Margaret Mead's observations led her to make a distinction between the "lap child," the "knee child," and the "yard child" in a number of non-Western cultures (described by Edwards [2002]), elaborated on in Chapter 6. The infant lap child is fed, held, and carried by the mother, and the "knee child" or toddler continues to stay close to the mother even after a new baby occupies the mother's lap. Once the child is weaned and able to move about, however, he or she joins a group of children who play together. These yard children may be supervised by an adult, but the shift to the peer group means that the close relationship between child and mother is weakened.

We can contrast this situation to a Western family where close relationships are sustained over an extended period, and where adults may be both encouraging the child's autonomy and responding to the child's desires. These cultural differences suggest that "self-assertion" may be a greater issue for the Western parent than for those non-Western cultures described by Mead and other anthropologists (Edwards, 2002). This also raises some very interesting questions. If toddlers in all cultures have a strong concern with control, how will this concern be played out in different cultures in relationships with parents and other adults? In relationships with other children? On the other hand, if "self-assertion" is not so much of an issue as for the United States, will the child's needs and concerns also differ? Taking culture into account, we must look at even the most primary developmental relationships with a critical eye.

In my courses on social development, I offered a classic series of films on children. One was the Robertson (1952) film *A Two-Year-Old Goes to Hospital*, documenting the separation of a 2-year-old girl from her parents during an extended hospital stay, and providing a vivid portrayal of a child's reactivity and self-regulation within family relationships. A second was *Four Families*, a 1959 National Film Board of Canada production filmed in India, Japan, France, and Canada, and narrated by Margaret Mead (Low, 2002). Two of the most memorable events in the *Four Families'* film were the baths given an infant in an east Indian village, and an infant in rural Canada. In India, the child was washed matter-of-factly, held by the arm in a standing position as water was poured over the baby's head. In Canada, the infant was comfortably seated in a carefully prepared small tub of water. As the bath progressed, the Canadian infant grabbed at the washcloth the mother was using. The mother tried to remove the washcloth from the baby's grasp, the child resisted, and an actual tug-of-war developed between the mother and the infant. Mead commented on how strange this interaction seemed, and how it might reflect Canadian children's training in independence. I didn't realize it at the time, but aspects of the children's selves were likely being shaped during these bath times and were captured in this film.

Effortful Control and Self-Regulation

Toddlers and preschool-age children are opening up to a world outside the family. They are also relating to this world based on their models of the self, the ego self, and their development of effortful control. As knowledge about the self develops, and the self is seen as an agent who can will action and experience frustration, major changes are seen in children's behavior. Temperamental effortful control, which develops strongly after the age of 2, allows children to both cooperate with their parents and to pursue their own goals with planfulness and persistence.

Preschool-age children in Western culture have historically practiced self-control in the games they play. A simple early game is Ring around the Rosey, where children sing and dance in a circle; when they reach the song line "All fall down," each child intentionally falls to the ground. In Red Rover, Red Rover, children run and throw themselves against the clasped hands of members on the opposite team, attempting to break through the line. Children act as both agents and objects in Red Rover, controlling when their runs begin and using their bodies as objects to break through the line and win the game. As children grow older, they also act as judges using explicit knowledge of justice and fairness, observing the actions of others, and applying the rules of the game. Piaget (1932) argued that young children's concern with the "rules of the game" are extended to include the rules of morality—things the child should or shouldn't do—although in Chapter 7, I argue that important aspects of children's morality develop well before their explicit knowledge of rules.

In other games, children practice self-control through the inhibition of action. In Mother, May I?, an action is prepared, but inhibited until the child has requested and received permission from the child in the "mother" role: "You may take two giant steps." "Mother, may I?" "Yes, you may." In this game, the younger child is very likely to take the two giant steps without asking or without waiting for the mother's permission. Other games stressing self-control include Red Light–Green Light and Concentration (Conner, 2007). When we were children, Mother May I and Red Rover were neighborhood games played by a range of ages of preschool- and school-age children, and organized by children's groups rather than adults.

Another popular game is Simon Says. The child is told to perform an action like rubbing his or her tummy, but may not perform it unless the command is preceded by "Simon says, rub your tummy." The younger child is frequently "caught out" performing the action when the phrase "Simon says" has not been said. These children's games both strengthen children's construct of self and allow practice in inhibiting and activating motor actions. Tools of the Mind (Bodrova & Leong, 2006) is a preschool program for young children that also emphasizes the importance of children's social play to fostering cognitive and social development. Evaluation research on this program suggests that the Tools of the Mind program, stressing pre-school social play and role taking, promotes children's development of self-regulation (Diamond, Barnett, Thomas, & Munro, 2007).

Children's games have been adapted to the measurement of effortful control in children. In 1984, Margorie Reed, Diana Pien, and I adapted the Simon Says game to the laboratory, using it to assess the development of children's ability to voluntarily inhibit their actions (inhibitory control; Reed, Pien, & Rothbart, 1984). In this study, children were 3½–4 years of age. Instead of using the words *Simon says,* we asked the child to perform an action such as "Touch your nose" whenever the command came from one puppet, but to inhibit the action when the command came from another puppet. We also used a pinball game, where the child was asked to hold back the plunger for varying amounts of time, inhibiting the release of a marble until permission was given. We could measure how long the child inhibited release, and for some children, it was a very short time. Perfor-mance on these tasks was greater over the 6 months of age from 3½–4, but even when corrected for age, performance on the Simon Says and pin-ball measures were highly related (Reed et al., 1984). Adaptations of these tasks have now been used to measure children's inhibitory control and self-regulation (e.g., Carlson, 2005; Kochanska et al., 1997).

In a later study, children were asked to follow the instructions of one stuffed animal, but not another (Jones, Rothbart, & Posner, 2003). At 3 years, even though children showed they understood the rules, they were only able to inhibit the forbidden response 22% of the time. Children who were about 12 months older, however, could do so 90% of the time. The older children also showed evidence of having detected their own errors by slow-ing down on the next trial after an error was made. The detection of errors and response to them is another capacity based on the executive attention network (Posner & Rothbart, 2007a).

We also wished to observe whether language would be used by chil-dren to aid in inhibiting their actions, as proposed in theories stressing verbal self-regulation (Vygotsky, 1962). The children in our study, however, used very little language (Jones et al., 2003). Instead, they used physical strategies like holding down one hand with the other, or sat on their hands to prevent performing an action. Effortful control, the ability to inhibit a predominant action in order to perform a subdominant action, is developing during this period and appears to develop as implicit knowledge, before children tie it to the language used for self-regulation.

Effortful control develops rapidly over the years 2–4, continuing until after adolescence (Rothbart, Posner, & Kieras, 2006; Rothbart & Rueda, 2005). By the age of 30 months, children begin to show consistency of performance on different effortful control tasks and considerable stability of these capacities is found after this age (Kochanska et al., 2000). Effortful control also includes the ability to inhibit the choice of a small reward now in order to receive a larger reward later, in delay-of-gratification tasks (Mischel, 1968). Children's capacity to delay gratification shows considerable stability over development, and is related to their adolescent performance on academic tasks and control of their negative emotions.

As children use inhibitory ("stop") and activational ("go") control to solve problems, they are practicing voluntary or self-willed intentions to control situations, and effortful control provides the basis for this behavior. After development of the self-construct, the changes in children's ability to regulate their own behavior also allow for major shifts in personality development and the development of self-control. Instead of being driven only by their positive and negative emotional reactions, children can now exercise control of their own actions. Fearful children can now approach the object of their fear; easily frustrated children can inhibit angry outbursts; and children will be able, if not always willing, to follow the do's and don'ts of social rules. These examples illustrate the child's control of undesired behavior, but it is important to remember that effortful self-control can be directed toward less desirable ends such as opposing others, intentionally breaking rules, or deceiving others. Motivation provides the goals and effortful control supports the effective means to pursue those goals, whether seen by others as good or bad.

Threats to the Constructed Self

With the development of language, the child can also consider his or her own self in a declarative or explicit way. In Case's (1991) terms, "Because children can now take themselves as explicit objects, i.e., as objects of reference, their implicit sense of themselves should also become something they can focus on directly, label, and communicate . . . (e.g., 'I'm not a bad boy; I'm a good boy! Don't say I'm a bad boy. Dat makes me sad.')" (p. 225).

Children now take pride in their successful activities and experience shame and embarrassment when they believe others disapprove of them. Children also develop personal responsibility for their actions. They are applying intentions to the *ego self* ("I didn't mean to do it") in deciding their own responsibility. When a child perceives he or she has done something bad or broken a rule, negative judgments of the self can lead to distress and self-punishment.

Explicit or declarative knowledge can also be linked to how the self is related to other selves and to judgments of others and self-judgments. As Ausubel and Sullivan (1970) describe it, "After this point is reached, self-reactions at a new abstract level become possible; these include identification with persons, goals and values, incorporation of standards, competitive behavior, and, finally, self-judgments, guilt feelings and conscience" (p. 256). These are all *extensions of the self*, aspects of the child's developing structures of meaning and personality.

Sander's (1969) issues involve the infant and toddler years, but the understanding of the self and the child's developing personality will continue to increase in complexity with development. Beliefs about the self and others will also continue to form important meaning structures. One aspect of this process is described by Ausubel and Sullivan (1970) as *devaluation*. The toddler often seems to believe that whatever he or she demands will occur, and when it doesn't, anger is a likely result. As children learn more about their lack of personal power to achieve what they desire, on the other hand, at least some children will realize that their power is limited. They may also recognize that adults hold much greater power than they, that adults may be following their own agendas and pursuing their own goals, and that these goals are not always in agreement with the child's agenda. Ausubel and Sullivan suggest that self-devaluing cognition can occur between about 2 to 4 years, and we would expect more temperamentally negative children and children with higher perceptual sensitivity to be more sensitive to it. These children may also turn to pleasing adults with the expectation that adults will protect them.

Stipek, Recchia, and McClintic (1992) found that just before the age of 2, children also begin to show evidence of appreciating adult standards (what the adult expects of them) for their behavior, and to show distress when they do not meet those standards. Stipek et al. observed that when toddlers were successful at a task, they were more likely to turn to adults for approval; when they failed at the task, they tended to turn away. Children also appeared to anticipate the reactions of adults to their actions, showing a desire to please them. Kagan (1984) found that young children became distressed when they found themselves unable to perform a task that had been modeled by an adult, and Kochanska (personal communication, 2005) found that children with greater temperamental perceptual sensitivity also showed greater sensitivity to adult standards. Self-devaluation can mark the beginning of some of the most powerful of coping methods and socialization influences, including the child's tendency to identify with more powerful figures and/or to oppose or avoid others seen as more weak.

The Narrative Self

Language provides further evidence of the development of self- and ego-self-cognitions ("I," "me," "mine," etc.), and provides information about the child's place in the world through adults' and children's narratives or stories. Many children will use the personal pronoun, "I" at about 2 years (Nelson, 2007), and over the next several years, the child will be developing a language-based view of the self. Children can then describe themselves to others and to themselves. Language allows for greater emotion regulation in the young child, as the child is able to communicate desires in words rather than being limited to the expression of emotions (Kopp, 2009). Using language, the child also comes to develop a *narrative self*, in which the self is placed within historical events and in relation to the acts and the inferred thoughts and emotions of others. The narrative or autobiographical self provides meaning structures that extend the scope of self-understanding back into the past and forward into the future (Nelson), and the meanings in the stories are often linked to emotions and evaluations.

The narrative self places the child within a set of stories that further (explicitly) define who he or she is. Constructs of self are developed, or rather, *co-constructed*, with important adults in the child's social world (Nelson, 2007). Even early in life, parents may greatly elaborate the declarations or simple scripts offered by their children, adding information about the events, emotions, intentions, goals, and desires of the actors. Here is an excerpt of a conversation between a 2-year-old and her mother (New York's Chrysler building is where the child's father works):

C: Mommy, the Chrysler building.

M: The Chrysler building?

C: The Chrysler building?

M: Yeah, who works in the Chrysler building?

C: Daddy.

M: Do you ever go there?

C: Yes, I see the Chrysler building—picture of the Chrysler building.

M: I don't know if we have a picture of the Chrysler building. Do we?

C: We went to . . . my Daddy went to work.

M: Remember when we went to visit Daddy? [We] went in the elevator, way, way up in the building so we could look down from the big window?

C: Big window.

M: mmhm

C: When . . . we did go on the big building?

M: mmhm, the big building. Was that fun? Would you like to do it again? Sometime.

C: I want to go on the big building. (Nelson, 2007, p. 194)

Here, meanings are added to the child's story by the mother and then further elaborated by the child. The mother recalls the elevator and looking down from a big window. She adds the idea of fun, to which the child responds by expressing a desire to go back to the building.

Some mothers are more highly elaborative than others in developing narratives and in other verbal interchanges with their children, and often this talk involves developing meanings about novel events and/or the child's emotions (Fivush & Reese, 1991, as cited in Nelson, 2007). In Nelson's terms, these *meaning structures* include "a temporal and causal sequence—this happened because that happened—and an evaluation—I was happy, sad, felt good, and so on" (2007, p. 195), creating a story of what happened and the child's role in it. Parents differ in how much they elaborate the child's language, and middle-class parents are especially likely to offer elaborations (Hoff-Ginsberg, 1991; Nelson, 2007). Relations have also been found between temperament and mother-elaborated language. More distress-prone infants of 6–8 months, for example, tend to receive less elaborated language from their mothers (Vernon-Feagans et al., 2008).

What is jointly discussed by caregivers and children also tends to be remembered by the child (Haden, Ornstein, Eckerman, & Didow, 2001; Tessler, 1986) so that the stories will influence children's memory and structures of meaning. The child thereby comes to see the world as involving a self who is a character, embedded in an elaborated past and an anticipated future. By the late preschool years, children can distinguish between the inner self and the outer self, and have a developing understanding of "presenting the self" to others (Nelson, 2007; Selman, 1980; see Figure 5.1). By the ages of 5–6, children are able to distinguish between the *inner, private self* and the *outer presentation of self.*

By middle childhood (7–8 years), children are aware of the kind of person their parents and others wish them to become (Higgins, 1991) and by adolescence, conflicts between the inner self (who the youth believes he or she really is) and the self seen as wanted by others, can lead young people to engage in "false-self behavior," including "not saying what you think" and "changing yourself to be something that someone *else* wants you to be" (Harter, 1998, p. 581). With an understanding of the differentiation of inner and outer selves (Figure 5.1), the child may come to feel that he or she, the parent, or another person is a phony, presenting an inauthentic self. This, like all aspects of self-concept development, would benefit from studies in different cultures, where the concept and experience of the authentic self may differ.

It is important to recognize, as Nelson (2007) argues, that explicit or declarative meaning structures do not necessarily supersede the previously developed implicit meaning structures related to the emotions and temperament. Indeed, the implicit meanings that continue to be held may *not* be consistent with the child's current beliefs and self-constructs. Once private and public self-aspects are distinguished, questions about who we *really* are also become possible. Are we really the person we present to others and ourselves? What if we are aware that the stories we tell, and the self we present to others, are not in keeping with who we would like to be? How do we react when someone else tells us how we are feeling, but in our perception, we are not feeling that way at all?

The Self Is Social

Just as the infant co-constructs an implicit world of meaning in interactions with others (Chapter 4), the explicit or declarative self develops in social settings. Here the child's representations of the self and ego-self will also be co-constructed with others (Bennett & Sani, 2004). We also learn who we are through others' reactions to us—and these reactions can be positive, neutral, or negative. They can also be implicit or explicit. Cooley's (1902) concept of the *looking glass self* was adapted by George Herbert Mead (1934) to indicate that we see reflections of who we are in others' reactions to us, or at least in the reactions we believe they have about us. When others' reactions are positive and loving, we see ourselves as worthy of love. When they are negative, we feel more worthy of shame. These can all be represented in implicit knowledge (e.g., in feelings of guilt or shame), and if the child is not sensitive to these events, he or she may be relatively unaffected by them. Language, however, adds a new explicit understanding of the parent's words that are critical, derisive, and unloving. Even the child who did not notice disapproving facial expressions of the parent at an earlier time is likely to put together a critical view of the self from the parent's words.

As we come to describe others, we also learn to describe ourselves, and typically use the same categories to describe the self and others. These categories and judgments are reflected in the *conceptual* self-construct or set of beliefs about the self (see Figure 5.1). We learn from the stories told us by others and our co-constructed understanding ideas of who we are, what we do, and what we feel and think. We also gain practice in acting out society's scripts and roles, learning from the behavior of adults and older children, and from the media, including television, film, books, and the Internet.

This learning is assimilated to what is called here the *primary meaning structure*, the model of the self or self-construct, along with the child's constructs of others. The ego self and its cognitive supports also provide meanings for us over time and in changing environments. Our organization of meanings may lead us to feel like the stars of our own life drama, with others playing leading or supporting roles. Significant others are part of the stories we develop and the models we have for ourselves, others, and our life. Capacities of effortful control will also allow older children to control their own thoughts and feelings, becoming to some degree the director of their actions. We may also attempt to direct others, by telling them what to say and do. Of course, others have different scripts, in which *they* play the starring role and interpret the behaviors of others; the scripts of two members of a relationship may often conflict, and anger can result if one partner does not play out the script intended by the other.

Although the narrative self involves extensions of the self in time, the extended self also includes the people we identify with, the objects and ideas we produce, the objects we own, and the other persons and groups that we experience as part of the extended "I." These extensions may be called *identifications*. We take pride in these aspects of self, but when they are threatened there is a threat to the integrity of the self as well. When an extended part of the self is threatened we attempt to protect and defend it, and the emotions we experience can be intense. In the past, developmental psychologists have discarded the concept of identification and instead used the concept of imitation; I believe it would be helpful to reassess and rehabilitate the identification concept.

The Idealized Self

Other approaches to dealing with self-devaluation have been described in Karen Horney's (1937, 1945, 1950) and Ausubel and Sullivan's (1970) theories of personality. In Horney's view, we set for ourselves an idealized self that we attempt to support through information gleaned from our parents and others. Often our self-idealization is extreme and impossible to attain. This means that in everyday experiences, children are likely to be receiving information that they are *not* living up to the person they wish to be. When this happens, the idealized self-model is challenged, the child's security is threatened, and anxiety or anger can result. To prevent these emotions and to avoid conscious realization of having fallen short of one's ideal, coping strategies are directed toward protection and defense of one's view of the self, and this coping often involves others.

Horney (1945) identified three types of adaptations or coping strategies that involve other people: moving toward others, moving against others, and moving away from others. The links between these coping strategies and temperament (affiliativeness, externalizing, and internalizing) should be clear. The first of these adaptations can involve the child moving into the orbit of a powerful adult or adults, identifying with them and using their perceived power to strengthen the child's own self-image. Horney saw identifications as one aspect of *moving toward* others. These identifications are not limited to other individuals. A person may identify with groups, religions, sports teams, political parties, languages, or nationalities. Identifications are meaning structures that may or may not be conscious, and threats or injuries to the objects of identifications can lead to retaliation and defense via one's own anger and aggression. Moving toward others may also include dependency and approval seeking in the child or adult.

The second orientation to self-threat, centered on anger, hostility, and aggression, is described in Horney's (1945) terms as *movement against* others. Through projection, children may shift the responsibility for their own actions or thoughts to others. Here, the source of the problem is seen as existing outside the self, avoiding the anxiety that would have been felt from experiencing one's own self-failure. The self is seen to be in the right and others in the wrong, and often the indignation and even hatred felt against others has a strong moral tone. When threat is removed from the self and shifted to others, the person may also be willing to engage in violence against the "bad," "oppressive," or "evil" group. *Movement against* can also involve negative identifications with others, when one wishes to be as different as possible from the other person.

A third orientation in Horney's (1945) view involves *moving away* from others, physically, mentally, or both. This strategy can allow freedom from unhappy interchanges, but it can also result in living within narrowly confined limits and in feelings of loneliness. Although a person may specialize in one of these three orientations, it is likely that over the course of time, a person will use all three. What is most striking about these personality orientations, however, is their emotional power. This power may stem from their close relation to protecting the meaning structure of the self, which in turn may derive its power from the evolutionary imperative for self-preservation.

Affiliative Meaning Structures

I have talked about temperament in terms of the child's emotional reactivity and sensitivities: sensitivity to reward, to punishment, to having made a mistake. Another sensitivity is linked specifically to our involvement with others. Sensitivity to the reactions of others can be seen in infants' reactions to the mother's "still face." In the still-face procedure, the mother is asked to maintain an unexpressive face and not respond to her infant's actions or entreaties (Tronick, Als, Adamson, Wise, & Brazelton, 1978). This procedure can result in the infant's attempts to regain the mother's attention, and often leads to infant distress or self-soothing when these attempts fail. In older children and adults, we can observe sensitivity to social rejection (Mischel & Ayduk, 2004). Because humans are affiliative, and because the support of others is evolutionarily vital to our self-protection, the threat that others will reject us and that we will be left alone is very powerful. Indeed, imaging studies have found that social rejection activates the physical pain areas of the human brain (Eisenberger, Lieberman, & Williams, 2003).

In Chapters 2 and 3, I considered affiliativeness as a dimension of temperament, with the disposition toward closeness being stronger for some children than for others. The enjoyment of close relationships with others may also be linked to distress at their absence via abandonment or rejection. Tendencies to fear or anger will also contribute to the person's sensitivity to rejection. In addition, because the model of the self is built socially, one of the ways we support our own model is by getting confirmation of that model from others. Rejection or the threat of rejection leads us to question whether the self we imagine ourselves to be (e.g., likable, good-natured, easy to get along with) is correct, adding further to its power as a threat. Mischel and Ayduk (2004) give an example of a person high in rejection sensitivity (RS):

> RS is a chronic processing disposition characterized by anxious expectations of rejection (Downey & Feldman, 1996) and a readiness to encode even ambiguous events in interpersonal situations (e.g., partner momentarily seems inattentive) as indicators of rejection that rapidly trigger automatic hot reactions (e.g., hostility–anger, withdrawal–depression, self-silencing). . . . Probably rooted in prior rejection experiences, these dynamics are readily activated when high RS people encounter interpersonal situations in which rejection is a possibility, triggering in them a sense of threat and foreboding. (p. 118)

As the possibility of a future rejection or memory of a previous one is repeatedly experienced and consolidated over time, a person's attention can become quite narrowly directed toward the possibility of rejection. In adults, social rejection produces both pain and strong activation of the anterior cingulate (ACC), suggesting an important link between RS, physical pain, and executive attention (Eisenberger et al., 2003). To protect the self-model from rejection, defensive coping (e.g., anger; rejecting the other to prevent the other's rejection of the self; viewing the other as incompetent, as an enemy, as a person of little importance; attempts at repair; identifying with a powerful other) may occur to fend off expected rejection.

As in the case of the child's fear toward the uncle, a person's RS may not extend to everyone. Although RS can extend to a wide range of relationships, it can also be more specific. For example, children may become sensitized only to rejection by their peers, but not to rejection by adults or siblings. RS may be *so* specific that it is limited to sensitivity to rejection from a single person (e.g., one's mother or father, a boyfriend or girlfriend, a spouse) or a single kind of situation, such as giving or receiving care, exchanging gifts, or making telephone calls. Strategies for coping with the threat of rejection (rejecting the other, anger at the other, attempts at approval seeking) can involve a whole array of social orientations, and the orientation adopted can also vary from one perceived rejecter to another. Thus, seeking approval may be done differently in the school than in the home.

Sensitivities to rejection and hurt are particularly likely to develop within intimate relationships, such as the family. In the nuclear family, the child may become sensitive to abandonment, to the loss of parental love, or to the loss of personal control. As the child moves beyond the family, sensitivities that have developed in the family may be carried over, so that when the child feels threatened or rejected, he or she may use strategies consolidated in the past. Thus, the experience of early criticism and rejection, which is likely to have its strongest impact on children who are temperamentally prone to distress, can result in long-term consequences for children's development.

The idea of sensitivity to particular kinds of social events can be extended to other situations and responses; one of which is sensitivity to hostility in others. Dodge and his associates (Dodge & Coie, 1987) studied sensitivity to hostility from others in aggressive and nonaggressive children. Aggressive children are more likely to see behavior that is ambiguous in its motivation as involving hostile intent (see also Orobio de Castro, Veerman, Koops, Bosch, & Monshouwer, 2002). A personal example of sensitivity may be helpful here. When I was 3 or 4 years old, I very much enjoyed answering the phone for my parents. On one occasion, however, the person at the other end of the line yelled at me (at least this is how I remember it) and said that only adults, not children, should be allowed to answer the phone. I was a fearful child, and this experience of punishment colored my later feelings about not only answering the phone, but also making phone calls. Even today, I make phone calls only when I think they are necessary and answer the phone only when no one else is available to do it and I think it might be important. I have spoken with a number of other adults who see phone calls as threatening, and who prefer less personal and intrusive means of communication. Indeed, I have learned that phone phobia (defined as a persistent, abnormal, and unwarranted fear of the telephone) is now being diagnosed and treated. In addition, however, I have used effortful control to schedule regular calls to family members, suggesting that even phobias can be self-adjusted.

Mischel and Ayduk's (2004) analysis of RS and my example of telephone sensitivity describe anxious or defensive sets, but of course, children's experiences with others will also be ones of acceptance and pleasure. When this occurs, the child will be less likely to be on guard about rejection and will be less self-protective. Instead, his or her attention can be directed more broadly, allowing for greater awareness of the state and needs of others, and related to a sensitivity for acceptance rather than rejection.

More distress-prone, fearful, and irritable children may be more likely to develop RS, and indeed personality neuroticism is related to RS in adults (Brookings, Zembara, & Hochstetlerb, 2003). After experiencing high levels of rejection, however, even a surgent child can become sensitive to rejection. Surgent children are more likely to be sensitive to positive experiences, and in the telephone example, may not have been at all bothered by what the stranger said or how she said it. A cold, rejecting childhood, however, can nevertheless shape the meaning structures of many children. In particular, rejection affects the child's beliefs and understanding of others and the self. Even though a child may be temperamentally positive and approaching, a devalued self-construct and sensitivity to rejection may develop.

When repeatedly experienced, as in the nuclear family, the activation of meaning structures becomes more consolidated and more difficult to change. These meaning structures may include actions, emotions, or thoughts. When these structures are distress-related, how might connections be weakened? In Eastern traditions, this is done partly through diminishing the importance of the ego-self so that situations and people become less threatening. Mental discipline and meditation further weaken the links between thoughts and emotions and between thoughts and action tendencies. Western therapy similarly works through a person's patterns of reaction, allowing the person to reconsider previously consolidated meanings, and offering new and alternative frameworks of meaning. The issues discussed in therapy often deal with the person's significant relationships.

Taking a developmental view, however, one would wish to give children the kinds of experiences that allow them to form more positive meanings and favorable expectations in the first place.

How might this be accomplished? One approach to more positive child rearing is Birth To Three (a different organization than Zero to Three), a parent-support program based in Eugene, Oregon. This program was founded by two of our temperament project team members who were parents themselves and by the parent of an infant participant in one of our early temperament studies. Birth To Three offers information to young parents who often find themselves alone with a new infant as did my parents, my husband and I, and many others. It offers the social support of other parents with infants of the same age, and a curriculum based on recent research findings in developmental psychology (Rothbart, 2007b). When an issue in the child's development arises, parents realize that they are not facing it alone and they are able to benefit from other parents' experiences as well as by the Birth To Three curriculum offered by the group leader. The group leader also offers videotapes and printed materials based on what has been learned about child development.

One aim of the program is to train parents not to only react automatically to the child's behavior, but to stop and adopt a conscious, problem-solving approach. Basically, this involves watching what one does, thinking about the meaning of one's actions in declarative terms, making a decision based on one's values to change that behavior, and practicing a different set of behaviors until they become automatic. It is interesting that in the past, programs have attempted to teach children who are low in self-regulation how to stop, look, and listen, without much good effect, whereas now *parents* are encouraged to do the same. Another aim of the Birth To Three program is to build positive relationships within the family. One of the major goals of Birth To Three is to equip the child and members of the family with more positive structures of meaning. I return to details of this program in Chapter 9.

Self-Esteem

Feelings of positive self-worth are highly valued in our society. Self-esteem has been a topic of interest in child development for many years, and Harter (2006) suggests that even young children display self-esteem in their behavior. She asked nursery school and kindergarten teachers to describe each child in their classes. A second group of teachers then sorted the descriptions into categories ranging from high to low self-esteem. This sorting described the high-self-esteem child as one who "trusts his or her own ideas, approaches challenge, initiates activities confidently . . . is eager to try doing new things, describes self in positive terms . . . is able to adjust to changes, comfortable with transitions, tolerates frustration and perseveres, and is able to handle criticism and teasing" (Harter, 2006, p. 515). The low-self-esteem child is described in this way: "Doesn't trust his or her own ideas, lacks confidence to initiate, lacks confidence to approach challenge, is not curious, does not explore, hangs back, watches only, withdraws and sits apart, describes self in negative terms . . . gives up easily when frustrated, reacts to stress with immature behavior, and reacts inappropriately to accidents" (p. 515).

These teachers' judgments were not related to other measures of the children's competence, but the descriptions appear to overlap with temperament dimensions of fear, anger, surgency, and soothability, and with the effortful control that is involved in children's perseverance, emotion regulation, and effective coping. They also reflect the child's general and more specific experiences of security or threat with others, including other children. In Chapter 6, I consider children's coping as it develops out of temperament, suggesting that temperament works in conjunction with our sensitivities to self-devaluation in influencing how we protect ourselves and react to others.

SUMMARY

In this chapter, I have considered personal meaning structures, including the development of models of the self. The chapter illustrates how basic temperamental dimensions such as fear, anger, approach, and affiliativeness become incorporated into the meaning structures that will help to shape the personality. These meaning structures need not be general, but can be specific to the child's experiences with particular others and particular situations. While this chapter stresses normal personality development, extreme versions of some of the coping strategies described in Chapter 9 are related to disorders of personality. For example, high and unrealistic self-regard may lead to narcissistic personality disorder, and failures of effortful control when combined with strong negative affect may predict other personality disorders. In the next two chapters, I consider how the social environment, including peers, teachers, and culture, can influence personality, and in Chapter 10, I consider temperament and the development of psychopathology.

CHAPTER 6

Coping and Culture

In 1931, Katharine Bridges published a book based on observations of nursery school children that would bring her influential theory of emotions in infancy into the preschool years. In her first observations of children in the McGill University Nursery School, she noted:

> The most striking differences observed during the preliminary experiment, and indeed at any time, were individual rather than age differences in behaviour both social and emotional. Some children "went their own way" and left others alone, while others seemed as if they had to be always in the crowd. Some children "hung around" the adults for attention, others spoke to the grown-ups only when necessary, and still others opposed almost every suggestion or request made to them by an adult. Some children cried frequently, others scarcely at all. Some children rushed about and laughed with delight, others sat quietly or stood about, making as few movements as possible and smiling only faintly. Some shouted and squealed frequently, others fought, and others whined in a complaining way. (p. 11)

At this point in a book on temperament, these observations should not be too surprising. They depict not only temperamental differences, but also differing ways of coping with the nursery school experience. Just as there are patterns in temperament, there are patterns in the child's adaptations to the social and physical world. For example, if we observe nursery school children over time, we will note that some of the children who are laughing with delight one minute might be fighting with other children in the next, or that other children might approach an adult when they are frightened or tired, but otherwise play alone. In this chapter, we consider the child's adaptations to the wider world, and culture's contributions to these adaptations.

CHILDREN'S COPING

Young children can often be observed simply enjoying the world, the self, and others. Their behavior is linked to the emotion of joy, one of the few emotions that is not concerned with attempting to change or control anything. In fear, we attempt to avoid danger; in anger/frustration, we attack obstacles; in sadness, we imagine how things might have been different; in anxiety over separation, we seek union. The emotion of joy, on the other hand, is often seen in the child at play, unself-conscious and enjoying what he or she is doing. Much learning goes on during play, and in role taking and games, the child is also able to practice effortful attention and control (Singer, Golinkoff, & Hirsh-Pasek, 2006).

Not all of the child's life is joyful, however. Children are also asked to adapt to new and challenging situations, and temperament influences the degree to which these will be experienced as stressful. Early in life, there will be adjustments by the child to these experiences, many of them related to temperament (Rueda & Rothbart, 2009). Early coping strategies include hesitancy, avoidance, and withdrawal; angry resistance, approach, and aggression; and affiliative or help-seeking dependency on others. Once used, the child's coping strategies can be carried forward to future situations. If a previously prepared adjustment is not acceptable to a new setting, it may lead to new problems and challenges.

Temperament and Coping

Just as children's temperament leads to specific reactions as it is applied to a given situation, in the specification of temperament, their coping often involves different strategies in different situations, depending on the child's temperament and what is possible in the setting. Nevertheless, coping styles that cut across situations and are consistent over time are also observed (Compas, 1987; Skinner & Zimmer-Gembeck, 2007). Researchers have factor analyzed coping questionnaires, for example, identifying "families of coping strategies" (Skinner, Edge, Altman, & Sherwood, 2003). One study identified four general approaches to coping: (1) avoidant coping, involving escaping or denying the disturbing situation; (2) distraction, involving oneself in another activity or thought to keep from thinking about the disturbing situation; (3) support seeking, using social support to solve the problem and reduce negative emotions; and (4) active coping, engaging in problem solving, seeking help, or information, and making a positive reappraisal of the situation (Ayers, Sandler, West, & Roosa, 1996).

As we have noted, individual differences in temperament are linked directly to behavioral tendencies (e.g., approach or withdrawal from a novel object or situation, attack on the object of the child's frustration, or a surgent approach to a potential reward). Temperament thus directly influences the structure of the child's early adaptations to life. I begin this section by reviewing some of the behavior tendencies that are part of early temperament and provide a basis for coping. Although coping is often defined as regulation under stress (Compas, Connor-Smith, Saltzman, Thomsen, & Wadsworth, 2001; Skinner, 1999), I will look at coping more broadly as behavior patterns directed toward dealing with both environmental challenges and rewards.

One approach to coping involves temperamental surgency in the tendency to approach novel and challenging situations, as well as rewarding ones. More fearful children will be more likely to withdraw from novel and challenging situations, and to take time before they approach. Children prone to anger/frustration may be especially likely to engage in aggression, and fearfulness will oppose acting on those impulses.

Affiliation is likely linked to seeking comfort and support from others. In our longitudinal study, infants who showed more fear or anger/frustration were more likely to show a pattern of seeking help when they were 7 years old (Rothbart, Ahadi, et al., 1994). Temperament preferences for high or low levels of stimulation are also likely to lead to different adaptive strategies. A child who is easily overwhelmed will try to keep things more quiet, whereas a child who requires high levels of stimulation to experience pleasure will attempt to seek out and create excitement. Challenges outside the home, such as a noisy and intense day care experience for an easily overstimulated infant, or demands for extended quiet time at a school desk for a stimulation-seeking older child, may also lead to problems.

Finally, effortful control offers an approach that can serve the goals of emotional tendencies or can be used to exercise control over those tendencies. Effortful control can be used to inhibit impulsive action, to activate a behavior that the child would otherwise not engage in (e.g., coming to dinner from play), the reappraisal of events, detection of errors, and planning for future goals. Overall, we would expect that effortful control would be related to active coping, and our review of research later in this chapter suggests this is the case. For the moment, however, let us look at a very rich observational study of preschool-age children's strategies for coping.

Murphy (1962) and her associates observed 2- to 5-year-old children of a midwestern town who had had been studied as infants in Escalona's (1968) laboratory. The children were observed in naturally occurring situations and during testing in the laboratory, and one of the most striking aspects of their behavior was their use of coping strategies. Murphy defined *coping* as "The steps or sequences through which the child comes to terms with a challenge or makes use of an opportunity. Adaptation is the result" (1962, p. 60). Murphy also defined *competence* as the skills achieved by the child, including his or her competencies in coping. Murphy argues that we need to understand each child's "own manner of dealing with pressures and threats, potential or actual. This way of thinking involves awareness of the individuality, spontaneity, even creativity characterizing the new patterns of response we see . . . as well as the gallant persistence and repetitive efforts which are often necessary in the struggle toward mastery" (p. 7).

Murphy (1962) stresses that what is a challenge for one child may be no problem for another. The amount of stimulation that is easily tolerated by most young children, however, may be more than some children can handle. It also may not provide enough excitement for others. Children's management of stimulation and regulation of their own reaction to it are important aspects of coping. Some children appear to need to turn down the volume or intensity of experience; others need to turn it up. For some more easily overstimulated children, environmental challenges can be severe, but coping is seen in all children.

The infants we observed in our laboratory managed the excitement of a mechanical toy by closing their eyes to shut out the sight of it, partially closing their eyes, looking away, covering their eyes, protesting, pushing away the threatening toy, turning to their mother for support, or attempting to leave the situation (Rothbart, Ziaie, & O'Boyle, 1992). For more surgent and extraverted infants, we observed approach and seeking of excitement, vigorous self-stimulation, and attempts to evoke arousing reactions from others. Some of the infants clapped their hands or even picked up and kissed the highly arousing mechanical toy. Even in infancy, the children were showing "the gallant persistence and repetitive efforts which are often necessary in the struggle for mastery" (Murphy, 1962, p. 7).

Murphy (1962) observed children's coping strategies at an outdoor party that included children from the study who did not know each other. At the party, the more surgent children (approximately one-third of the girls; two-thirds of the boys) rushed in and took part in all of the social activities offered. They swallowed the lemonade offered them in a few quick gulps and joined the party without asking for adult permission, "taking for granted that this new world was theirs to enjoy and explore" (p. 98). Other children used a more cautious approach. They would first survey the situation and then stay within a small, safe area before venturing out. Some of these more cautious children sipped their lemonade very slowly, looking over the tops of their paper cups to observe the situation. Murphy noted that some of the children appeared to do this anxiously, but others appeared to be quite comfortable. The more comfortable children were simply gathering more information about the scene before approaching.

Some children further postponed joining the group by going into a nearby garage that had been equipped with toys. Some played by themselves in this way-station for a while and then went out to join the party. Others resisted any attempts of adults or other children to tempt them out. The more hesitant children who did come out appeared to be more comfortable when adults were directing games rather than when the children were unsupervised. A few children completely refused to participate. One child "simply stood, looking close to tears, and after some delay said, 'I don't want to go to the party'" (Murphy, 1962, p. 111).

Although Murphy's (1962) observations dealt mainly with the adjustments of shy and cautious children, surgent children also face challenges. These include injuries due to risky behaviors (Schwebel, 2004), and other children's retaliations to acts seen as aggressive, overexuberant, loud, and socially insensitive. These behaviors can affect the child's acceptance or rejection by other children in the playgroup. Later in elementary school, they can also affect the reactions of teachers as well as peers. More outgoing children face fewer problems in initiating an approach in a new situation. However, self-control may be challenging for them, as when they are asked to sit still at a desk for long periods. For more surgent children, developing adequate self-regulation will be particularly important.

Murphy (1962) also observed how children evaluated their own skills when given psychological tests. Some children would repeat incorrect responses without showing any concern about having made errors. Others denied any failure. Other children dealt with the threatening test materials by pushing them away, carrying them off, hiding them, or treating them roughly. Some children rejected the more challenging tests, and others offered to switch roles with the tester, assigning the tester the more difficult tasks. Some children prepared for potential failure with warnings to the tester like, "If you give me trouble, I'll go home" (p. 214).

When we observe children engaging in coping or defense in a situation, we can infer that they are troubled by or sensitive to a potential outcome or thought that is negative to them. Here the sensitivity is to having made an error (suggesting the child is not perfect) or being seen as a failure (another unacceptable possibility). In Murphy's (1962) study, at least a third of the children used active escape, attempting to leave the room, or used passive coping, simply going through the motions of the task without attending to it. Other coping responses included refusals, protests, silence, refusing to do anything at all, or objecting to repetitious tasks, declaring a task to be done when it wasn't, or rejecting the materials.

When my husband began graduate school, he was training in clinical psychology, and one of his assignments was to give an intelligence test to a young child. This test had the requirement that the child make several consecutive errors before the test could be ended. Mick came home from the testing situation visibly shaken. His chief impression of the test was the extreme anxiety shown by the child about her performance. Given the recent environment of testing in the schools, a study of children's coping with test taking and with the possibility of error, may help us put less pressure on children to pass tests and instead create an environment that encourages learning.

Studies of Temperament and Coping

Lengua and her colleagues have related 8- to 12-year-old children's temperament to their patterns of coping with stressors such as divorce (Lengua & Long, 2002; Lengua, Sandler, West, Wolchik, & Curran, 1999). Children higher in temperamental negative emotionality viewed events as more threatening, suggesting that they were more subject to stress than less reactive children. Their coping was also more likely to be avoidant, including withholding of action and not thinking about upsetting information. Positive emotionality (surgency), on the other hand, was related to lower appraisals of threat and more active coping. Children's attentional regulation was also related to more active coping, including direct problem solving, decision making, seeking understanding, positive reappraisal, and optimism. Active coping methods tend to address the problem directly rather than to avoid it.

Eisenberg and her colleagues have similarly found that negative emotion was linked to less constructive coping, and attentional control to more constructive coping (Eisenberg et al., 1993). In adolescents, positive emotionality has been related to active coping (Wills, DuHamel, & Vaccaro, 1995), and in adults there are connections between negative emotion and avoidant coping (Bolger, 1990) and between self-regulation and active coping (Fabes & Eisenberg, 1997). In adults, personality neuroticism (negative emotion) has been associated with wishful thinking, emotion-focused coping, and withdrawal (Connor-Smith & Flachsbart, 2007).

The use of planning and preparing for upcoming events suggests that coping does not occur only in the moment of the experienced challenge or opportunity. Coping is often preparatory. Coping strategies develop in interactions, but planning, decision making, and implementing an action allow the child to prepare for upcoming events. Children who position themselves at the edge of nursery school activities are selecting a different set of experiences than the children who rush to the center of social action and excitement.

Preparatory Coping

Coping strategies can be initiated well before the beginning of a potentially stressful event. For example, children are likely to choose environments that are best adapted to their temperament. Scarr and McCartney (1983) call these adaptations "niche picking." As children become more personally responsible for their own choices of environment and experience, temperament can increasingly affect their choices. Because of niche picking and other preparatory coping techniques, we might follow a more fearful and a less fearful child over the course of a day, and not notice any differences between them in their expressions of fearful behavior. Here, the more fearful child may be operating in selected safe, familiar places and engaging in fewer risk-taking activities, whereas the less fearful child does not need such precaution.

Temperament also supports the development of more complex coping strategies than simple avoidance, defense, or approach. A child who experiences high distress to strangers, for example, may offer to help in the kitchen during a party. Helping relieves social pressure for interaction while allowing the child to remain part of the social scene. A more surgent child who has experienced pleasure in interactions with strangers in the past is likely to show more confident approach and to be actively mingling at the party. With adaptations like these, the child's use of temperament-related coping mechanisms may magnify initial temperament differences through experience. The more surgent child becomes more adapted to higher and higher levels of excitement, whereas the more fearful child uses more protective methods. To the extent that a coping strategy works, it is likely to be repeated. Helping in the kitchen, however, may put the child in close enough connection with the social activity that he or she can venture out on a future occasion.

How Others React to the Child's Temperament Shapes the Child's Coping

Scarr and McCartney (1983) have noted another effect of temperament on coping: children's temperament leads to reactions from others that can shape the child's subsequent action. Thus, a child with a positive and outgoing disposition may receive greater support and affection from others, even in a high-risk environment (Werner, 1985). In situations where children are at high risk for neglect or abuse, Radke-Yarrow and Sherman (1990) found that some children were protected if their characteristics met the needs of the parent. Children's acceptance by adults can then lead them to feel there is something special or important about themwselves, building a more positive view of self. This idea is very similar to Thomas and Chess's (1977) "goodness-of-fit" argument. Thomas and Chess found that the presence of just one supportive adult, who may or may not be the parent, can have a positive influence on the child's development. This person may be an aunt, a grandparent, or even an adult living down the hall in an apartment building.

Adult reactions can also lead to the child's selection of less positive coping methods. When a toddler lashes out in frustration, the parent's response may be punitive, leading to retaliation from the child, which leads to further retaliation from the parent. As a coercive pattern develops, each partner to the interaction responds to pain from the other by directing punishment to the other. Coercive cycles can also reinforce aggressive coping in the child, especially when the parent then has enough of the exchange and drops out of the interaction (Patterson, 1980, 1982). In the home, coercive cycles can also develop with siblings, and outside the home with peers and even with teachers.

Coping, like other habitual orientations that develop under the influence of temperament, can be specific to a particular setting, a particular relationship, or a particular setting and a particular relationship. We can think of the coping strategies available to the child as a kind of tool kit. Some coping strategies are used and consolidated in particular situations, but can easily be generalized to related situations. Preparatory coping can also be adapted to different settings in advance of the event. Birth To Three also offers parents a tool kit for interacting with their children.

The temperament characteristics of one's partners in the relationship can also influence children's coping. For example, the temperamental characteristics that two siblings bring to their interactions have been related to their aggressive coping toward each other. Stoneman and Brody (1993) found that the highest negativity and conflict were observed when both siblings were high in activity level, or when the older child was more active than the younger. The lowest levels of negativity and conflict were observed when both siblings were low in activity. Conflict was also high when older siblings were high in activity and younger siblings were low in adaptability.

Once a child develops comprehension of being judged by others, the child's sensitivity to error or criticism becomes an issue (Stipek, 1995). When parents and other significant people are highly critical, the child may become sensitive to failure and develop coping strategies to deal with these threats to the self. One way children defend against negative information about the self is by thinking and acting as if they are better than others, showing paradoxically high self-esteem to protect against low feelings of self-worth.

Further Influences of Adults on Children's Coping

When adults intervene, children's coping patterns will also be influenced. Patterson, Littman, and Bricker (1967) found that in U.S. preschools where teachers intervened when conflicts developed, there was less development of aggression in the children over the course of the school year. In other cultures, older siblings take on caregiving roles with younger siblings, often strengthening the nurturing skills and qualities of the older child (Whiting, 1963). Social arrangements for children affect their adjustments, and these differ across cultures and over historical time within a culture. Later in this chapter I consider some of the links between culture, socialization, and the child's temperament.

How do parents help their children face new and challenging situations? Caregivers can take advantage of the fact that objects or events that are frightening are also often intriguing. Thus, even though avoidance may be the child's first response, there will exist latent approach tendencies that can be strengthened. When fearful children are given control of a noisy vacuum cleaner, for example, their fears of it may decrease or disappear. Children's fear of dinosaurs or snakes may lead them to want to learn more about archaeology and herpetology, including the big words associated with them. Parents can support these interests, allowing children to master material that previously scared them. Parents can also talk about and accept the feelings the child is experiencing, rather than denying or suppressing them. When there is emotional support and encouragement, the child's openness to the environment is strengthened. Parents can also support their children by providing a script for the child to follow in a threatening situation, for example, suggesting to the child that he or she can go over to another player on the soccer field and ask the child if he or she likes soccer.

Taking the child's fears and sensitivities seriously is important. One of our sons at about 4 years of age refused to go to bed because he was afraid a vampire might come after him. My husband argued that there is no such a thing as a vampire and that he was perfectly safe. This approach did not work, and our son became even more fearful. When I told my husband I was going to bring some garlic (a well-known "vampire preventative") to our child's room for protection, my husband was concerned, thinking I might be making the boy an emotional invalid. After I had shown our son the garlic and placed it under his pillow, he nevertheless slept well. He never asked for the garlic or complained about a vampire again.

Another approach is to make achievement situations less threatening and more clearly open to the child's effort. In our culture, early independence training and emphasis on personal performance is often related to the child's belief that anything less than perfect performance is linked to a flaw in the self. When children view their performance as reflecting on their own ability or lack of ability, they can become very upset about the possibility of error or failure (Dweck, 2000). Errors then have only one meaning; that the child does not measure up. If, on the other hand, the child is encouraged to use information about errors to increase *effort* toward achieving a goal, the child may accept errors without having them reflect on the self. In this quite different view, when you run into problems, you work harder. Being a hard worker can also be taken as a personal quality of merit, but it allows children to persist in situations where they might otherwise have been threatened, and used self-defense or withdrawal.

Social Environment and Coping

Until now, our discussion has assumed that active coping is the most appropriate response to a challenging situation, in keeping with our culture's general emphasis on independent action of the individual. However, the active approach may not be successful in some settings. Tolan and Grant (2009) note that a given coping method may be more or less effective depending on the setting. In settings of urban poverty, active coping with violent events predicted increased aggression and risk of harm to the child (Rosario, Salzinger, Feldman, & Ng-Mak, 2003). Avoidant coping, on the other hand, was associated with more positive outcomes. Tolan and Grant (2009) suggest that "adopting a more realistic and less personally demanding view that 'there is little one can do to change things' may serve individuals better when facing great stress than to insistently attempt to change circumstances beyond their control or to consider a given event's occurrence and impact as one's personal responsibility" (p. 67). Hindu Vedanta teachings similarly stress the importance of recognizing that one often has little control over the outcomes of events. This point of view eases feelings of responsibility in stressful situations, while at the same time supporting and encouraging one's appropriate action.

Group Child Care and Temperament

In the United States and other countries, many infants are now enrolled in group care, and by the age of 3, many more children will be attending nursery school. Children who are introduced to group care as infants may remain in day care for years. Gunnar and Quevedo (2007) describe the child's transition to day care as involving "the entrance into a complex and challenging environment that demands the emergence of social skills including control of inappropriate behaviors, adapting communication to the listener's point of view, interpreting emotional cues, and maintaining play themes over transitions" (p. 158). All of these are major issues and real challenges to the child. Murphy (1962) and her associates used more familiar terms to describe some of the uncertainties of 3- to 4-year-olds starting nursery school: "Who will take care of me? Who will help me? Will I be able to do what is expected? Will I be able to control my feelings and actions or will I get scolded or punished? Whom can I love and who will love me?" (p. 67). These concerns may not be posed verbally or even recognized consciously, but they are issues children face when they enter a group care situation (Crockenberg, 2003).

Group care creates stress reactions for many children. During periods of stress, the adrenal cortex secretes steroid hormones, including cortisol and corticosterone (Carter, 1986). These hormones help provide the energy needed to support action in challenging situations. They promote glucose production for energy, and recruit an anti-inflammatory response to counteract possible injury and disease. Gunnar and her colleagues have extensively studied cortisol reactivity in relation to temperament and children's group care experience (Gunnar & Cheatham, 2003).

Young children (2–4 years) in group care show increases in cortisol levels over the course of the day, suggesting daily increases in stress reactions, but 5- to 8-year-olds in group care do not. Younger children who are being raised and tested at home also do not show these increases (Dettling, Gunnar, && Donzella, 1999; Dettling, Parker, Lane, Sebanc, & Gunnar, 2000). The challenges of group care also appear to be experienced differently for children with differing temperaments. Children who are easily overstimulated and sensitive to distress at low-intensity levels can have a difficult time in group care if the level of stimulation is high.

Gunnar and her associates (Dettling et al., 1999, 2000) used cortisol levels as indicators of stress in connection with group care. Children who were higher in temperamental negative emotionality and lower in inhibitory control showed greater increases in cortisol levels over the course of the day than did less distress-prone, more regulated children. This was found in both full-day child care centers (Dettling et al., 1999) and home day care settings (Dettling et al., 2000). In home day care, the quality of care was also measured by the amount of focused attention given by caregivers to individual children. With higher-quality care there were lower increases in cortisol levels.

Gunnar (1994) sees children's coping activities as mediating their cortisol reactions. For example, one way for children to control their own stress is by using caution in approaching groups of children. Shy children at first tend to avoid active interchanges, staying at the sidelines and putting off the experience of stress in interactions (Gunnar, 1994). More outgoing children tend to approach stress-related interchanges rapidly, and these children show effects of stress in their cortisol levels early in the school year. Later in the school year, more fearful children will tend to venture out; their social interactions will then be related to heightened cortisol levels (Gunnar, 1994).

Group care has also been found to increase children's aggressiveness, and once again, this occurs in interaction with children's temperament. Hagekull and Bohlin (in press), found that temperamental unmanageability as reported by mothers and fathers at 10- to 20-months of age predicted children's day care aggressiveness at age 4. Day care quality also affected the children's aggression. When more manageable children were in higher-quality care, they were less aggressive than those in lower-quality care. In less manageable children, however, aggressiveness occurred in both settings and was not related to quality of care.

CULTURE, SOCIALIZATION, AND TEMPERAMENT

Culture is defined by Mascolo (2004) as "a dynamic distribution of meanings, practices, and artifacts throughout a linguistic community" (p. 83). Meanings here refer to systems of categories, values, and emotions linked to particular thoughts, feelings, or behavior. These provide structures of meaning for the child, with the values and emotions often developed implicitly. Practices refer to the routines, scripts, and skills that are practiced in or required by a culture. Many of these are learned at an implicit level. The third is artifacts, the physical representations of culture, in tools, books, media, and other influences on the person. Specific settings within the culture may stress cultural learning to a greater or lesser degree. For example, the school might value independent thought and action, while autonomy is less valued in the home. Both settings may promote compliance.

Why do we wish to study culture along with temperament and development? There are a number of very important reasons: First, research in differing cultures gives us a real-world laboratory for testing whether the structure of temperament is similar even when child-rearing strategies and cultural values vary. This research has not been easy to do and it requires scrupulously translating questionnaire items and laboratory tests from one language and culture to another (Super et al., 2008). Because temperament includes emotional reactivity, and because the primary emotions are similarly displayed and understood in different cultures (Ekman, Sorenson, & Friesen, 1969), we have expected that the structure of temperament would also be similar across cultures, and this appears to be the case. Studies using the CBQ and other temperament scales in the United States and other cultures have replicated the structure of temperament in different cultures (Ahadi et al., 1993). To the extent that the Big Five and FFM measures of personality also reflect the structure of temperament, as I discuss in Chapter 8, they have also been consistent across numerous cultures (McCrae, 2001).

Although we are interested in similarities of temperament structure in different cultures, we are also interested in how the expression of temperament is shaped by culture. The qualities seen as "difficult" in children, for example, at least partially depend on culture. Super et al. (2008) studied temperamental qualities seen as difficult by parents in seven different cultures: Australia, Italy, the Netherlands, Poland, Spain, Sweden, and the United States. Although parents in most of the countries saw negative emotionality as "difficult," parents in Italy were much less concerned about the expression of negative emotion. Instead, they saw children who were not outgoing and approaching (shy children) as difficult.

Research on toddlers in non-Western countries even suggests that some of the issues we have associated with different developmental periods will vary from culture to culture (Edwards, 1995; Harkness & Super, 1983). As decsribed before, Margaret Mead and Beatrice Whiting (see Edwards & Liu, 2002) have described the lap child (infant) as becoming the knee child (toddler), the yard child (preschooler), and then the community child (the school-age child). Edwards (1995) describes toddler development in a highland Mayan community, Binacarta, as follows: "The transition from infancy to early childhood is not typified by resistant toddler demanding and asserting control . . (the familiar 'No! I can do it!'), but instead by watchful, imitative children who acquire toilet training and other elements of self-care with a minimum of fuss" (p. 47).

In Binacarta and a number of other Third World cultures, the toddler is not being constantly attended by the parent or other caregiver during waking hours, as is seen in Western culture. Instead, after weaning, and when they are able to get about, children join a playgroup (Edwards, 1995). Adjustments to the child's peers are thus required at an early age, and much of the child's socialization will occur in the peer group. In this setting, the major issue for the young child in relation to the mother occurs when another infant is added to the family, and the older child no longer receives close attention from the mother. This event may be reflected in dejection and listlessness in the displaced child. Differences in developmental issues and transitions may thus differ considerably from those described earlier in this book. The question of how culture, temperament, and developmental change influence each other is an exciting one, and will require further observation and analysis across a wide range of cultures.

Over the past 2 years, I have also become aware of an approach to the mother and her newborn infant that has in the past been part of the culture of child rearing in many non-Western cultures, including the Sikh tradition (Kim-Godwin, 2003). After the child's birth, the mother and infant will stay in the home together for the first 40 days of the child's life. Friends bring the mother food and clean her house, but they do not spend a great amount of time with the mother and baby. One goal of this arrangement is to allow the mother to simply be with her infant for an extended period. During this time the mother is not distracted by her usual responsibilities, and is able to develop a strong relationship with the child. In this setting, postpartum depression appears to be rarely observed. It should be noted that this practice may work at developing an attachment between the child and mother at a deeper level than usually described by attachment researchers. In Eugene, Oregon, this practice is being followed by several new mothers; it would be interesting to see whether this experience would lead to even more security in the child than is usually found.

Studying temperament in different cultures also broadens our view of personality far beyond the content of the Big Five and the temperament traits. For a fuller understanding of personality, we include both cognitive processes in personality and the dynamics of children's reactions and adaptations to situations. I have discussed the meaning structures that are basic to the personality, and I now identify aspects of personality seen to vary across cultures.

Personality, as we have seen, develops through interchanges in a social world. The child develops and consolidates ways of acting and thinking while observing and interacting with other members of the culture (at first, with parents and siblings). Ways of acting and thinking are also influenced by the material artifacts of culture including the media: tools, books, television, advertising, and so on. Goodenough (1981) identified a number of the ways in which culture affects personality that go beyond the Big Five personality traits. These influences are linked to cognitions of self and others, and to the development of skills and coping strategies. In Goodenough's view, culture influences an extensive list of items, which I discuss below:

1. The *categories* that we use to represent events, as reflected in our language and schooling.
2. The *propositions* or *explicit knowledge* we come to possess.
3. Our *beliefs* (propositions for which we do not have satisfactory evidence, but believe to be true).
4. Our *values* and *goals*.
5. Our *awareness of the rules* and *values* of groups (including aspects of temperament and personality that are valued or discouraged by the group culture).
6. Our *standard procedures* for accomplishing our goals.
7. The *scripts, routines*, and *standards of behavior* we habitually follow.

In addition, culture provides or influences:

8. The *physical means* for acquiring knowledge: books, television, tools, the Internet, and so on.
9. The stories or *narratives* that we tell about events and our role in them.
10. The *skills* we wish to develop.
11. The cognitive model of *self* we develop and project into the social world.
12. Our cognitive *models of significant others* and of relationships.

Categories and Evaluation

Earlier in the book, I addressed how temperament provides biologically based structures of meaning for evaluating and responding to the world. These mechanisms include our sensitivity to reward and related approach, sensitivity to threat and related fear and anger, and sensitivity to change related to orienting. All of these structures are part of our genetic heritage. Individual differences in the sensitivity of these systems in turn influence the adaptations we make to situations. Each structure may include a cognition (e.g., "This is dangerous"), an evaluation (e.g., "This is bad for me"), and motivations (e.g., to freeze, flee, or fight). Emotional appraisals operate in infants and young children long before they have developed concepts of emotions or words to describe them. Through experience, emotional structures become specified and adapted to particular situations, particular occasions, and particular people, as in the example of the children who differed in their responses to their uncle.

Temperament is further adapted to form more specified personality structures. Thus a child may become upset by one person but not another. Other aspects of personality, as indicated in the 12 points above, include categorical and propositional knowledge, beliefs, habits, narratives, and skills, all of which are influenced by experience, and many of which have been strongly influenced by temperament. An example of the influence of a category is seen in the following joke. Kreplach is a tasty Eastern European dish made up of ground cooked meat and onions wrapped in a packet of dough and then boiled, fried, and put into soup. It is a dish similar to wonton or ravioli.

A Jewish mother has a problem with her son—he refuses to eat kreplach. Although most children (and adults) find it very tasty, her son hates it and will not touch it. His parents and others describe to him how nice kreplach is to eat and how delicious it is, but the child is adamant. His parents take him to a child psychologist. The psychologist tells the mother that there is an easy solution to the problem: she should introduce the ingredients of kreplach to the child one at a time. As the child accepts each new addition, he will be able to finally accept the kreplach when it is put together. When they return home, the mother takes her son to the kitchen and sits him down to watch her prepare kreplach. First, she shows him a small mound of dough and a plate of chopped meat she has prepared. "Look," she asks, "is there anything wrong with this food?" "No, mom," smiles the boy. Then she puts the meat in the center of the dough; the child accepts it. She folds over one corner. "Is there anything here to be worried about?" "No, mom." She folds over the second corner and then the third; all goes well. Finally, she folds over the last corner, and the child screams, "Oh no, kreplach!"

Here the child's kreplach category was not reached until the mother's final step, but when it arrived, the cognition (kreplach), the child's evaluation (hate it), and the motivation (to avoid it) appeared at once. Moreover, the kreplach construct has little to do with the real-world construction of the kreplach. Not many constructs are connected to such passionate emotion and motivation, and others seem to be completely separated from emotion. As we see in Chapter 7, however, our evaluations and motivations have a great deal to do with what we learn and how we learn it.

Categories are very important in the transmission of culture and the behavior of groups. When groups are separated by category boundaries, even if the category boundaries are not meaningful, there are strong tendencies to show more favorable attitudes to the group one belongs to (also called the in-group) and potential to disparage the other group (also called the out-group). These tendencies can lead to unfortunate consequences as nations, races, and religions relate to each other (Rothbart & Lewis, 1994). I explore in Chapter 11 how different levels of influence, including the influence of social groups, can affect the person and vice versa.

Standards of Behavior

Besides learning in the family and school, we learn from the media, religious institutions, our peers and colleagues, and part of this learning involves the propositions or beliefs we come to hold to be true. Values and goals, which pervade the socialization process, are also important in personality functioning. Because values and cultural standards are often associated with what we "should" do, we may experience embarrassment and punishment from others and/or the self if we do not follow them. Cultural standards prescribing how things are done are important influences on personality, because they can lead to habits that differ considerably from culture to culture. Even conventional standards often take on a "should" quality. Schwartz (1978) gives the simple example of "sitting" in a classroom:

> We do not have to look very closely to see that each student is behaving quite differently at some level of physical or anatomical specification. And yet, even though no two behaviors are physically alike, all the students are "sitting." . . . A slight transgression—for example, someone sitting on their seat in the lotus position—might make the observer aware of a difference; he might even experience some slight anxiety or discomfort and may raise an eyebrow or edge away as a minor sanction. . . . Transgressions of cultural standards are seen in the transgressor's awareness, discomfort, anxiety, shame, and anger; they may show up in external responses by others to the behavior in the attention it arouses, the sanctions it may elicit, or in its perception as familiar or unfamiliar. (pp. 426–427)

Cultural standards can lead to pressure on the individual from other group members, and even to interpersonal aggression within and/or between groups. When a person feels rejected by other group members, it is difficult not to feel as though the self has failed in some way and that the person has not "measured up." The ancient Greeks' use of ostracism in the citizen's banishment from the city–state was considered one of the harshest forms of punishment. Although modern forms of group ostracism appear to be less extreme, they retain considerable power through the human need for affiliation and belonging and the person's sensitivity to social rejection.

Culture and the Self

Some of the most powerful meaning structures in personality involve the person's construction of the self, including how rigid that construction is, how well it is adapted to reality, the defenses we use to maintain the self-structure, and the coherence of the self-structure as revealed in our thoughts, emotions, and actions. The extended self is another meaning structure important to the personality, with stories of the self extended backward (Why did that happen to me?) and forward (What might happen to me?) in time. Identifications with others and with particular ideas and beliefs will further strengthen (or weaken) the construct of the self. Children's self-constructions can help them feel secure and well cared for, but threats to one's self and one's objects of identification may lead to threats to the very integrity of self. These threats may be in turn tied to defensive reactions, including defense of our identifications and beliefs (Cramer, 2006). Self-structures can differ from culture to culture (Markus & Kitayama, 1991) and from one historical period to another depending on the goals, values, and needs of the groups to which the child belongs, but we expect the basic influences of temperament, cognition, and the child's historical experiences to contribute to this structure.

Scripts, routines, and customs influence the traits we develop in dealing with members of our family, friendship groups, work groups, or professions. This suggests that for any individual there are multiple sources of culture that can conflict and change over time. Mascolo (2004) argues that

> in a society there are enclaves of meaning and practices with which a given individual has little direct contact (for example, practices that exist within industry, an inner city, the national government) . . . the idea that cultures are dynamic implies that they are not fixed entities. The elements of culture—its members, practices, technologies, and artifacts—change over time. (p. 84)

A good deal of variability may be allowed within families for enacting scripts and routines. For the teacher, the work manager, and members of a profession, however, routines and roles are often more highly specified.

Through them, the culture influences the goals a person pursues and the ways a person goes about achieving those goals or expressing his or her values. Although culture is responsible for influencing or directly teaching many of our categories and propositions, the kreplach joke reminds us that not all cultural messages are imparted successfully to a given child, and that the child is busy extracting personal meaning from the events he or she experiences (Kohlberg, 1976).

In fact, temperament and the appropriate behavior as specified by the culture do not always agree. This shows up in traditional gender roles that specify the appropriate behavior for men and women, and boys and girls. Traditionally, for example, girls have been allowed to be more shy than boys. One of the most interesting recent approaches to culture and temperament involves children's shyness, to which I now turn.

Shyness and Culture

Shyness is probably the most studied trait in connection with culture and temperament, but many other characteristics could also be studied, such as argumentativeness, sensitivity to criticism, or social skills. In the study of shyness, Buss (1986) distinguished between early-developing temperamental shyness (seen before the age of 2 years) and later-developing shyness (3–4 years or older). In addition, Asendorpf (1989, 1991, 1993) identified different paths toward shyness. One is more temperamental, corresponding to Buss's early-appearing shyness; the other is a learned shyness that appears to be related to children's previous rejection by members of their peer group (Asendorpf).

Asendorpf (1989, 1991, 1993) studied kindergarten-age children and found that temperamentally shy children (that is, children who responded to strangers with social fear) tended not to join in active group activities at the beginning of the school year. A number of these shy children, however, adapted successfully to group life over the kindergarten year. Some of the more extraverted children, who had rapidly approached other children at the beginning of the year, developed learned shyness and withdrawal over the course of the school year. Asendorpf suggests that these children may have experienced disapproval of peers in the classroom that led to their withdrawal.

This important research suggests that punishment from peers can influence a child's development of shyness even when there is not a temperamental disposition toward it. Peer reactions are not the only ones that can promote the development of shyness in a child who is not temperamentally shy. If a child has had several bad experiences with strange adults, for example, or was taught by the parents that strangers are dangerous and that he or she must not talk to strangers, the child also may develop a shy demeanor.

Asendorpf (1994) found that children's IQ and social competence were related to decreases in observed shyness and teacher-reported shyness between the ages of 4 and 10 years. Although IQ is not a direct measure of effortful control, the link could mean that effortful coping can influence shyness over time. Asendorpf (1993) also followed two groups of children, those who had shown early shyness and those who developed shyness while in school. Children in the latter group, who had developed shyness while in school, were more likely to show low self-esteem in adolescence than were the temperamentally shy children. We do not know the extent to which these observations are specific to Germany, where Asendorpf carried out his research, in that temperamental shyness is seen more positively in Northern Europe than in North America (Kerr, 2001). In the next section, I consider views of shyness that differ in different cultures. Shyness appears to be influenced by the value placed on it by the culture, and also by the culture's gender roles. Here I discuss culture as defined by the person's country of origin, but there are many other ways to study culture, as in the cultures of families, organizations, gangs, and academic departments.

In North America, people who are shy tend to be judged as less talented (Jones, Cavert, & Indart, 1983), less physically attractive (Jones & Carpenter, 1986), less friendly, less likable, and less poised than nonshy people (see review by Kerr, 2001). Kerr (2001) suggests that these findings reflect a culturally shared negative evaluation of shyness in North America. I have also noted above that shyness is associated with ratings of difficulty in Italy (Super et al., 2009). In other cultures such as China, however, shyness or reserve was, at least up to the 1990s, positively valued. Research on children in Canada looked at the popularity of shy children in two cultures. Preschool-age children who were shy and reserved were more popular among Chinese Canadian children, whereas non-Chinese shy children were *less* popular and more often rejected by non-Chinese Canadian children (Chen, Rubin, & Sun, 1992; Rubin, Chen, & Hymel, 1993).

In the home, Chinese mothers also seemed to place a higher value on shyness and reserve than non-Chinese mothers (Chen, Rubin, & Li, 1995). When Chinese children were more shy and inhibited, their mothers reported having more warm and accepting attitudes toward them; when non-Chinese children were more shy and inhibited, their mothers expressed less warmth and acceptance of them. In the United States, shy children tend to have a low estimation of their own social skills and are more prone to depression and loneliness than less shy children (Boivin, Hymel, & Bukowski, 1995);

shyness in Chinese children, on the other hand, is related to more positive feelings about the self (Chen, He, & Li, 2004). Since the early 1990s, however, shyness may have become more devalued in China. Chen, Cen, Li, and He (2005) found a lowered evaluation of shy behavior in Chinese elementary schools; this evaluation was linked to lower peer acceptance. Chen et al. (2005) point to economic and political change in China as promoting more assertive and less reserved individual behavior.

In some of our earliest work with the CBQ (Ahadi et al., 1993), we looked at the factor structure of temperament in China and the United States, finding considerable similarities in structure. The only major difference was a contribution of the smiling and laughter scale to the effortful control factor in the United States and a Japanese sample, and to the (expected) surgency factor in China. We have also found that U.S. children higher in effortful control showed more smiling when they receive an unwelcome gift, that is, one they had previously rated as undesirable (Kieras, Tobin, Graziano, & Rothbart, 2005). Thus, there may be a link between socialized smiling and effortful control in cultures where the expression of positive emotion is encouraged.

Overall, Chinese children showed more negative emotion than children in the United States. We also found that children higher on effortful control in the United States scored lower on negative emotionality, whereas there was no relation between negative emotionality and effortful control in the Chinese sample (Ahadi et al., 1993). Children high in effortful control in China, however, tended to be lower in surgency and thus higher in shyness. There was no relation between effortful control and surgency in the United States. These findings fit with the idea that the structure of temperament is similar across cultures, but that effortful control may be used to strengthen those behaviors that are more valued by the culture and to weaken behaviors that are devalued.

Cultural approval or disapproval of shyness has also varied depending on whether the child is a girl or a boy. In Great Britain, Stevenson-Hinde and her colleagues found that mothers were more positive about shyness in their girls and less positive about shyness in their boys (Stevenson-Hinde, 1989; Stevenson-Hinde & Hinde, 1986). Mothers' attitudes were particularly negative toward older boys who were shy (Stevenson-Hinde & Shouldice, 1993), suggesting that shyness becomes even less acceptable in boys as they grow older. Stevenson-Hinde and Hinde (1986) also found that shy girls tended to show better adjustment than nonshy girls, whereas shyness was related to poor adjustment in boys.

Culture and gender are also related to adult shyness. In the United States, when shy boys grow up they tend to marry later than do nonshy boys (Caspi, Elder, & Bem, 1988). Very shy boys also become parents later and establish a career later than nonshy boys. Very shy girls, on the other hand, marry at about the same time as nonshy girls, but are less likely to develop a career and more likely to give up their career when they marry or have a child (Caspi et al., 1988). We need to be wary of applying this finding today, however, because of recent historical change in gender roles in the United States.

Swedish adults show some interesting differences from adults who have grown up in North America. In Sweden, shyness is not seen as a negative quality and shyness does not seem to be used in employment decisions (Kerr, 2001). In Sweden, shy boys pursue careers just as early as nonshy boys, although they still tend to marry later and to have children 3–4 years later, in a pattern similar to that of the United States (Kerr, Lambert, & Bem, 1996). Swedish women, however, are generally not as encouraged to pursue careers in academia, and shy Swedish women are much less likely to earn a university degree than nonshy women. Both shy and nonshy girls marry at about the same time in both cultures.

Cultural research thus suggests differences across cultures and over historical time in the value of shyness. With an understanding of the structure of temperament, we can better view the contributions of culture, even if cultural values change over time. There is also a reciprocal influence: With knowledge of cultural influences, our understanding of the development of personality is enhanced. The biological equipment that constitutes temperament appears to be similar across cultures, even though the cultural standards, expectations, and narratives about the self, the world, and others will vary from culture to culture.

By the time children become well-socialized members of society, their biologically based temperament will have been shaped through repeated interchanges with members of the culture and repeated exposure to the media, including books and television, into a set of habits, values, goals, and representations of the self. Children will also develop a view of what is good and what is bad as influenced by temperament, the views of significant others, and the culture. Even for those children who have not been well socialized as members of the larger community, the values of smaller face-to-face groups are likely to have an effect. Children in delinquent peer groups, for example, try to excel in behavior valued by that group, even when those values are not socially acceptable ones for the wider culture (Dishion & Patterson, 2006).

Finally, globalization and worldwide media production allow cultural practices to be transformed or hybridized through the rapid influence of one culture on another, giving opportunities for a wide variety of personality outcomes. Hermans and Kempen (1998) noted: "Such multiple identities as Mexican schoolgirls dressed in Greek togas dancing in the style of Isadora Duncan, a London boy of Asian origin playing for a local Bengali cricket team and at the same time supporting the Arsenal football club, Thai boxing by Moroccan girls in Amsterdam, and Native Americans celebrating Mardi Gras in the United States" (p. 1113).

Culture has its effects on the individual, and multiple cultures from very different geographic locations can thus influence how people see themselves and others. This situation also allows for a much greater range of "niche picking" for the person in search of a better temperament–culture match. My own identity has been positively broadened through my husband's Jewish heritage, the great richness of my international colleagues' lives and work, and most recently, through the study of the Hindu philosophy of Vedanta.

SUMMARY

This chapter has considered the adaptations a child makes to the wider world of childhood, specifying some of the contributions of culture to this development. Several kinds of coping patterns have been identified, including avoidant coping, distraction, support seeking, and active coping. Studies of temperament and coping have linked negative emotionality to the avoidant strategies, positive emotionality to active coping, and attention regulation to the active coping strategies that are seen as the most adaptive in our culture. The effectiveness of a coping strategy, however, will depend on the amount of control the child can reasonably have over their own behavior and the events he or she experiences. I also considered culture as a vital influence on personality. Temperament structure appears to be similar in different cultures, but cultural meanings, practices, and artifacts can influence a wide variety of personality outcomes. I considered in detail the quality of shyness; the value of shyness differs across cultures and often differs between boys and girls. A child's temperament qualities thus may or may not be adapted to cultural expectations, and the resolution of culture–temperament mismatches may have long-term consequences. In this chapter, I have considered some of the ways culture and temperament can interact. In Chapter 7, I focus on temperament's influence on the development of conscience, competence, and learning within cultures.

CHAPTER 7

Conscience and Competence

As part of a program for the parents of infants and young children, Birth To Three parents are asked to pack an imaginary suitcase. In it, they are to include all the things they hope their child will carry with them when they grow up and leave home. Parents often hope that their children will be carrying the qualities of caring, compassion, and kindness. They also hope their children will be able to develop skills for work, contribute to society, and thrive in their relationships with others. Love and work, the focus of these parental wishes, were seen by Freud as the cornerstones of our humanity, and these are the topic of this chapter. In this chapter, I consider how temperament contributes to the development of conscience and the skills of life.

DEVELOPMENT OF THE MORAL EMOTIONS AND CONSCIENCE

The ancient Greek philosophers, including Plato and Aristotle, argued that living a virtuous life gives a person a special kind of happiness (Homiak, 2007). This moral happiness is not passively received pleasure, as when people are given what they desire; instead, it is the product of moral choice and action. In Plato's *Republic*, a moral education was seen to prepare a young person to make right choices and actions. Aristotle argued that developing the ability to think, choose, and act in a moral way gives a person both self-

162

regard and enjoyment. "He comes to like his life and himself and becomes a real self-lover" (Homiak, 2007, p. 2.4). Those who do not engage in moral choice and action, however, love themselves only, "in the sense that they love material goods and advantages. They desire to secure these things even at the expense of other people" (p. 2.4).

Later Western philosophers like Kant and Hume adopted a more rule-based view of conscience, stressing the moral value of laws, duties, and obligations rather than the positive moral virtues identified by the ancients. More recently, however, moral philosophers (e.g., Anscombe, 1958) have once again emphasized how everyday choices allow a person to live a moral life. This trend in moral philosophy is in keeping with developmental psychologists' study of *prosocial* motives and behavior (Eisenberg, Fabes, & Spinrad, 2006). It is also in keeping with the recent development of a "positive psychology" (Seligman & Csikszentmihalyi, 2000). Positive psychology goes beyond the study of problems between people to include the study of interpersonal skills, forgiveness, the capacity to love, and the civic virtues, including tolerance, nurturance, civility, responsibility, and the work ethic. This list is familiar from the contents of Birth To Three parents' suitcases for their children.

How do children learn to be good? How do they learn to make the right choices? Taking a temperament point of view, some children will have certain kinds of moral learning, like the development of conscience, come easier than will others. Because the development of empathy and conscience contributes so much to our society, it is important to recognize that children who differ in temperament may take different developmental paths, or trajectories, to achieve them (Kochanska, 1995).

Although some theorists believe that understanding and following rules is the prerequisite to higher levels of morality (e.g., Kohlberg, 1969), the signs of prosocial and caring action are actually seen well before the development of the body self, extended language, or the learning of rules. As early as 12–18 months of age, children show positive concern and give help in response to others' distress (Zahn-Waxler, Radke-Yarrow, Wagner, & Chapman, 1992). These reactions have been found in young children's behavior toward siblings, peers, and strangers (see review by Eisenberg, Spinrad, & Sadovsky, 2006).

Caring behavior is also seen in other animals, including the great apes (Preston & de Waal, 2002). Chimpanzees can be seen to console individuals who have been hurt in a fight with another animal, and to "make up" or reconcile after a conflict (de Waal, 2001). Zahn-Waxler et al. (1992) observed that not only did young children show concern about the distress or hurt of someone in the family, but that the family dog would sometimes come to the distressed person, hovering over them or putting its head onto the distressed person's lap. In the ancient world, "healing dogs" were employed with the sick (Meier, 1989), and the contributions of pets to adults' mental and physical health have also been demonstrated (e.g., Banks & Banks, 2002; Friedman, Katcher, Lynch, & Thomas, 1980).

EMPATHY

One important contributor to caring behavior is empathy, previously discussed as part of the temperament dimension of affiliativeness. People high in affiliative tendencies care about others and their welfare; they are concerned about what happens to others. These concerns provide a basis for empathy and action toward helping others. Empathy itself is closely related to compassion, that is, the awareness of the suffering of others and the desire to alleviate that suffering.

Empathy can be observed at several levels. At its simplest level, empathy occurs when an observer experiences the same emotion as the person they are observing. In a more sophisticated form, empathy involves concern for others combined with attempts to make the other person feel better that go far beyond a simple matching of emotion. When one of our sons was very small, he would try to rub away signs of distress in my face by smoothing out the wrinkles in my forehead. Children may bring a favorite toy to the person who is upset, for example, offering a stuffed bear or doll to an adult in distress. The child may also offer help, or kiss the spot that has been hurt, as his or her caregiver has done when the child was injured (Radke-Yarrow & Zahn-Waxler, 1984).

There is evidence of matching or contagious effects of distress in newborn infants. When one infant in the newborn nursery cries, there is a spread of distress so that soon, other infants will also be crying (Sagi & Hoffman, 1976). Martin Hoffman's (1979) theory of moral development begins with the observation of this contagious reaction, which he calls "global empathy." The word *global* here means that infants do not yet differentiate themselves from others; distress spreads as an automatic reaction. These and later contagious processes of emotion may involve the activity of "mirror neurons," where one person's behavior leads to a matching activation of brain circuits in the person observing that behavior (Decety & Jackson, 2004; Gallese, 2001).

Over the second year of life, the child is becoming able to differentiate between feelings of the self and feelings of the other, and to be more appropriate in what he or she offers to ease the discomfort of others (Hoffman, 1979, 2000). By the age of 2, children are using emotion words as well. A more complete cognitive understanding of others' feelings, however, does not appear to develop until about the age of 4 (Baron-Cohen, Tager-Flusberg, & Cohen, 2000). At this age, children can perform tasks indicating an understanding of other minds, and can express beliefs about the beliefs and mental states of others. Theory of mind itself, however, is linked to self-regulatory temperament (Carlson & Moses, 2001).

Parents often encourage their children to learn empathy, caring, and compassion. For example, children's empathic distress is used by parents to stop the child from causing harm to others (Hoffman, 2000) in a process called "inductive reasoning." Here, parents explain why the child should not be doing things that could cause harm or hurt to others, using questions like "How would you feel if Max did that to you?" Inductive reasoning can serve to call up the child's own distress and match it to the other child's potential upset. This allows children to anticipate others' distress prior to their own performance of a possibly hurtful act, and to inhibit that act. If parents use more directly punitive measures, however, children may become more concerned about avoiding the parents' detection of the prohibited act than inhibiting the hurtful action. Induction can also generalize across settings as children show an internalized tendency to control their own actions. Ultimately, it can lead to the application of the "Golden Rule," treating others as one would wish to be treated.

With development of the self-construct, two other moral emotions appear: guilt and shame, which can be seen as aspects of personality due to their connection with the self concept. In guilt, the child recognizes that he or she has done something that is not allowed or seen as wrong, resulting in feelings of distress and self-blame. These feelings can lead to confession and acts to undo the effects of the previous action, as well as inhibiting the act in the future. When a child ruminates about a guilty act, the child may also become caught up in negative thoughts and feelings about what he or she had done.

Shame, a close relative of guilt, refers to the feeling that the self is bad, unworthy of the approval of others or one's own self-approval. Shame is similar to guilt in that it involves negative emotions, but it also comes with a judgment that the whole child is unworthy. Feelings of shame can result from parents' and others' rejection of the child. Shame is a social emotion, and clinicians have sometimes linked it to the child's reaction to the rejecting face of the caregiver. A child feels shamed when he or she feels that others think badly about the self; the child judges the self through the eyes of others and finds him- or herself wanting. The threat of shame to the family due to the wrongdoing of a member is used in some cultures to develop internalized control in the child (Benedict, 1947). If children believe their improper acts will bring shame and suffering onto members of the family, they will have strong reasons to avoid these actions.

Fear and Empathy; Extraversion and Prosocial Behavior

In our longitudinal study of temperament, children who were more fearful in the laboratory during the first year of life also were reported by their parents at age 7 to be higher in empathy, guilt, and shame (Rothbart, Ahadi, & Hershey, 2004). Our measure of empathy involved chiefly the tendency to "feel with" others. Other researchers, however, have reported that children who are high in negative emotion are more likely to feel personal distress to others' distress, and may make relieving their own distress a priority over giving help to others (see review in Eisenberg et al., 2006). Children higher on temperamental extraversion, on the other hand, were more likely to *act* prosocially.

These studies, reviewed by Eisenberg et al. (2006), most often involved children's prosocial action in a laboratory or a school situation. Here, fearfulness would be related to the child's feeling distress in response to others' distress, but the child's fear would also tend to inhibit action, including prosocial action. In this way, the more fearful child may feel a desire to help, but be inhibited from doing so when in a fear-producing situation. If the event occurred in a familiar and safe situation such as the home, with the person hurt also being familiar, fearful children may be better able to help. We would thus expect differences across situations in more fearful children's prosocial action.

If more surgent tendencies contribute to actively helping others, even in novel or threatening settings, can a more surgent child who is also not very sensitive to negative emotion come to behave in an empathetic way? In this case, the child needs to *learn* cognitively which situations require which kinds of behavior, such as commiserating when a person has been hurt, or asking other people how they are feeling and whether they need help. This kind of training may be more likely to occur for girls, who are especially encouraged to develop empathic skills, and who display greater empathy than boys (Hoffman, 1975). One way to think about cognitive influences on empathy is that, just as there are a number of methods for teaching a child to read, there are also a number of methods for training empathy. One method (induction) makes use of the child's own feelings; another uses knowledge and practice to train prosocial action. The first approach may be the easiest, because it takes advantage of children's emotional dispositions.

When fear inhibits action, however, it may lead to an inhibition of helping or to strategies for protecting the self from experiencing the distress of others. The cognitive approach for instructing emotionally less sensitive children depends more on the use of language. Children who make a priority of reducing their own distress might also be taught strategies to subvert their own fearful inhibition while encouraging helping others.

Can all children be taught empathy? An extreme lack of empathy is seen when caring about others is low to nonexistent, and where deficiencies in fear lead to difficulties in perceiving another's hurt. Psychopathy, a mental disorder involving uncaring, aggressive, and antisocial behavior includes a core trait called *callous–unemotional* (Frick et al., 2003). This trait involves tendencies to manipulate others and to lack empathy, anxiety, and guilt. The callous–unemotional trait can be measured in childhood and is related to children's deficiencies in becoming distressed by effects of their hurtful behavior on others (Pardini, Lochman, & Frick, 2003).

Children who are high on the callous–unemotional trait also are low on fearfulness, and psychopathic adults also show low levels of fear (Glenn, Raine, Venables, & Mednick, 2007). Children and adolescents high in callous–unemotional characteristics also show reduced amygdala activation to pictures of fear expressions (Marsh et al., 2008), suggesting an insensitivity to signs of hurt in others. Callous–unemotional children show strong tendencies to engage in aggressive and antisocial behavior (Frick & Dickens, 2006), and appear to be highly resistant to the effects of parenting in correcting these tendencies (Wooten, Frick, Shelton, & Silverthorn, 1997).

For children who were described by parents and teachers as low on the callous–unemotional scale, more positive parenting was related to fewer conduct problems (Wooten et al., 1997). Children high on the callous–unemotional scale, however, were high on conduct problems whether parenting was positive or not. This pattern was replicated by O'Connor and Dvorak (2001) in a community sample, and by Oxford, Cavell, and Hughes (2003). We need more research, however, on how the callous–unemotional trait develops and its sensitivity to intervention.

Effortful Control and Empathy

Effortful control makes important contributions to the experience and expression of empathy. In a study of children's empathy toward a child depicted in a film, effortful control was related to children's expressions of concern and sadness when a child was shown being hurt, as well as their feelings of sympathy for the hurt child (Guthrie et al., 1997). Children lower in effortful control showed more signs of anxiety and tension during the film. High effortful control was also related to parents' reports of empathy and sympathy in their children (see review by Eisenberg, Smith, Sadovsky, & Spinrad, 2004). Effortful control gives the flexibility of attention that allows the child to shift from focusing on the self to focusing on the other, moving beyond contagious personal distress to understanding the state and needs of the other person. Thus, when sensitivity to the negative emotions is combined with temperamental effortful control, both empathy and prosocial behavior are likely to be promoted. Effortful control can also be used to regulate negative emotion, bringing it down to a level where directing attention to the other person is possible.

Effortful control is also related to peers' ratings of children's prosocial behavior and to preschool teachers' ratings of children's agreeableness, including their sharing, helping, and being nice (Eisenberg et al., 2004). Children at age 3 who showed high negative emotionality and low self-regulation were seen by parents and teachers as being less friendly, caring, helpful, cooperative, popular, and well behaved. In adolescence, these children were seen as lower in maturity, interest, enthusiasm, persistence, creativity, sense of humor, and activity (Caspi, Henry, McGee, Moffitt, & Silva, 1995). Belsky, Friedman, and Hsieh (2001) found that children's negative emotionality at 15 months predicted lower social competence at age 3; but only when the children showed lower attentional persistence—a component of effortful control. High effortful control also predicts high social functioning for school-age children, and does so more strongly for children who are high in emotional intensity (Eisenberg et al., 1997).

CONSCIENCE

In the 1990s, Kochanska (1993, 1995) began an important program of research that has greatly increased our understanding of conscience, temperament, and social development. Based on her theoretical reviews, Kochanska posited that temperamental fear and effortful control, the two major temperament control systems of early development (Rothbart, 1989b), would both contribute to the development of conscience. How might fear come to support conscience? Kochanska (1995) cited the work of Hoffman (1983) and Dienstbier (1984) on how children come to internalize standards. Their models describe how children learn to control their own behavior and to follow rules, even when no rule giver or enforcer is present. When more fearful children associate an upcoming act with likely punishment (including parent disapproval), they will inhibit the expression of that behavior. Even when a likely punisher is not present, the threat of punishment will be felt as though it had come from within the self. Thus, fearfulness can support the development of conscience. As in the case of empathy, however, the child must not become too fearful. If the child's distress is too great, any moral action will be linked to feelings of pressure from sources outside the child, so that feelings of being coerced will result. Thus harsh, authoritarian parenting might be too much for the more fearful child, whereas more gentle inductive reasoning may be effective in conditioning moral behavior, along with the child's perception that it is internally caused. In fact, the combination of fear and gentle parenting was found to be most effective in promoting conscience (Kochanska, 1995).

In Kochanska's research, children's fearfulness and their mother's control styles were found to work together in the child's development of conscience (Kochanska, 1997; Kochanska, Aksan, & Joy, 2007). The temperament trait of fearfulness predicted children's moral behavior in the laboratory at 2 and 3 years, and also predicted maturity of moral reasoning at ages 4 and 5. Conscience was measured in the child's following rules, complying with requests, refusing to cheat at games, and using more mature moral reasoning. Studies from laboratories other than Kochanska's have also found higher levels of conscience and greater emotions of guilt, shame, and empathy in more fearful or shy children (Asendorpf & Nunner-Winkler, 1992; Rothbart, Ahadi, et al., 1994). Fearful children's conscience is further predicted by mothers' use of gentle, non-power-oriented discipline, which can serve to keep the children's fear of punishment within tolerable limits. Kochanska and her colleagues also found that nonfearful children appeared to follow a different pathway to conscience, linked to a positive, goal-oriented partnership between parent and child. This can involve parents telling the child what to *do* rather what not to do. These findings have been recently replicated by Kochanska et al. (2007).

Social psychology also contributes to models of the development of conscience. One interesting finding from this research is that offering weaker external reasons for an act often has a stronger influence on behavior than offering stronger external reasons for the act (e.g., Greene & Lepper, 1974). Even in the preschool years, children appear to think about why they have acted in a particular way. If they view their action as occurring because of some outside reward or punishment, they are less likely to think they "wanted" to do it. Offering rewards for children to do what they otherwise would have done by preference also results in their diminished interest in the activity (Greene & Lepper). Thus, the parent needs to be careful about providing too much external justification (e.g., punishment) for the child's action, especially when the child is sensitive to negative emotion. We would also expect surgent children, more sensitive to reward, to be more influenced by external rewards. It is interesting, however, that our more surgent older child was especially sensitive to the idea that he was being "bribed" to do something; he would much rather do it for internally generated reasons. Other children accept bribes with pleasure, and may come to expect them.

The conscience associated with fear is built on a response to threat; in empathy, that threat comes from the possibility of hurting another person. Once effortful control becomes available, however, more neutral and nonemotional control is possible. Fear is a less powerful predictor of conscience in older children, and increasingly, effortful control comes to predict stronger conscience. High effortful control also predicts greater empathy and prosocial behavior (Eisenberg et al., 2004), as well as lower aggression. Kochanska et al. (1993) also found that high effortful control and low impulsivity in girls was related to their greater discomfort to wrongdoing.

There is also some evidence that fear provides an early basis for the development of effortful control. Aksan and Kochanska (2004) found that children who were more fearful as infants and toddlers were more likely to show high effortful control during the preschool years. Kochanska suggests that because fear is associated with the inhibition of action, fearfulness may give the child the time needed to develop planfulness and effortful control. Fear may also provide the motivation for being good and following rules, and the fearful child may also especially want to please the parent. Effortful control in turn will facilitate the child's following the rules.

Overall, Kochanska, Tjelokes, and Forman (1998) have found that children's effortful control is a powerful predictor of children's conscience that becomes increasingly important with age. Effortful control and executive attention include a number of qualities that promote moral education. The first is the ability to inhibit forbidden action and to activate appropriate action. The second is the ability to plan ahead. The third is the ability to detect errors, related to children's sensitivity to having done something wrong. Effortful control also allows flexibility in problem solving, so that the child can consider and choose among different ways of avoiding or dealing with moral infractions. These could include confessing wrongdoing or making plans to avoid the behavior in the future.

Although these examples all stress the child's ability to inhibit actions, effortful control also includes the ability to plan and to activate positive behavior, via activational control (Kieras, Tobin, Graziano, & Rothbart, 2005). There is thus an important difference between inhibitory control and effortful control, with the latter including attentional, inhibitory, *and* activational control. Finally, flexible attentional control is important in the development of empathy, allowing the person to shift attention from one's own feelings of distress to the other, being able to evaluate the outcome of one's own behavior toward the other and its meaning to the self.

Aksan and Kochanska (2005) have recently developed a structural model for the development of conscience in children. They analyzed behavioral measures of conscience in 33- and 45-month-old children and identified two factors. The first involves *moral emotion*, including guilt and empathic distress; the second is *rule-compatible conduct*, in which the child complies with the mother's and experimenter's rules. Children were highly stable on these measures from 33 to 45 months of age. Correlations between moral emotion and rule-compatible conduct were also higher at 45 months, suggesting that there is increasing coherence among measures of conscience and stronger links to effortful control as children develop. Moral emotion will be seen earlier than rule-compatible conduct, and one child may find it easier to develop conscience using the moral emotions and another by following the rules, using cognitive guides to action and feeling.

How might a child also come to moral feeling by following rules? I have already considered how the child who lacks sensitivity to others' feelings may nevertheless learn how to act in empathy-related situations. In fact, a very interesting aspect of children's socialization is "learning how to feel" in different situations and toward different people (Saarni, Mumme, & Campos, 1998). There are potential problems with this approach, however, when there is conflict between the child's authentic feelings and what he or she is instructed to feel. We might also expect that when the child is encouraged to do helpful acts, he or she will be reinforced by the positive feelings that occur when one "does good".

Personality Structure and Moral Development

Morality itself is a complex phenomenon. The human conscience sometimes can be characterized as an inner social order including a number of sources of moral judgment. There is, for example, an inner policeman warning of probable transgression and punishment if you behave badly, and an inner prosecutor and judge who set the scene for self-punishment and feelings of guilt. Meanwhile, an inner defender works to cognitively reframe the situation so that both the police arrests and judge's verdicts are directed against someone else rather than the self. How might such a complex moral structure be internalized? Kohlberg (1969) cites George Herbert Mead (1934) describing the child at play:

> The child plays that he is offering himself something, and he buys it; he gives himself a letter and takes it away, he addresses himself as a parent, as a teacher; he arrests himself as a policeman. He has a set of stimuli which call out in himself the sort of responses they call out in others. A certain organized structure arises in him and his other which replies to it, and these carry the conversation of gestures between themselves. (Mead, 1934, pp. 150–151)

Kohlberg (1969), unlike other developmental psychologists of the time, felt that identification was an important concept. He argued that as the child takes on the roles of others, he or she develops higher levels of thinking about morality. Just as the child is developing a concept of self describing who he or she is, what he or she does, and what he or she is like (Damon & Hart, 1982), the child is also mentally and often physically acting out the roles of internalized others: who they are, what they do, and what they are like; and these roles become consolidated within the child's self-structure. In a complex society like ours, there may be many internalized self-structures with varying degrees of communication with each other. In a colloquium at Oregon many years ago, Daniel Kahneman talked about the multiple rabbis within the mind, each offering a different counsel; we can in this way feel at several minds about an issue. All our internal roles are structures of meaning, but they may or may not be integrated within the person. One of the challenges facing the person on a road to maturity is developing integration and coherence of the self.

Summary

The development of the person's empathy and conscience is a major goal of a well-functioning society. Empathic morality is seen in other animals and is observed in human development well before the child has developed rule-based cognitions. Early conscience is related to the moral emotions of fear, guilt, and empathy, the internalizing negative emotions. Because children differ in their sensitivities to these emotions, some children will "learn" conscience earlier and in a somewhat different way than others. Conscience will eventually involve increasing layers of learning and influence on the child's behavior, including rule following, the exercise of internal judges, and an understanding of why the self (and others) do what they do (Pfaff, 2007). This analysis goes beyond the scope of this book, but it will be important in the future to study how these layers of meaning and understanding are related to each other as the child develops.

DEVELOPMENT OF COMPETENCE AND MOTIVATION

I now turn to the second large item in the child's suitcase, the child's development of competence and achievement in school and society. Competence refers to abilities that support effective performance. Competence is usually not a general quality: We may be relatively competent in one area (e.g., school achievement), but less competent in others (e.g., developing and maintaining friendships or gaining and holding power). How are competence and temperament related to each other? One way is through the influence of temperament on what we practice doing and on how long and how intensely we practice.

Just watching an expert is exciting: an athlete, a physician, a plasterer, a professor, a short-order cook. It always gives me joy to see someone who is good at what he or she does. Becoming an expert, however, requires practice (Posner & Rothbart, 2007b). Herbert Simon argued that to become a chess master, for example, about 50,000 hours of practice are required. When a person has become an expert in an area, he or she has stored a large body of accessible memories on the subject. These memories often include the relations among items, more specific item information, and motor skill knowledge. Practice is needed for the development of most competencies and for practice to occur, motivation for practice is needed. Several temperamental dispositions influence the development of children's practice in developing competencies and expertise.

Temperament provides building blocks for the development of motivations toward mastery, competence, and expertise. When we are positively motivated to engage in an activity, we take pleasure in what we are doing. When our motivation for action is related to fear of punishment for not doing well, on the other hand, we may feel anxious and driven by internal or external forces to perform. In the development of skills and knowledge, as in the development of empathy, there are different paths to competence. Some children will be more inclined to practice and may find a given accomplishment easier to achieve than others, who may become discouraged in the effort. Other children will work chiefly to please their parents and others. Although children differ in their initial approaches to practice depending on temperament, we all have the potential for the joy that comes from improving thought and action.

Many competencies are developed through schooling, and there has been an increasing awareness of how temperament-related qualities prepare the child for success in school. Hyson (2008) cites the National Education Goals Report on what constitutes the child's aptness for learning: "(1) Openness to and curiosity about new tasks and challenges; (2) initiative, task persistence, and attentiveness; (3) approach to reflection and interpretation; (4) capacity for invention and imagination; and (5) cognitive approaches to tasks" (Kagan, Moore, & Bredekamp, 1995, p. 23). Children's positive and approaching tendencies can contribute toward "children's *enthusiasm*—their interest, pleasure, and motivation to learn—and their *engagement*—their attention, persistence, flexibility, and self-regulation" (Hyson, 2008, p. 45). Although these goals show an emphasis on the positive, we also know that many schools depend on fear as a goad to children's learning.

Openness to events and information is also very important to learning. Any child has the capacity to approach tasks with openness, and it is easy to see the openness of infants and young children. Nevertheless children can also be put into a threatened, defensive, or discouraged position. Indeed, even a child who is positive at the beginning of an undertaking has the potential to be put under threat before it is completed. Harter (1998) found that as children grow older, they become less motivated by intrinsic interest and more motivated by the desire to give the teacher what he or she wants. If parents and teachers want high performance on tests, the child may become more concerned about achieving high test performance than in pursuing learning or mastery goals. When children pursue *learning* goals, they tend to believe that through persistent effort, success is possible (Dweck, 2000). Other children may believe that their performance is chiefly a reflection of their innate ability, so that any lack in performance will reflect badly on the self. This belief directs the child toward achieving *mastery* goals, and may put children into a defensive stance, where they try to protect the idea that they *are* truly able. They may also try to devalue skills they do not appear to possess.

The idea that personal effort can lead to success supports a more open and self-regulated stance for the child. Dweck (2008) has developed a program based on what we have learned about the plasticity of the brain ("Brainology") to encourage middle school children to think about how they can change their own brain's structure through effort and practice. This approach allows children greater control over what they practice and removes the stigma of early failure, changing it to an opportunity to shape the brain. This approach is in keeping with the idea that mistakes provide information that can be used toward future competence. Overall, the program emphasizes learning goals rather than self-protection goals in thinking about one's own learning. In preliminary evaluations, the program has shown positive effects in the classroom (Dweck, 2008).

Effectance Motivation

We now consider how the emotions and related motivations can support or undermine learning, and note that although effortful control is not linked to specific motivations, it can be applied in the service of a wide variety of emotions, goals, and motivations. Effortful control allows the activation and inhibition of action, the control of emotion, planning for goals and outcomes, and persistence in thought and action. All of these skills support the development of competence. In general, greater effortful control is related to positive outcomes and to the development of competencies. When the person takes a more protected or defensive stance, however, effortful control can also be directed toward limiting the child's or adult's experiences. A fearful person, for example, may live a highly organized and protected life to avoid threat. Effortful control can provide the means for this organization, even though the result of the controlled life is a general limitation of experience.

White (1959, 1963) identified *effectance motivation* as a disposition to actively engage the environment with the purpose of influencing it. When White first proposed effectance as a motive, most psychologists viewed motivation as the result of rewards and punishments, based on bodily needs like hunger and thirst or the avoidance of threat. White (1959) pointed out that nonhuman animals show effectance motivation, as when rhesus monkeys will do work in order to have access to interesting and challenging environments (Butler, 1954, 1957). Infants and young children also clearly derive pleasure from manipulating materials and situations during play (Lillard, 2005). Even young infants will engage in play that does not require contingent rewards from others; there appears to be pleasure in acting itself. White (1963) saw children's play as evidence of mastery pursued for its own sake, not in the pursuit of social reinforcements and rewards.

Some competencies seem to be products of our own internal desires and wishes, as when the young infant works to sit up or roll over; these accomplishments are often associated with signs of pleasure (Rothbart, 1973). In the laboratory, even young infants reveal expressions of pleasure, fear, frustration/anger, and boredom as they interact with objects (Rothbart et al., 2000). The emotions children display are linked to their patterns of exploration of objects, and the emotions expressed in object exploration are in turn tied to individual differences in temperament. These act as primary motivations for early effectance or mastery motivation (Barrett & Morgan, 1995; White, 1959, 1963). Later in development, motivations may include attempts to please parents, teachers, or peers, to fit in or excel in a social setting, or to satisfy one's own self-related standards and goals. We have called these secondary motivations (Rothbart & Hwang, 2005).

Mastery Motivation

Mastery motivation, a similar concept to effectance motivation, was defined by Morgan and his associates as a "psychological force that stimulated an individual to attempt independently, in a focused and persistent manner, to solve a problem or master a skill or task that is moderately challenging to him or her" (Morgan, Harmon, & Maslin-Cole, 1990, p. 319). Messer (1995) pointed out that mastery motivation can be decomposed into the psychological processes that contribute to the selection, engagement, and sustained interest in an object or activity. Children differ in (1) their choices of objects or activities, (2) how readily they engage with them, and (3) how long they remain focused on the activity in the face of distractions. I now consider each of these processes.

Selection and Engagement in an Activity

Temperament contributes to our choice of activities, depending on our preferences for high- versus low-intensity situations and activities. Persons who are more easily overstimulated tend to choose activities lower in stimulation; those less easily stimulated may choose activities that involve higher-intensity stimulation (Strelau, 1983, 2008). Temperament also contributes to how rapidly we engage in an activity. In the laboratory, children high in smiling and laughter and surgency engaged with objects more rapidly and generally showed less caution with novel or exciting toys (Rothbart, 1988; Rothbart et al., 2000). In our studies of temperament in college students and adults, measures of surgency and orienting sensitivity were related to higher scores on the Big Five personality dimension of openness to experience (Evans & Rothbart, 2007). Temperament is thus related to openness to a wide range of ideas, experiences, and emotions. When a person takes on a defensive or threatened stance, however, the openness is likely to be shut down.

Overall, children high in surgency, low in fear, and low in effortful control may more readily launch into new situations or activities. This rapid approach is adaptive when the action is not a risky one. When the situation is risky, however, approach can lead to negative outcomes; the more surgent and fearless child may engage too rapidly. Strong fear and/or low surgency/extraversion are related to cautious behavior that is appropriate when danger is present, or to an overly inhibited approach when it is not. More fearful children in their choice of activities may also tend to avoid novel situations and experiences altogether, missing the opportunity for mastery. In Jack and Jeanne Block's theory of the developing personality, the rigid overregulation of impulses related to fear is called *overcontrol*, whereas the unconstrained release of impulses is called *undercontrol* (Block, 2002; Block & Block, 1980). Both extremes can lead to problems in adaptation but *resiliency*, related to effortful control, can allow children to flexibly switch from approach to caution or vice versa, as the situation requires.

During the preschool years, the potential for achieving effects and developing new competencies is greatly increased, as can be seen in a Montessori school (Lillard, 2005). By school age, children are motivated to make friends;

to protect themselves from outside threats, and to pursue competence in the schoolroom, where their grades and test scores give them a running account of their performance. In the classroom, a teacher can readily observe differences in how children approach school activities: "At the crafts table, for instance, she will see behavior ranging from picking things up quickly and using them firmly, through all grades of tentativeness and uncertainty, to hanging back or turning completely away" (White, 1963, pp. 74–75).

Persistence

Persistence is probably the most frequently studied aspect of children's mastery motivation. How long will the child sustain interest in an object or activity? How long will the child repeat attempts at making an object "work"? Positive emotion is related to how long 2-year-olds sustain engagement in activities. Spangler (1989) found that when children showed positive emotion, either playing alone or with their mothers, they remained engaged in activities for longer periods. In our laboratory, we studied how long 13-month-old infants maintained attention toward a toy before pushing it away or discarding it. Infants who smiled more and whose mothers reported more general smiling and laughter sustained interest in toys for a longer period, whereas children who showed more distress sustained interest for a shorter time (Rothbart & Hwang, 2005). In a second study, infants' smiling was specifically related to their *active* involvement with objects, that is, to the amount of time infants spent manipulating toys while looking at them, but not to how long the child simply looked at toys without manipulating them (Rothbart & Hwang). Active involvement has been linked to infants' gaining information about an object; passive looking by itself is unrelated to increases in information (Ruff, 1986).

Positive mood is also related to mastery motivation and creative action in adults. Erez and Isen (2002) induced positive and neutral moods in adults, and found that those in a positive mood performed better on an anagrams task, showed greater persistence, and reported higher levels of motivation than those in the neutral condition. Participants in a positive mood condition also had greater expectations of success and evaluated the rewards they were offered for good performance more positively.

Interest, identified by Izard (1991) as a positive emotion, is reliably related to children's performance. This is seen in a meta-analysis of studies involving children in grades 5 through 12 (Schiefele, Krapp, & Winteler, 1992). The review included 121 studies performed in eight different countries. Interest was consistently related to children's achievement, and was more strongly related to achievement for boys than for girls. Another interpretation of these findings is possible, however. Interest may lead to achievement, but achievement may also lead to heightened interest, whereas failure may lead to decreased interest in an activity.

Problems in the relation of temperamental extraversion/surgency and achievement have also been identified. Shiner (2000) studied 8- to 12-year-olds who were seen again as teenagers and young adults. Extraversion at 8–12 years was related to children's academic achievement at the time, but when the children had reached high school and college their earlier extraversion predicted later *lower* achievement. Shiner suggests that the more social orientation of extraverted high school and college students may create conflict with the solitary activity that is often required for school achievement in high school and college.

Although young children often experience direct pleasure in mastery, older children may take other motivational paths toward action. They are influenced by their own self-evaluations, their views on how others evaluate their performance, their ego involvement in the task, their long-term goals, and their feelings of competence in a particular area (Harter, 1980). Persistence, discouragement, or defensive coping strategies are thus increasingly influenced by the child's views of the self. Whereas mastery motivation can be influenced by children's direct experience of success or failure, with development, children become strongly influenced by the goals and evaluations of others (Harter). These goals and evaluations can also be internalized.

If a basic tendency of the child is toward influencing the environment, how does it happen that so many children's feelings of efficacy and attempts at mastery appear to be so low? Freedom of movement contributes to children's feelings of efficacy, and parents and the physical setting may hinder efficacy by not allowing opportunities to play and to observe. Developing a more closed, defensive stance can also prevent the child from learning. As in other aspects of personality, a closed stance need not be widely applied; it may be related to a single task on a single occasion, as we see below. The great French author Simone de Beauvoir (1958) describes her childhood freedom to move about and follow her interests:

> At my aunt's, as at my grandfather's, I was allowed to run freely over the lawns and touch everything. Scratching at the earth, playing with lumps of clay, stroking leaves and flowers, polishing horse-chestnuts, popping seed pods, I was learning things that are never taught by books or official syllabuses. . . . Everywhere, in the green water of the ponds, in the waving grasses of the fields, under the thorny hedgerows and in the heart of the woods were hidden treasures that I longed to discover. (pp. 24–25)

Opposing this kind of approach and pleasure-related motivation, however, and sometimes suppressing approach are fear, frustration, and feelings of insecurity that are related to a more defensive and "closed" stance. As noted above, this stance need not be applied to situations generally; it may be related to a single event. De Beauvoir (1958) recalls a trip to the beach with friends of her family when she was 8 years old:

> It was the first time I had been away from my sister. . . . I found the sea boring; the baths filled me with horror; the water took my breath away. . . . The truth was that, separated from my family, deprived of those affections which assured me of my personal worth, cut off from the familiar routine which defined my place in the world, I no longer knew where I was, nor what my purpose was here on earth. I needed to be confined within a framework whose rigidity would justify my existence. . . . I was afraid of changes. (p. 62)

The two situations as experienced by de Beauvoir point up an opposition between open and defensive stances in other areas of adjustment. Cacioppo and Berntson (1994) have argued that there is a negativity bias in human functioning, so that when both positive and negative motivations are activated, the defensive system will prevail over the reward-related system. Their argument makes evolutionary sense: a threat may prove dangerous to life itself, and would thus require priority over pleasures. This position suggests that fear, anger, sadness, and discomfort, when activated, will prevail over approach, affiliation, and openness. In addition, threat, shame, guilt, humiliation, and negative self-judgment may prevail over the positive emotions and evaluations as the self-model develops.

Ito and Cacioppo (2005) have also noted temperamental differences in both a negativity and a positivity bias. When children are strongly criticized or pressed to achieve in the home or school, negative reactions to achievement may also develop, whatever the original temperament of the child. One coping strategy to deal with threats to the self is identification with others who seem to possess qualities of competence. These identifications can be with real people, celebrities, or with heroes and heroines of books, stories, movies, and television. Adults also make strong identifications with sports teams, nationalities, political movements, political figures, religions, and languages.

Fear and Mastery Motivation

Late in the first year, some infants demonstrate fear reactions that are seen in their inhibited approach to unfamiliar and intense stimuli (Kagan, 1994;

Rothbart, 1988; Schaffer, 1974). This inhibited reaction is predicted by the infant's crying and motor reactivity to stimulation at 4 months (Calkins et al., 1996; Kagan, 1994). Fear also controls other impulses. When fearful control occurs, there is likely to be an absence of approach, a more tentative approach, or actual avoidance of the object. This hesitancy can provide the time necessary to analyze a problem or plan the next step of action, but it can also lead to avoidance of possible failure and the rigid overcontrol of behavior (Block & Block, 1980; Kremen & Block, 1998). Anxiety reflected in enhanced attention to threats (Derryberry & Reed, 1994, 1996; Vasey, Daleiden, Williams, & Brown, 1995) can also lead to rumination on problems that in turn can lead to further inhibition. In Chapter 3 we discussed the neural basis for how initial fearfulness can, with traumatic experience, develop into more generalized anxiety.

Fear and Ego-Related Anxiety

Fearfulness is seen in young children's inhibition of approach toward new situations and challenges (Kagan, 1994, 1998). Once the child's concept of self develops, however, evaluations of the self can lead children with a wide range of temperamental endowments to become anxious about the possibility of failure, and/or to take a defensive stance and resist evidence that they have failed (cf. Ausubel, 1996; Ausubel, Sullivan, & Ives, 1980). A fearful temperament may strengthen these effects. Harter (1980), for example, reported signs of fearful children's decreased interest in challenging tasks and their behavioral withdrawal when they expected to be observed and evaluated by others.

By 2 years of age, there is increasing understanding of the self as a separate entity who can experience being in control of events, and Bronson (2000) notes the toddler's increasing awareness of the possibility of being in control. The 2-year-old often forcibly attempts to influence events, and resists being controlled by other people. Attempts to exercise control in a world that often does not allow it may become a lifelong enterprise (Adler, 1946). However, 2-year-olds have few self-regulatory skills and very little patience. When they are not allowed control, or their attempts to control are not met with success, they often respond with anger, crying, or temper tantrums (Kopp, 1992). White (1960) noted that when children's effectance motive is frustrated, children will attempt various coping measures. Viewing children's reaction to frustrations as a kind of coping gives us a somewhat different view of some of the behavior of toddlers: During this period, White wrote, the child's "stubbornness, parsimony, and orderliness are completely of a piece. They are ways of preventing oneself from being pushed around by the environment, [and happen] when there is a relative feeling of incompetence in relation to the environment, especially the human one" (p. 290). Control over one's own behavior will be developing during the preschool and school years, along with the executive attention system and developing capacities of effortful control.

Independent achievement is highly valued by adults in the United States. As children develop representations of themselves, they become more vulnerable to and anxious about not succeeding in valued areas (Harter, 1998). Children's temperamental susceptibility to fear can heighten these reactions, but all children are potentially vulnerable. Children whose feelings of self-worth are strongly linked to their individual performance, perhaps because they view their parents' love and acceptance as contingent on it, will be more anxious about failure than children whose positive image does not rely on pleasing others (Ausubel, 1996). Under the influence of socialization, even a temperamentally positive and approaching child can become vulnerable to anxiety about the possibility of failure, and react to a feeling of inferiority through actions that may seem to be its opposite, for example, arrogance and expressions of self-importance (Adler, 1946).

Goals valued by the parents, society, and eventually by the child (e.g., personal attractiveness, wealth, or individual achievement), become part of the self-image of the socialized child. Block (2002) views the self's goals and related gratifications and threats as *personality structures*. In Block's view, "personality structures are marshaled to give priority to avoidance of immediate threats to the viability of the individual. With that constraint, the system is further disposed also to gratify the individual and enhance long term viability" (p. 183). Block's reference to priority being given to immediate threats is similar to the conclusion of Cacioppo and Berntson about the dominance of negative reactions (1994).

Children with vulnerable concepts of self will be subject to frustration, defense, and depression when their positive self-evaluations are threatened (Harter, 1998). Individuals will also differ in the strength of their ego-related structures of meaning, including their self-concepts, goals, and identifications in others, and each of these structures creates opportunities for both reward and anxiety (Block, 2002). Self-knowledge and knowledge of others are closely linked: How we see others gives us a template for viewing ourselves, and how we see ourselves gives us a template for viewing others. Typically, valued qualities are seen to be more evident in the self and our friends than in others, and defense and protection of the self-image is likely to occur when information threatens the self or those with whom we identify (Leary, 2004).

One's self-image can provide the basis for intense persistence in an activity, but it can also lead to avoidance of achievement attempts, as when students maintain they do not care about an activity when failure in that area would threaten the self-image. The child may also derogate the threatening activity or view an outside person as being responsible for imposing it on him or her. These are two among many ways of avoiding bad news about the self (Leary, 2004). When circumstances do not allow the person to fend off bad news, as when a spouse dies or a partner leaves, there often results a painful need to reconstruct the model of the self and the self-image, and depression may result (Guidano, 1987). Again, these influences go far beyond temperament, but they allow us to see how later-developing evaluations can powerfully influence all of us, whatever our original temperament.

Effortful Control and Self-Regulation

If our actions were limited to temperamentally based approach, inhibition, and avoidance tendencies, we would be unable to approach the things that were feared or avoid the things that were rewarding. Nevertheless, it is possible to oppose our reactive tendencies. We (Posner & Rothbart, 1998, 2007b; Rothbart & Bates, 2006) have proposed that individual differences in effortful control, based on development of the executive attention system, provide the child with the self-regulation and flexibility needed for these events to occur. Effortful control gives us the capacity to approach the things we fear and avoid the actions we would otherwise find rewarding. Like the emotion systems, the attention networks of the human brain are the result of evolution. They allow us to access a wide range of information, to consciously select which information to focus on, and, depending on our goals, to control our own behavior and emotion.

Effortful control, as measured in scales of inhibitory and activational control, attentional focusing, perceptual sensitivity, and low-intensity pleasure, is related to laboratory assessments of the efficiency of the executive attention system in children and adults (Kanske, 2008; Rothbart & Rueda, 2005) and is also related to children's performance on problem-solving tasks (Rothbart et al., 2003). Children's performance on a tower-building task and a nesting cup-stacking task, both of which required involvement in the task, detection and correction of errors, as well as persistent action toward the goal, were related at 24-months to their mother's reports of higher effortful control. By the age of 30 months, children's performance was related to both high effortful control and low levels of impulsivity. Effortful control allows the child to inhibit immediate action, search for appropriate actions and opportunities, resist distractions, detect and correct errors, overcome obstacles, and continue working until the goal is achieved (Rothbart & Rueda). As these skills become practiced, becoming more automatic, they can be combined with other skills to make further goal-related competencies possible.

One notable aspect of effortful control is the ability to persist at a task. Bramlett, Scott, and Rowell (2000) used teacher ratings of children's persistence versus withdrawal and parent ratings of children's activity on the Temperament Assessment Battery (TAB; Martin, Drew, Gaddis, & Moseley, 1988) to predict children's academic competence. Children's temperament, particularly the trait of persistence, predicted their academic competence, and teacher ratings of temperament were better predictors of classroom behavior and academic status than were parent ratings.

Teachers also have well-developed ideas about the qualities of a teachable student (Keogh, 1989). These qualities include low activity and reactivity, high attention span, high approach, and adaptability. The teacher–child relationship is also related to how well the child's temperament characteristics match this list. Martin (1989) found that children who were distractible and low on attention span received more criticism from teachers. In a study by Pullis (1985), if teachers thought a child was capable of self-control but not practicing it, they were more likely to use punitive and coercive discipline with the child. Finally, Guerin et al. (2003) found that low levels of activity and distractibility and high levels of persistence and adaptability were related to children's learning, happiness, and appropriate behavior in class (Guerin et al., 2003).

One of the most interesting aspects of temperament and the school situation is that the school and classroom create a press for different temperament characteristics at different times of the day and different settings. When children are asked to move from one activity to another or to sit at their desks for long periods, they will be affected in ways that depend on their temperament. Including knowledge of temperament in education curricula (Rothbart & Jones, 1988) and considering the physical structure of the classroom (Keogh, 2003) for children are important issues to consider. Keogh's (2003) book, in particular, is a helpful source for teachers and school administrators who wish to match the individual child to their school experience.

Effortful control is also involved in the inhibition of immediate approach with the goal of a larger reward later, in what Block (2002) has called "hedonism of the future," and Mischel (Mischel, Shoda, & Rodriguez, 1989) has called "delay of gratification." It is also related to activational control, that is, to carrying out an action that is likely to lead to personal discomfort and would otherwise be avoided. This allows the person to act "on principle." In most cases, effortful control is not a basic motivation, but rather the means to accomplishing desired ends. It is similar to the attentional capacities underlying Block's construct of ego resiliency. Ego resiliency involves the flexible ability to shift levels of control depending on the situation. In Block's view, "the problem of psychological development is to move toward resiliency, or, less optimally, to find a life recess wherein resiliency is not seriously or continuously required" (p. 185).

Locus of Control

We can now relate temperament to an aspect of personality closely linked to achievement. Locus of control refers to a person's perception that outcomes are brought about through his or her own efforts, rather than as the result of chance or the actions of others (Rotter, 1966). Locus of control, like other personality constructs, develops out of interactions between children's dispositions and experience. What a person comes to believe about the controllability of outcomes depends in part on effortful control, the ability to carry out flexible and adaptive responses through the use of attention and self-regulation (see Declerck, Boone, & Brabander, 2006). Effortful control will allow for more quickly attained mastery, the production of desired outcomes, and hence will support the belief that one is in control. Thus, high levels of temperamental effortful control are likely to influence the development of locus of control perceptions.

The environment is also critically important in the development of perceptions of control. Some environments pose greater challenges and offer less support for children's self-regulation. For example, poverty conditions offer little support for the child's perception that he or she is a controller of outcomes. Parents and teachers may also discourage the child's autonomy by making their love and attention conditional (Assor, Roth, & Deci, 2004). Children's expectations about outcomes will be thus be based on both temperament and experience.

When the locus of control is viewed as internal, a child will be more likely to take on challenges that further promote mastery, creating positive cycles of engagement and learning. Thus, locus of control will be an outgrowth of basic temperamental processes in interaction with situations, but once developed, it can set into motion patterns of behavior that will influence ongoing development. Even with a history of success, however, children who are highly susceptible to negative emotion may experience self-doubt and threat to the self-image. This doubt may in turn be related to worry that the child will not be able to meet future expectations and to the adoption of a protective or defensive stance.

Let us now briefly return to the school situation and the qualities that schools may wish to foster in all children, regardless of their temperament. Although a child may be easily discouraged or quick to take on a protective or defensive stance, the potential for other, more positive reactions is real and can be fostered. We might then wish to encourage a more positive and open stance to learning, involving "children's *enthusiasm*—their interest, pleasure, and motivation to learn—and their *engagement*—their attention, persistence, flexibility, and self-regulation" (Hyson, 2008, p. 45), along with their willingness to expend effort.

In fact, we might wish to pack a suitcase of our own, full of the characteristics that would characterize a developed intelligence. Jackson (2002) offers these qualities: "a host of personality dispositions, habits, and attitudes—among them patience, persistence, open-mindedness, careful observation, unflagging attention to detail, reflection, experimentation, imagination, an abiding faith in one's own capacity to pursue the truth, an enduring delight in that pursuit, and even—all cautious properties aside—an undying love of it" (p. 81). Few children are likely to achieve all of these qualities but there is much we can do to encourage intelligence and a broad range of valued expertise.

Finally, I recently heard an inspiring talk at the University of Oregon. The speaker was a physicist who specialized in the study of extreme cold, very close to absolute zero. He was making a visit to the University, and had offered to give a free public lecture. His talk and demonstration attracted all kinds of people from Eugene, and it was a marvel. He showed such excitement in what he was studying and such pleasure in demonstrating to us what happens when materials become very cold, that I could not help but think of him as a physicist at play in the fields of the Lord. Some of us are able to achieve this kind of pleasure in what we do, but approaching this point does not require us all to become physicists. Working hard at what we do, feeling that our work has meaning, learning how to do it well, and applying ourselves to it without wanting to change what we are doing is likely an unreachable goal, but it is very much worth pursuing.

SUMMARY

In this chapter, I have considered two major tasks for the child in society: the development of empathy and conscience, and the development of competencies and achievement. Some of these tasks will be easier for one child than another, in part related to temperamental differences. However, a skill like empathy can be mastered through both more emotional an more cognitive routes. A positive attitude toward learning is something that a child of any temperamental disposition can come to possess. It is the job of the parent, teacher, and community member to make sure that as many children as possible will become open and self-regulated with learning and mastery goals in mind. In Chapters 9 and 10, I consider temperament's influence on psychopathology and antisocial behavior, remembering at the same time the possibilities for more favorable outcomes.

CHAPTER 8

⁓

Stability and Change from Child to Adult

The great American humorist and student of human nature Mark Twain became convinced that his life and the lives of others were governed by the laws of temperament and circumstance. In describing one of his life's major turning points, for example, he pointed to a circumstance (his finding a $50 bank note on the street), which in combination with his surgent temperament, led him to take off for South America on a trip to the Amazon:

> By temperament, I was the kind of person that *does* things. Does them, and reflects afterward. So, I started for the Amazon without reflecting and without asking any questions. That was more than fifty years ago. In all that time, my temperament has not changed, by even a shade. I have been punished many and many a time, and bitterly, for doing things and reflecting afterward, but these tortures have been of no value to me; I still do the thing commanded by Circumstance and Temperament, and reflect afterward. (Twain, 2000, original 1910, p. 482)

And at a time of grief on December 27, 1909, just after the death of his much-loved daughter Jean, he asks:

> Shall I ever be cheerful again, happy again? Yes. And soon. For I know my temperament. And I know that the temperament is master of the man, and

186

that he is its fettered and helpless slave and must in all things do as it commands. A man's temperament is born in him, and no circumstances can ever change it. My temperament has never allowed my spirits to remain depressed long at a time. That was a feature of Jean's temperament, too. She inherited it from me. (Twain, as cited by Paine, 1912, p. 1552)

Mark Twain felt that temperament could not be changed, and that it dictated one's responses to life's circumstances. In this book, however, I have put forward a more complex view of temperament and personality. First, we have noted that the components of temperament themselves change during maturation and development. In particular, the self-regulatory system of effortful control shows strong development, especially during the preschool and early school years, but continuing to adulthood. In Chapter 3, we also found that gene expression and proneness to distress can be modified by experience and stress. Third, we have seen that personality is influenced through the life experiences of the individual, including experiences in specific situations and with specific other people. Finally, if the environment of a person does not create a press for a given temperament reaction, it will not occur. Overall, these principles stress that temperament and personality are shaped by experience, but looked at in another way, we might be only specifying what happens when Mark Twain's laws of temperament and circumstance interact.

This chapter begins with a review of research on the stability and instability of temperament. In Chapter 2, I reviewed the stability of individual differences in temperament during the early years, and in this chapter, I consider predictions from the early years to adulthood and look at general changes in personality in adulthood. Personality can change, even in the later years of life, and the self-regulatory components of temperament may contribute to this change. I also relate the structure of temperament to the broad personality traits in the Big Five and the FFM.

What is stable and what is changeable in individual temperament, and how does change in personality occur? Because of the many influences on behavior, "It depends" may be the most appropriate answer. Stability and change depend on the balance between systems of temperament, the person's coping strategies, and how he or she interacts with the events of his or her life. I suspect that this will continue to be the answer to this question in the future, but that we will be better able to specify what "It depends" means in detail, as we learn more about the influences on development.

I begin, however, by repeating the point that just because a process is biologically based, this does not imply that it is immutable and impervious to change. Indeed, many of the capacities we are born with actually serve the function of change and adaptation to the environment. We inherit the structures that we use for learning and changes in understanding, and for regulation and self-control. For the most part, the broad traits of temperament show moderate stability over time and are linked to closely related traits of personality. Nevertheless, there will be different developmental paths to personality outcomes that are influenced by both temperament and the person's thoughts and cognitions.

Consider the miser, for example. The hoarding and stinginess of a miserly person are likely to stem from a protective stance toward money and possessions, and to be related to a mistrust of others who might wish to take advantage of the person or to steal his or her money or property. The miser protects his or her possessions by both saving and nongiving. The miser's protective stance may be related to temperamental tendencies toward the negative emotions, but it may also be strongly influenced by culture. When members of a culture are given reasons to believe that others cannot be trusted and that one's wealth must be carefully protected, they may engage in miserly behavior. They may also develop mistrustful thinking about the motives and intents of others, which can in turn lead to increased experience and expression of negative emotion in the person. Balzac's (1833) novel *Eugenie Grandet* describes both the complete miser (Eugenie's father) and Eugenie, a woman whose difficult lifetime is shaped by her father's miserliness. Still, Eugenie is able to give from her vast inherited wealth to charity, even though she continues to live a life of frugality that closely matches the life of her parents.

TEMPERAMENTAL STABILITY AND CHANGE

Because temperament itself develops (Rothbart, 1989b), new systems of organization (e.g., smiling and laughter, frustration, effortful control) come "on line" over time. Whenever a later-developing system regulates action and emotion, it can also change the expression of those characteristics. When this happens, there may be little continuity between traits at an earlier and a later age, and this will be especially true during periods of rapid change.

This can be seen in reviews of the stability of temperament and personality such as the one by Roberts and DelVecchio (2000). They examined lifetime stability of individual differences, beginning with studies of temperament and personality in infancy. Estimated across-time correlations for the period 0–2 years, 11 months, were .35; for 3–5 years, 11 months .52; for 6–11 years, 11 months, .45; and for 12–17 years, 11 months, .47. The lower stability between infancy and early childhood is found during the period when the two major temperament control systems, fear and effortful control, are coming on line. Development of fearful inhibition is seen late in the first year and effortful control develops rapidly during the preschool years. Thus patterns of behavior during and following the preschool years would be expected to show more stability over time, and this is the case. Beyond childhood, levels of stability continue to increase through adolescence and young adulthood, not peaking until after the age of 50 (Roberts & DelVecchio).

Stability from Infancy

Nevertheless, links have been found between reactivity in infancy and adult personality and adjustment. The Uppsala Longitudinal Study in Sweden (Hagekull & Bohlin, 2008) found that mothers' reports of infants' reactivity at 10–15 months such as the intensity of the infants' reactions to a bright light, loud sound, and to a new food, predicted self-reported temperament and personality when the participants were 21 years old. Reactivity predicted adult neuroticism, and internalizing and externalizing problems. Children's activity and sociability (surgency) at 20–48 months predicted lower neuroticism and higher extraversion at age 21. Shyness at 20–48 months predicted higher internalizing at age 21.

Highly Stable Aspects of Temperament

After their appearance over the early months, some aspects of temperament show stability over long periods. The characteristics of surgency (extraversion) and fearful social inhibition (introversion), which inhibit one another, show considerable stability, as Mark Twain may have anticipated. These patterns were seen in some of the earliest longitudinal studies. In the Fels longitudinal study, scores on "spontaneity" (surgency) versus "social interaction anxiety" (social inhibition) showed stability over long periods for both girls and boys (Kagan & Moss, 1962). Bayley and Schaefer (1963) also found that the most stable and persistent disposition between infancy and 18 years was "active, extraverted" versus "inactive, introverted" behavior. Finally, Honzik (1965) found that the two most stable dimensions between 21 months and 18 years were "introversion" versus "extraversion" and "spontaneity" versus "excessive reserve." Recent studies of children's shyness (social inhibition) have also shown considerable stability from early childhood onward (Asendorpf, 1993; Gest, 1997). Pfeifer, Goldsmith, Davidson, and Rickman (2002) have also found stability of both outgoingness and inhibition.

Kagan (1998) and Kagan and Fox (2006) have reviewed research on behavioral inhibition (fearfulness/social anxiety), and found considerable stability of this tendency, along with some change. Caspi and Silva (1995), for example, followed a group of 3- to 4-year-old children until they were 18 years of age. Children who were highly approaching and confident at ages 3–4 (described as outgoing, eager to undertake tasks, making an easy adjustment to challenging situations) were, at age 18, higher on social potency (greater leadership and lower shyness) and lower on control (more impulsive). Children who were inhibited at ages 3–4 (fearful, with problems in sustaining attention) were, at age 18, more highly fearful, very low on aggression, and low on social potency.

Another temperament-related dimension that shows considerable stability over time after ages 3–4 is the ability to delay gratification, one of the aspects of effortful control. The ability of 4-year-olds to wait for a larger reward, rather than claiming a smaller reward immediately, predicts the children's attentional and emotional control in high school as reported by their parents (Shoda, Mischel, & Peake, 1990). The number of seconds that preschool-age children could delay while waiting for the larger rewards also predicted their attentiveness and ability to concentrate as adolescents. Children who had shown less delay in preschool were reported to be more likely to go to pieces under stress and to show lower academic competence, even when intelligence was controlled (Shoda et al.). Children's delay as preschoolers also predicted their goal-setting and self-regulatory abilities when the participants had reached their early 30s (Ayduk, Mendoza-Denton, Mischel, & Downey, 2000). Other studies have reported predictions from self-control at ages 3–4 to adulthood. In Caspi and Silva's (1995) research, preschool-age children who were "capable of reserve and control when it was demanded of them" (p. 492) showed greater leadership and lower shyness at age 18. Children who were irritable and showed little self-regulation at ages 3–4 years were high on negative emotionality at age 18.

Caspi et al. (2003) studied 1,000 children at age 3 and related their preschool qualities to their self-reported personality at age 26. Their findings indicate that child temperament, especially after the appearance of effortful control, provides a clear basis for the developing personality. *Undercontrolled* 3-year-olds, who were high in surgency and negative emotionality and low in attentional control, showed more neurotic and alienated tendencies as 26-year-old adults than did other groups of children. *Confident* and surgent children tended to be confident and unfearful as adults. More shy and fearful (*inhibited* and *reserved*) children were high in caution and fearfulness and low in social potency as adults. More extremely *inhibited* children were high in constraint (a mixture of fearfulness and self-control) and low in positive emotionality. As adults, the inhibited children also reported a lack of social support. The relation between inhibition and later lack of social support may be in keeping with Scarr and McCartney's (1983) idea that temperament can lead to differences in how others respond to us. The shy person may make fewer friends than the nonshy person, but may also be less likely to *perceive* social support, even when others might see it as present.

Children who develop the control systems of fear or effortful control earlier in life may have quite different experiences than children who develop them later (Rothbart & Derryberry, 1981). For example, a child who is fearful and sensitive to potential dangers from infancy onward may spend more time just watching and making sense of events than the less fearful and inhibited child. The child who develops fear-related inhibition later, on the other hand, is likely to have approached a greater number of potentially threatening objects or situations, often finding that they were in fact safe.

Changes in Early Childhood

Now we turn from stability of individual differences from infancy and early childhood to overall changes in temperament early in development. How is it possible to have both stability and change? In Chapter 1, I introduced Shirley's (1933) argument about how one can find both stability of temperament and change in temperament with development. She described how Virginia Ruth, the most irritable infant, and James Dalton, the least irritable infant, maintained their rank in comparison with the other children, but also changed over time by decreasing in their irritability, just as the group of infants had done overall. For those interested in further reading, McCall (1990) has made a clear and very helpful presentation of how individual stability and group change can occur.

I have previously discussed how infants increase in their positive emotion, activity, and soothability over the first year of life. I have also discussed the onset of effortful control and its development during the preschool and early school years. Increases have been found, for example, in inhibitory control and attention shifting between ages 4 and 12 (Murphy, Eisenberg, Fabes, Shepard, & Guthrie, 1999). There are also changes in positive and negative emotionality over this period. Vaughn, Sallquist, et al. (2009) found that both positive and negative emotional intensity declined over a 6-year period beginning with children ages 5–8. Greater emotional control is expected as children enter school, and effortful control may regulate both kinds of emotional expression. Bates et al. (2010) suggest that "initially higher levels of extraversion and negative emotional reactivity in infancy and early in childhood (or at least their outward expression) may be reined in by increasing self-regulatory abilities as children get older."

Stability from Middle Childhood

Shiner and her colleagues recently studied the stability of personality by following 8- to 12-year-old children until they were 20 years of age. Twelve-year-olds' mastery motivation, surgent engagement, and self-assurance related to early temperament, predicted their positive emotionality at age 20, but childhood achievement and positive social adaptation did not predict later positive emotion (Shiner, Masten, & Tellegen, 2002). Children with lower school achievement and greater conduct problems at ages 8–12, however, were higher in negative emotionality as adults. Childhood mastery motivation and surgent engagement predicted lower adult negative emotionality.

Interpersonal skills and anger/aggressiveness have also shown some stability from childhood to adulthood. Kubzansky, Martin, and Buka (2004) found that 7-year-old children's behavioral inhibition (shyness) did not predict their adult functioning, but their anger predicted adult hostility/anger, and children's lack of interpersonal self-regulation predicted low adult interpersonal sensitivity. Asendorpf, Denissen, and van Aken (2008) also found stability from ages 4–6 to 23 years for children who were aggressive. These children showed greater delinquency and anger problems as adults. Children who had been highly inhibited at ages 4–6, however, did not see themselves as inhibited as adults, and showed no greater internalizing problems in adulthood than did less inhibited children. This lack of stability of inhibition is interesting, and further reviews of research in this area may shed light on these findings. These reviews need to take into account culture (for example, Asendorpf's work was done in Germany, where shyness is more acceptable than in North America). It will also be of interest to document the different kinds of coping strategies used by shy children to make positive adaptations.

Temperament and the Factor Structure of Adult Personality

In Chapter 2, I discussed the structure of temperament in infancy and childhood. Over the past 30 years, research by personality psychologists has yielded its own factor structure in broad dimensions extracted from a wide set of personality traits (Digman, 1989; Goldberg, 1990). The number of factors extracted from large sets of personality items ranges between three and seven, and the most common estimate of the number of personality factors is currently five. On the basis of this number, it has been argued that there are five basic broad dimensions of personality. The Big Five taxonomy (Digman, 1972, 1989; Goldberg, 1990; John & Srivastava, 1999) and the five-factor model (FFM) of personality (McCrae & Costa, 1987) are the two major trait models of personality today, and the most commonly used labels for the five factors are extraversion, agreeableness, conscientiousness, neuroticism, and openness. The Big Five personality model was derived by carrying out factor analyses of large numbers of adjectives describing personality traits; the adjectives were originally taken from the dictionary (Digman, 1989; Goldberg, 1990). McCrae and Costa's FFM is based on longer questionnaire items.

The Big Five personality tradition followed the idea that the most important aspects of individual differences in personality would be found in the words we use to describe others and ourselves. By factor analyzing long lists of adjectives from the dictionary, it would be possible to identify the basic dimensions of individual differences in personality. Big Five research began with thousands of adjectives used to describe the self and others. Through repeated culling of adjectives with similar meanings and factor analysis of the remaining adjectives, the original thousands of terms were reduced to a small set that often described five broad factors of personality (Digman, 1972, 1989; Goldberg, 1990). Items from the Big Five scales developed by Gerard Saucier (2002), called the minimarkers of the Big Five, are listed in Table 8.1. Costa and McCrae's (1994) FFM, in addition to using longer items, contributed lower-level scales or facets contributing to the broad factors. The FFM factors and their facets are also listed in Table 8.1.

Extraversion adjectives in Saucier's (2002) minimarkers range from the terms bold, energetic, and extraverted to quiet, reserved, shy, bashful, and withdrawn. *Agreeableness* ranges from sympathetic, kind, and cooperative to unsympathetic, rude, cold, and fault finding. *Conscientiousness* adjectives range from organized, thorough, and responsible to careless, disorderly, and slipshod. Neuroticism ranges from tense, anxious, and moody to stable, calm, and unemotional. Finally, *intellect/openness* ranges from wide interests, imaginative, and intelligent to commonplace, simple, and shallow.

In Costa and McCrae's (1994) FFM, each of the five broad personality dimensions was further divided into lower-order *facets* of personality. The five factors and their facets are (1) Extraversion, with facets of warmth, gregariousness, assertiveness, activity, excitement seeking, and positive emotionality; (2) Agreeableness, with facets of trust, straightforwardness, altruism, compliance, modesty, and tender-mindedness; (3) Conscientiousness, including facets of competence, order, self-discipline, dutifulness, deliberation, and achievement striving; (4) Neuroticism, with facets of anxiety, angry hostility, depression, self-consciousness, impulsiveness, and vulner-

TABLE 8.1. Adult Temperament and Personality Scales

Adult Temperament Questionnaire (Evans & Rothbart, 2007)	Big Five (Saucier, 2002)	Five-factor model (Costa & McCrae, 1992b)
Non-aggressive negative affect 　Fear 　Sadness	Neuroticism 　Envious, fretful, jealous, moody, temperamental, touchy versus relaxed, unenvious	Neuroticism 　Anxiety, angry hostility, depression, self-consciousness, impulsiveness, vulnerability
Effortful control 　Activation control 　Attentional control	Conscientiousness 　Efficient, organized, practical, systematic versus careless, disorganized, inefficient, sloppy	Conscientiousness 　Competence, order, dutifulness, achievement striving, self-discipline, deliberation
Extraversion/surgency 　Sociability 　High-intensity pleasure 　Positive affect	Extraversion 　Bold, energetic, extraverted, talkative versus bashful, quiet, shy, withdrawn	Extraversion 　Warmth, gregariousness, assertiveness, activity, excitement seeking, positive emotions
Orienting sensitivity 　General perceptual sensitivity 　Affective perceptual sensitivity 　Associative sensitivity	Intellect/openness 　Complex, creative, deep, imaginative, intellectual, philosophical versus uncreative, unintellectual	Openness to experience 　Fantasy, aesthetics, feelings, actions, ideas, values
Affiliation 　Emotional empathy 　Empathetic guilt	Agreeableness 　Cooperation, kind, sympathetic, warm versus cold, harsh, rude, unsympathetic	Agreeableness 　Trust, straightforward, altruism, compliance, modesty, tender-mindedness
Aggressive negative affect 　Frustration 　Social anger	— — —	— — —

ability; and (5) Openness to Experience, including facets of fantasy, aesthetics, and openness to feelings, actions, ideas, and values.

　Another important difference between the two models is that the Big Five scales are almost all bipolar, that is, they range from one dimension at one pole (e.g., agreeable) to its opposite extreme (e.g., disagreeable), with scales ranging from an extreme in one tendency (affiliativeness) to an extreme in an opposing tendency (aggression). The FFM dimensions, on the other hand, tend to be unipolar. With a unipolar scale, tendencies are not forced into opposition. Can a person be both agreeable and disagreeable? In our model, the answer is yes. A person may be quite agreeable in social settings, but also quick to anger and hence disagreeable on the job. Can a person be both extraverted and inhibited? Yes. A child can show extraversion in the home (a situation experienced as safe), while being inhibited in more threatening situations.

The Big Five/FFM models of personality traits share an interesting history with temperament research (Digman, 1996). At the turn of the century, Webb (1915) studied factors describing temperament and character, and in the 1930s, Cattell (1933) identified four factors of temperament based on college students' ratings of familiar others. Both Webb and Cattell identified a *w*, or Will, factor that shares similarities with Effortful Control and conscientiousness. Cattell also identified a Surgency (extraversion) factor, a Maturity factor (good-natured versus malicious), similar to the five-factor Agreeableness, and a Well-adjusted factor, including emotional versus unemotional qualities, similar to neuroticism. Of the many early trait researchers, Cattell's list of factors was most similar to the five factors of personality discussed today (Digman).

Between the 1930s and the 1980s, researchers were consistently extracting three to seven factors from personality tests, with five factors being the most common. In the late 1980s and early 1990s, Digman (1989) and Goldberg (1990) began to speak and write on the Big Five, and the FFM also was put forward by McCrae and Costa (1987). We and others also have found that factors extracted from temperament scales are highly correlated with and conceptually related to the Big Five and the FFM (Evans & Rothbart, 2007; Martin, Wisenbaker, & Huttunen, 1994; McCrae et al., 2000; Rothbart, 1989b; Victor et al., 2006). I now turn to this work.

Temperament and the Big Five/FFM

In our early research on adult temperament, Doug Derryberry and I (Derryberry & Rothbart, 1988) developed adult scales based on theories of temperament. These scales were later revised to form a broader temperament measure, the Adult Temperament Questionnaire (ATQ; Evans & Rothbart, 2007). Using factor analyses of self-reports collected from college students and from a large community sample ranging in age from 26 to 91 years, we studied the structure of adult temperament (Evans & Rothbart). This analysis yielded six factors that proved to be substantially correlated with Big Five and FFM measures. This factor structure has been replicated across different cultures, and has proven useful for studying influences of culture and gender on temperament. The broad temperament factors and scales of temperament are listed with the personality factors in Table 8.1.

Temperamental surgency includes enjoyment of high-intensity pleasure along with enjoyment of social interaction. Scores on surgency are strongly related to Big Five and FFM measures of extraversion, where items range from quiet and withdrawn to bold and energetic. Effortful control in the ATQ includes measures of activational control (the ability to perform an action when there is a desire to avoid it, e.g., getting out of bed when the alarm clock rings), and effortful attention (the ability to voluntarily shift and focus attention). Effortful control is strongly related to Big Five and FFM conscientiousness. High effortful control is also related to low FFM neuroticism, reflecting the opposition between attention and negative emotion described in Chapter 4.

In the ATQ, we found two factors involving negative emotionality: One measured fear and sadness, which we called Nonaggressive Negative Affect, and the other, frustration and social anger, which we called Aggressive Negative Affect. Both of these factors were related to Big Five neuroticism, which has content ranging from relaxed and unenvious to fretful and jealous. For the FFM, nonaggressive negative affect was most strongly related to neuroticism, with smaller correlations between aggressive negative affect and neuroticism.

One of the most interesting factors to emerge from our adult temperament analysis was the factor of Orienting Sensitivity and its relation to personality. Temperamental Orienting Sensitivity includes reactivity to low-intensity stimulation and having thoughts frequently come to mind (associative sensitivity). Orienting sensitivity was substantially related to Big Five intellect and FFM openness measures, which have items ranging from unintellectual and uncreative to complex and intellectual. FFM openness was also related to temperamental extraversion/surgency. Both Big Five and FFM agreeableness were related to higher temperamental affiliativeness, and they were also related to lower aggressive negative affect, but not to nonaggressive negative affect.

How do we interpret the strong relations between temperament and the personality factors? I believe they support McCrae et al.'s (2000) argument that the Big Five and the FFM are based on individual differences in temperament. McCrae and his colleagues argue that evidence from behavior genetics, individual differences in animals, stability of the five-factor structure of personality, and continuity of the structure across cultures supports the idea that the five-factor model is based on fundamental temperamental processes (McCrae et al.; see also Costa & McCrae, 2001). McCrae et al. also note that whereas temperament researchers tend to emphasize individual differences in basic psychological processes like attention and emotion, Big Five and FFM researchers define dimensions more in terms of their social effects. Both conscientiousness and agreeableness, for example, describe the kind of personal characteristics one might look for in hiring an employee. The differences in emphasis between temperament and personality actually complement each other, and overall, they allow us to extend our understanding of personality traits from social descriptors to temperament traits to underlying genetics and neurochemistry (Posner & Rothbart, 2007b; see also Chapter 11 of this book).

How might the Big Five/FFM develop out of early temperament? We would expect personality extraversion to develop from a core of surgency that can be observed as early as infancy. Personality conscientiousness, on the other hand, would be based on effortful control and the executive attention system that develops strongly during the preschool and school years. In addition to the capacity for effortful control, conscientious would be influenced by the person's motivation to follow society's rules. Personality neuroticism would be based on both aggressive and nonaggressive negative affect, but chiefly nonaggressive affect. Lower neuroticism would also be related to higher effortful control, reflecting the ways in which attention regulates the negative emotions and vice versa (Rothbart & Sheese, 2007).

Personality agreeableness would be based on temperamental low aggressive negative affect and high affiliativeness, reflecting its bipolar nature in the Big Five. Personality intellect/openness would be based on temperamental orienting sensitivity, which can be seen in early infancy. Later, orienting comes under more control of the executive attention system. How does early orienting become linked to adult personality terms like complex, deep, philosophical, and intellectual? How can a tendency toward openness be closed down? These will be exciting questions for future research.

Research within the Big Five tradition has also linked children's temperament to the Big Five model. Digman and Shmelyov (1996) studied teachers' ratings of 8- to 10-year-old Russian children on scales of both temperament and personality. Temperament scores were related to four of the Big Five personality measures: (1) merry/talkative versus constrained was related to extraversion; (2) angry versus soothable was related to low agreeableness; (3) impetuous versus focused was related to conscientiousness; and (4) afraid versus brave was related to neuroticism. None of the temperament scales used in Digman and Shmelyov's study were related to the Big Five measure of intellect/openness, but this is not surprising, since neither orienting sensitivity nor effortful control were assessed in this study. Our recent research on adults (Evans & Rothbart, 2007) and on children (Victor et al., 2006) further suggests that temperamental orienting sensitivity is related to personality openness.

In this view of individual differences, temperament differences can be seen to project onto a broad range of individual differences in personality. Temperament dispositions, personality traits, and coping mechanisms can also reinforce or oppose each other. Thus in the example of the miser offered earlier in this chapter, a tendency to negative emotion may promote the suspicious and defended condition of miserliness, and the condition of miserliness may promote the person's negative emotionality. In the future, molecular genetics methods will allow us to increasingly look for similarities and differences in personality related to temperament (genetics), environment and experience.

Because temperament can be studied from early infancy, we most often think of the developing personality as influenced by temperament. The example of the miser, however, suggests that influences can operate in the opposite direction, from personality to the expression of temperament. Personality traits like jealousy and paranoia, for example, will increase a person's negative experiences, regardless of the individual's temperamental dispositions. Indeed, neuroticism in its very name conveys the idea that negative information has been linked to concepts of the self and others. Negative thinking can thus be linked to neuroticism with or without a strong temperamental base for it, but a disposition to negative emotion is likely to strengthen negative thinking and its effects of neuroticism. Overall, cognitive and cognitive-behavioral approaches to psychopathology and psychotherapy and Eastern philosophies such as Buddhism and Vedanta suggest that through changing how we see ourselves and others, we can influence the expression of negative emotion (Beck, 1967, 1983).

Combined Temperament and Personality in Childhood

We now turn to a study of temperament and personality in childhood (Victor et al., 2006). This work grew out of a conference on the developing structure of personality (see Halverson, Kohnstamm, & Martin, 1994) where researchers set out to interview parents to study the structure of children's personality (Kohnstamm, Halverson, Mervielde, & Havill, 1998). Unlike the adult approaches to personality based on words from the dictionary, these researchers developed a child "dictionary" of individual differences from parents' free descriptions of their children. Parents were asked questions that included "What is your child like?" and "How is he or she similar to or different from other children?" Investigators in seven countries interviewed over 3,000 parents, and parent descriptions were coded into a standard format using a system developed by Dutch and American research teams (see Havill, Allen, Halverson, & Kohnstamm, 1994; Kohnstamm et al., 1998).

In research at Hampton University, supervised by the late James Victor (Victor et al., 2006), an additional step was taken. Victor used Costa and

McCrae's FFM and its facets (Costa & McCrae, 1992a) as a framework for sorting the mothers' descriptions into personality dimensions, leading to unipolar scales. Because items were based on parents' language, the items used in these scales were clear and understandable. At the same time, using the FFM to organize the mothers' descriptions allowed Victor to see which scales based on mothers' descriptions matched the FFM facets, and which did not. A number of traits were missing from the mothers' descriptions, and many of them seemed to be temperamental. Temperament traits of soothability, perceptual sensitivity, and effortful control (inhibitory control, perceptual sensitivity, attentional focusing, and attentional shifting/distractibility) were not found in the parent descriptions. For this reason, Victor and I used temperament scales from the CBQ (Rothbart et al., 2001) to supplement the personality scales that had already been developed, and to create a comprehensive measure of child personality and temperament (Victor et al., 2006) that could be used in other studies. Because the structure of temperament and personality was also of interest to us, we looked at the relations among these measures.

A comprehensive exploratory factor analysis (CEFA) was performed on items from mothers' questionnaires in a sample of 915 children 3–12 years old. We examined the structure of the combined personality and temperament measures, finding that a five-factor solution was the best fit for all analyses. The first factor, which we labeled *Externalizing Negative Affect* (ENA), included low agreeableness scales assessing self-centeredness, noncompliance/aggression, and manipulativeness, along with higher excitement seeking, assertiveness, anger/hostility, impulsivity, activity, and low inhibitory control. The second factor, which we labeled *Surgent Sociability* (SS), was made up of gregariousness/sociability, warmth, positive emotion, soothability, and activity. Because activity and gregariousness contributed to both externalizing negative effect and surgent sociability, we hypothesized that surgency in infancy and early life may branch into two kinds of personality organization—one (ENA) less socialized and the other (SS) more highly socialized, one (ENA) related to lack of control and angry affect, and the other (SS) to positive emotion and sociability.

This analysis takes us back to Gesell's (1928, as cited by Kersen, 1965) predictions about the little girl he called CD, who showed a surgent temperament from infancy to age 6 years. He argued that effective socialization combined with early surgency may allow control of her emotions and actions, supporting development of a "good citizen." Lower-quality environment and parenting, however, may incline the child toward externalizing negative affect and even delinquency. In molecular genetics research, we have found that children with the DRD4 genetic allele associated with attention-deficit/hyperactivity disorder, whose parents showed higher-quality parenting, were at age 2 more likely to show moderate levels of activity level and sensation seeking (Sheese et al., 2007). Children with the gene whose parents showed lower-quality parenting, however, showed high activity, risk taking, and stimulation seeking. Quality of parenting did not appear to affect measures of these behaviors in children without the DRD4 allele, who showed moderate levels of them.

The third factor, labeled *Internalizing Negative Affect* (INA) is similar to FFM neuroticism in that it includes anxiety, depression/sadness, dependency, and self-consciousness. Anger/hostility, however, is not present in this temperament factor. Instead, it contributes to ENA. As in our adult temperament research (Evans & Rothbart, 2007), two forms of negative emotion were identified. One involves more active and externalized emotion, including anger and unsocialized surgency/extraversion; the other form involves less activity and is more internalized, and includes the emotions of anxiety, depression, and feelings of self-consciousness. I have returned many times in this book to a distinction between externalizing and internalizing negative emotions. This distinction plays a major role in Chapters 9 and 10, where I discuss the development of behavior problems and psychopathology.

The fourth factor of our combined personality/temperament measure was labeled *Effortful Control*. Effortful control is composed of scales of order, diligence, inhibitory control, self-discipline, attentional focusing, and low distractibility/attention shifting. This factor was greatly strengthened by the addition of temperament scales (inhibitory control, attention focusing, and distractibility/attention shifting) added to Victor's scales of order, diligence, and self-discipline based on mother's descriptions (Victor et al., 2006).

Personality conscientiousness was strongly linked to temperamental effortful control as measured in inhibitory control, attentional focusing, and distractibility (Victor et al., 2006). Similar measures of personality have been given many other labels, including orderliness, self-control, constraint, achievement, superego strength, and will to achieve (Digman, 1989). Each construct carries different and sometimes complex connotations, but it is likely that each could be linked to temperament components, which in turn may be linked to executive attention and gene function (Posner et al., 2007). In the future, we will be able to move closer to understanding the processes underlying these important individual differences.

The fifth temperament/personality factor, *Openness to Experience*, is composed of four scales: aesthetics/creativity, openness to ideas, intellect/quick to learn, and temperamental perceptual sensitivity. As in our adult studies (Evans & Rothbart, 2007), we found a correlation between orienting sensitivity scales and Big Five openness in the children (Victor et al.,

2006). Openness was also strengthened by the addition of temperamental perceptual sensitivity to the other openness scales. In our previous infant research, perceptual sensitivity was part of the surgency factor (Gartstein & Rothbart, 2003). By early childhood, however, perceptual sensitivity was more strongly linked to temperamental effortful control (Rothbart et al., 2001), and by later childhood and adulthood effortful control is differentiated from openness, with each of them in a different factor. It will be critically important to gain an understanding of these findings using longitudinal research. I suspect they are related to the age at which executive attention gains control of orienting (Rothbart et al., in press) and whether a more open or protective coping stance is adopted by the person.

Shiner (1998) has made a major contribution to our understanding of individual differences in childhood by proposing a basic structure for personality in children. Shiner has proposed that there are two negative emotion clusters; one composed of fear, worry, and guilt, and one based on anger/hostility, our research supports this distinction (Rothbart et al., 2000; Victor et al., 2006). Shiner also proposed a personality dimension of dependency, and scales for dependency have also emerged from our research (Victor et al.). Part of our internalizing negative affect factor, dependency describes children who need others to do things for them, need help, tend to give in to others, and so on. Finally, a depression/sadness scale also contributes to the set of scales assessing internalizing negative affect. In Chapter 9, I argue that these two forms of negative emotion contribute to the development of internalizing and externalizing behavior problems.

In the future, Victor's temperament and personality model (Victor et al., 2006) can inform research on genes and parenting in predicting personality outcomes. These studies will be particularly useful if they can follow the same group of children across time and experience, to see how surgency may divide into its two major outcomes and to study links between perceptual sensitivity, surgency, and effortful control at different ages.

Stability and Change in Adolescence and Adulthood

I have previously discussed results of the meta-analysis of Roberts and DelVecchio (2000) on temperament and personality stability, noting increasing stability of temperament after age 3 until early adulthood. Before the age of 3, that figure is smaller. The stability of personality measures continue to increase as we grow older, peaking at about age 50 ($r = .75$), and then declining slightly. Bates et al.'s review (2010) has found similar stability over development. Caspi and Shiner (2006) reviewed research on individual stability and change, finding that individuals whose personality changed little from adolescence to adulthood were "more intellectually, emotionally, and socially successful as adolescents" (p. 337) than those who changed. They were also more adjusted (Block, 1971). Similar findings were reported by Asendorpf and van Aken (1991) on stability in resilient children, and Roberts, Caspi, and Moffitt (2001) found that traits of emotional stability, agreeableness, and conscientiousness were associated with stability. These findings are in keeping with a win–stay position, the idea that those with more adaptive and successful characteristics are likely to have less need to change.

Changes in Adolescence

Like the toddler and preschool periods, adolescence is a time of rapid change, both biological and social. During adolescence, young people increase in social dominance (Roberts, Walton, & Viechtbauer, 2006), decrease in shyness, and increase in negative emotionality (Ganiban, Saudino, Ulbricht, Neiderhiser, & Reiss, 2008). Adolescents are also higher in stimulation seeking (Zuckerman, Eysenck, & Eysenck, 1978), risk taking, and responsiveness to reward (Somerville, Jones, & Casey, 2010). Adolescents also show decreases in conscientiousness (Allik et al., 2004; DeFruyt et al., 2006), although this is not found in all studies (see review by Bates et al., 2010).

Research results reviewed by Somerville et al. (2010) indicate that although adolescents may understand the riskiness of a given behavior, they do not seem to be able to control the risky behavior when there is an immediate prospect of a reward. Thus, greater injuries, car accidents, homicide, and suicide occur during this period (Eaton et al., 2008). New models based on brain development have now been put forward to account for these changes. These models suggest that emotionality (amygdala activation) and reward reactivity (nucleus accumbens activation) increase during adolescence. This increase exaggerates adolescents' responsiveness to reward in a way that is not yet opposed by regulatory brain structures (increases in prefrontal structures lag behind reactive changes) (Somerville et al., 2010). The increased seeking of rewards and heightened emotional reactivity may be linked to the development of reproductive behavior and sexual maturation, with adolescents more influenced by gonadal hormones (Steinberg, 2004; Zuckerman et al., 1978). Exciting progress is currently being made in the study of adolescence, and research in this area fits well with models of individual differences in reactivity and self-regulation, both before and after maturational change. Coping strategies and influences of parents, peers, and communities will be important in this development.

Achieving Maturity

There is also evidence that, even when adults retain their rank order in a characteristic over time, there are general changes in temperament and personality as we age. Roberts et al. (2006) found that most changes occurred between ages 20 and 40, but change continued into old age. Agreeableness increases with age (ages 40 to 60), as does conscientiousness, assertiveness (up to age 40), and openness (up to age 60). Neuroticism decreases, leveling off at about age 60 (Carstensen, Pasupathi, Mayr, & Nesselroade, 2000). Slightly lowered gregariousness and openness have also been found, but only very late in life, at a time when disabilities can stand in the way of successful social activities. In Bates et al.'s (2010) review, evidence for decreases in extraversion is observed across cultures. How might change take place? Some changes appear to be related to the roles people occupy in adulthood in family and work. Participation in a stable marriage and having a committed career are linked to increases in assertiveness and conscientiousness and decreases in neuroticism in adult life (Roberts & Wood, 2006). In Chapter 10, Labouvie-Vief's (1999) model for adaptation with aging will further enrich our view of this period.

Karen Horney's (1950) view of change occurring even late in life is that "man has the capacity as well as the desire to develop his potentialities and become a decent human being, and that these deteriorate if his relationship to others and hence to himself is, and continues to be, disturbed. I believe that man can change and keep changing as long as he lives" (p. 19). Studies of personality change in adulthood support Horney's view (Roberts & Mroczek, 2008). In addition to changes supported by psychotherapy, other sources can lead to increased self-understanding. Eastern philosophies such as Buddhism and Vedanta argue that the models of the self we have constructed and carried into adulthood may not be the whole answer to who we are. Maturity allows us to observe ourselves. We can clarify and consult our values, and act to change our own behavior to agree with them. Here the person plays an active role in observing the self and moving toward becoming more authentic and integrated; in a word, more mature. Temperamental effortful control aids in our choosing and implementing goals and values; it likely also strengthens being able to observe what one does, how one thinks, and the emotions one experiences. Goals for change can then be implemented, so that a person can become more authentic and self-accepting.

Gale (1974) describes a mature person as one "who thinks positively about himself and others, is aware of and open to experiences, views himself as a significant part of a world in flow, recognizes and accepts his human strengths and frailties and those of others, develops and appreciates human values as the vital sources of behavior and growth, lives congruently with his values even in the face of opposition, and casts himself in the creative role of assuming the commitments and the involvements of his own becoming and that of others" (p. 13).

The general changes in personality observed in adulthood would support a movement toward maturity with less neuroticism and greater openness, conscientiousness, and agreeableness. Roberts and his associates suggest that changes in adulthood are linked to the qualities of maturity needed in the work site and the family (Roberts & Wood, 2006). However, the view of maturity described above suggests that we may be able to specify values related to maturity in more detail, relating it more directly to our experiences and self-understanding. Gale's (1974) description includes both general personality characteristics, and the values and goals that can be the elements of change. I have called this change "moral bootstrapping," and described it in greater detail elsewhere (Rothbart, 2009). A definition of maturity also allows us to investigate how psychotherapies and alternative programs for change may influence and increase maturity in participants of any age.

SUMMARY

In studies of stability in temperament, some characteristics (surgency, caution, effortful control) have shown stability from ages 3–4 onward. Stability of negative emotionality has been found in links between infant negative reactivity and self-reported personality in adulthood. In this chapter, I have made connections between the Big Five and the FFM personality models and their likely bases in temperament, finding that the organization of broad personality traits is quite similar to the structure of temperament. In adult research, we have found strong correlations between measures of temperament and Big Five and FFM measures, and our work on combined temperament and personality in childhood suggests some likely developmental pathways from temperament to personality. As might be expected at this point in the book, temperament also shows important connections with the development of behavior problems and psychopathology, and I consider these pathways to problem development in Chapters 9 and 10.

CHAPTER 9

⌒

Problems and Interventions in Development

How do problems in adjustment develop in young children, and who is chiefly responsible for them—the parents, for their lack of sensitivity, or the children for their "difficult" temperaments? There has been a strong tendency to see *either* the parent *or* the child as primarily responsible. Attachment theorists, for example, often argue that the mother's insensitivity is the source of the child's insecure attachment and related problems. However, in Chapter 4 evidence was reviewed that temperament in interaction with the child's experience makes a substantial contribution to attachment security.

Clinicians specializing in temperament, on the other hand, have seen the child's "difficult" temperament as the problem, to be managed by the parent. Earlier I considered how modern research on temperament began by assessing the temperament of the "difficult" child, and I have discussed problems with that approach. First, difficulty encourages a highly simplified view of temperament, when in fact temperament is composed of a number of separable dimensions. Second, it often does not recognize that "difficulty" is defined by social context, so that a characteristic that is difficult in one setting may be a virtue in another setting. Third, defining an infant or child as difficult is, surprisingly, blind to development. A difficult infant is not necessarily a difficult child and certainly need not become a difficult adult. Similarly, an "easy" infant does not necessarily foretell an easy

205

child or adult. Although the attachment and difficulty models may apply to some extreme cases, I believe they oversimplify the situation. Emotion and behavior problems most often develop out of interactions that involve both parent and child.

ADAPTATION AND ADJUSTMENT IN INFANCY

I begin this chapter by considering the development of problems in infancy, in part because this may provide a simple model for thinking about reactivity and regulation in relationships, and in part because of the rich research, theory, and clinical applications in this area. During infancy the relationship between parent and child is getting off to a start that may be relatively smooth or troubled, and this relationship will vary depending on the reactivity, coping, and adjustments of both child and parent. Later, the child's cognitive judgments and evaluations of the self and other, self-representations (including perceptions of one's body), conscious self-presentations, language, and thinking can create new challenges, vulnerabilities, and means of coping (see analysis of the development of depression by Hyde, Mezulis, & Abramson, 2008). By adulthood, all of these influences will be operating, and from the first days of the infant, they all may apply to the parent.

As an example of problems that can develop in the caregiver–infant relationship, let us consider the development of sleep disorders (see also Anders, Goodlin-Jones, & Sadeh, 2000). If you are a parent, you know that sleep problems are common in infancy; in fact, they are the most frequent problem reported by parents to the pediatrician (Anders et al.). During the first 2 years, problems with sleep will also be related to problems with feeding, anger, and clinginess (Schieche, Rupprecht, & Papousek, 2008). By the preschool period, problems with sleep are associated with general adjustment problems (Bates et al., 2002).

Sleep Problems

How might sleep problems develop? Infants at 2–3 months often need the support of the caregiver to go to sleep (Papousek, 2008; Schieche et al., 2008); parents may rock the child, hold the child close, carry the child around, or feed the child, among other soothing methods. Problems can originate, however, in those infants who at 2–3 months need a good deal of soothing from their parents to fall asleep. Because all infants typically wake once or more during the night (Anders et al., 2000), the infant will also require soothing during the night. After 3–4 months of age, the infant has gained a higher level of self-regulation and is less in need of parent soothing, and can learn how to fall asleep without parent support (Schieche et al.). However, if parents continue to use their sleep ritual involving direct soothing of the child, the infant comes to expect it. The evening soothing ritual that helped at 2–3 months may then be continued even when children might have been developing their own sleep strategies. Now that the infant expects soothing, he or she will also vigorously protest when the parents, now exhausted, try to give it up.

The infant's protest often leads the parents to return to their previous soothing rituals. Over time, the parents become increasingly exhausted, feel frustrated, and may experience anger and guilt about not being good enough parents. There is clearly a sleep problem here, but is the problem located only in the infant? Only in the parent? The problem has grown out of repeated parent–infant interactions at bedtime, and both have contributed to it. The child's temperamental distress proneness and low soothability make a contribution, as does the parent's desire to prevent the child's distress. Although parents had provided the regulation needed when the child's self-soothing was less available, their continued efforts may have contributed to problems.

Although I do not have space to discuss them here, problems in children's eating, clinging, anxious, defiant, and aggressive behaviors all develop within early relationships. They develop out of the child's temperamental dispositions in interaction with the parent's knowledge, confidence, and coping strategies for dealing with the situation (see Papousek, 2008). During development, each member of the interaction is adapting to the other, and some of these adaptations may themselves lead to problems.

In the Research and Intervention Program for Fussy Babies in Munich, Germany, where these observations were made, parents who need help with infant sleep receive counseling about development generally and about their infant's capacity for self-regulation (Schieche et al., 2008). Parents are also taught a "checking" strategy. The infant is put to bed after a soothing ritual; the parent then says goodnight and leaves the room. If the child cries or screams, the parent checks in at short regular intervals, offering soothing and reassurance to the child in words but not using any other soothing procedures, and then leaves. If the child cries again, the parent continues with the checking until the infant falls asleep. The purpose of this approach is to give the infant the opportunity to develop his or her own self-soothing strategies. Their application of the program created little stress for the parent or child, and most of it was experienced the first night. By the fourth or fifth night, children showed strong improvements in maintaining sleep, and the majority of infants showed continuing effects for the

3 months when they were observed. Even when children showed relapses, they tended to improve after a second counseling session, and overall only 8% of the infants failed to improve.

Another possibility in the relationship is that parents offer little soothing from the start. When the parent does not offer comfort, the child may not learn to see the parent as a source of soothing, trying instead to develop self-soothing strategies. These children may be less likely to turn to the parent for social regulation, but try to handle the situation on their own. Problems can also develop when the parent is highly intrusive and insensitive to the child's signals (Tronick, 2007). Here, the regulation offered by the parent may not fit the needs of the infant, or the social regulation may be offered at the wrong time. The temperament of the child, especially the child's proneness to distress and soothability, will likely contribute to both of these problems (Papousek, 2008), but the parents' contribution is very important.

Face-to-Face Interactions

Self-regulation and other-regulation can also be seen in face-to-face interactions between parent and infant during the day. Here, the parent reads (or fails to read) the child's signs of developing distress and attempts at self-regulation (looking away, self-soothing, etc.) and can use that information to help regulate the child, often by decreasing the intensity of the interaction (Brazelton, Koslowski, & Main, 1974; Stern, 1985). When reading the child works well, full distress is much less likely to develop, and the interaction can continue at a comfortable level. If the child's signals are so weak that they cannot be read by the parent, or if the parent tries but is not able to soothe the infant, the parent may be the one to be discouraged, becoming unavailable to the child. Problems in interaction are much less likely if (1) the child is not easily distressed, or (2) the parent knows about his or her infant's signals and how to read them.

The mood state of the mother can also contribute to problems in social regulation. When depressed mothers were observed in interaction with their infants, two distinctive patterns of behavior were observed (Tronick, 2007). *Intrusive* mothers handled their babies roughly, poked at them, spoke angrily to them, and actively interfered with their activities. *Withdrawn* mothers, on the other hand, appeared unresponsive and disengaged, offering little support of their infants. The infants of withdrawn mothers were likely to protest and become angry at first, but later in development begin to fuss and cry, showing a more helpless and nonassertive response. Over time, the children of withdrawn mothers were likely to develop "a disengaged and self-regulatory style characterized by self-comforting, self-regulatory behaviors (e.g., looking away, sucking on their thumb), passivity, and withdrawal as a way of coping with their state" (p. 285). These infants did not seem to expect their mothers to respond, and the infants may also have given up on assertive attempts at coping, since they were not effective.

Children of more intrusive mothers, who were less contingent in their treatment of the child, tended to respond to their mothers with anger. These infants may have learned that their expressions of anger sometimes *did* serve to limit their mother's actions. "To the extent that these coping behaviors are successful in fending off the mother these infants eventually internalize an angry and protective style of coping that is deployed defensively in anticipation of the mother's intrusiveness" (Tronick, 2007, p. 286). It is also likely that the infant's temperament makes a contribution to these adaptations.

The still-face situation was developed by Tronick (2007) and his colleagues as a model for the infant's interaction with a depressed and withdrawn mother. In the still-face situation, the mother first plays with her infant for 2 minutes and then is asked to become unresponsive to the infant for the same amount of time. She then plays with her child once again, and the interactions are videorecorded. During the still-face period, infants as young as 3 months show initial greeting of the mother, often with cooing and smiling, but become increasingly disturbed as the still face continues. Infants look away or suck on the hand or thumb in attempts at self-soothing. Infants may also extend their arms in pick-me-up signals in attempts to make contact with the parent, or try to escape from the situation, and physiological signs of stress are often recorded (Tronick).

Weinberg and Tronick (1994) indentified four coping strategies of 6-month-old infants to their mothers' still face. The first involved expressions of joy, vocalizing, looking at the mother, and self-stimulation, and was called *social engagement*. The second pattern included sustained looking at, scanning, and mouthing objects, and was called *object engagement*. *Passive withdrawal* involved facial sadness, fussing, and autonomic signs of stress. Finally, *active protest* included anger expressions, fussing, scanning, crying, the pick-me-up gesture, attempts to escape, and autonomic signs of stress.

These coping strategies appear to be related to temperamental reactivity and self-regulation. Object engagement is a form of self-regulation through orienting, whereas social engagement is likely related to surgent coping. The two kinds of coping involving negative emotion, active protest and passive withdrawal, are especially interesting to the student of temperament. In our research on the structure of temperament, we identified two kinds of negative emotions: the angry assertive or externalizing negative affect (likely related to active protest), and the nonassertive or internalizing negative affect (likely related to passive inhibition or withdrawal) (Evans & Rothbart, 2007; Victor et al., 2006). These emotions map well onto the patterns observed by Weinberg and Tronick (1994).

We know that interactions between parent and child are neither consistently happy, nor are they always marked by comfortable levels of arousal for both of the partners, even in the best of relationships. This means that interactions will show periods of both disruption and repair (Tronick, 2007). Disruptions of smooth interaction may lead to signs of distress and self-regulatory behaviors in the infant (looking away, self-soothing, etc.). If the caregiver reads these events as "Things are becoming uncomfortable for my child," the mismatch can be repaired as the adult quiets and looks away for long enough for the situation to quiet down. When the child's negative emotions, signs of self-regulation, or active attempts to engage the parent are successful, repair occurs and the infant is able to experience feelings of efficacy within the relationship (Crockenberg & Leerkes, 2000). The child is also gaining ability in sustaining engagement in an interaction in the face of stress.

The child's capacities for reactivity and regulation and the role of adults in promoting the child's self-regulation need to be taken very seriously by parents, child care workers, and teachers. If we can prevent long-term problems before they begin or repair potential problems when they are still tractable, the possibilities of positive development are increased (Papousek, 2008). One very early approach to prevention is described at the end of this chapter: the Birth To Three program for parents of infants and young children. Another approach to caregiver–infant problems uses brief therapeutic interventions based on ideas of reactivity and regulation (Papousek). Several of these approaches have been found to be helpful, and I present them briefly here.

Interventions for Problems in Parent–Infant Interaction

One approach to regulation problems is educational (Papousek & von Hofacker, 2008), stressing the importance of good communication between infant and caregiver. The parent is taught how to read the infant's signs and signals, and how best to respond to them. The parent learns the kinds of infant behavior to expect at different ages, and how to promote self-regulation in the child. The second approach bypasses the more abstract teaching of the first approach, and instead offers parents a concrete behavioral strategy for dealing with the problem. As discussed in Chapter 4, parents may be asked to imitate their infant who is often looking away, resulting in decreased stimulation for the child who seems overwhelmed. Alternatively, they may be instructed to get the infant's attention when the child is showing little engagement (Field, 2007). For sleep problems where the child calls out for the parent, the parent is encouraged to slowly reduce the amount of attention and soothing given the child, allowing the child to self-regulate and fall asleep (Schieche et al., 2008).

The third kind of intervention involves video recording a parent–child interaction, for example, recording a feeding session (von Hofacker, Papousek, & Wurmser, 2008). Later, the therapist reviews with the parent parts of the video where the parents' strategies seem to be working. Here, the parent is encouraged to continue these strategies. The therapist then discusses sections of the video where there are problems in regulation, and works with the parent to develop new strategies for regulation and repair. Discussing the videotapes also gives parents an opportunity to talk about their own feelings as they watch the scene. For example, a parent may see the child as rejecting, and then recall memories of parental rejection in their own childhood. This allows the therapist to bring up the "ghosts" of the parent's own history that may be contributing to problems of regulation with the infant and help to lay them to rest (Beebe, 2003; Fraiberg, 1980). One of the most exciting aspects of this approach is that parents can observe themselves, identify their own problems, and then work to change their behavior. The result can be positive for both infant and parent.

By the last quarter of the first year of life, the child has developed clear intentions and is able to pursue his or her wants and desires (Sander, 1977). Now the parent and child can engage in what is called child-directed inter-action (Cohen, Lojkasek, Muir, Muir, & Parker, 2002; Greenspan, 1995). In child-directed interaction, the parent is asked to allow the *child* to control the interaction. The child chooses toys and activities for play, and the parent follows the child's lead in play and conversation. This interaction is experienced positively by the child, and after a period of child-directed interaction, the child is more likely to comply with the mother's requests (Parpal & Maccoby, 1985). During child-directed play, parents need to devote their attention more directly to observing their child than they would normally do, responding to the *child's* needs rather than imposing their own expectations on the child. Parents can in this way learn more about their children's likes and dislikes, and the parent and child can become more of a team.

Child-directed interaction is also an important aid to therapy when the parents have been asked to set limits for their children. In applying limits, the parents let the child know when and where a behavior is appropriate and when or where it is not. Limit setting becomes especially important when the child enters the period of self-assertion (Sander, 1977). Papousek and von Hofacker (2008) suggest that when parents are asked to set limits on their children's behavior, "Each demand . . . must be balanced by a positive relational experience guided by the child's needs and interests and characterized by positive reciprocity, relatedness, and the parent's undivided attention" (p. 193). This is particularly helpful for the toddler period, when there are frequent parent–child conflicts, and where a combination of affection and guidance can lead to psychological growth in the child.

EMOTIONAL AND SOCIAL REGULATION IN CHILDHOOD

It is hard to gauge the point when we might talk about a problem of self-regulation as "in the child," but it may be when children have moved from the family out into the world, carrying their temperament capacities and their previously developed coping strategies with them. By the age of 3–4 years, strategies for regulation of the self and other have become part of the child's personality, as I have shown in Chapter 7. Nevertheless, social interactions in the home, school, and playground will continue to shape the child's adaptations, especially as new challenges appear.

Later in development, parents continue to play an essential role in both providing social regulation and encouraging self-regulation. They can help the child recognize the negative emotions, talk about them, and deal openly with them (Kopp, 1989; Thompson, 1994). If the parent is emotionally unavailable, however, or denies the presence of negative emotion in the child, the child will miss learning about emotions and how to regulate them (Fabes, Poulin, Eisenberg, & Madden-Derdich, 2002; Jones, Eisenberg, Fabes, & MacKinnon, 2002). In addition, when caregivers chiefly offer comforting to the child, the child may come to use distress as a strategy to receive attention from adults. Patterns of distress and comforting can also be seen in later relationships, including sibling interactions, friendship, marriage, and other intimate relationships.

Problems in social regulation can be seen in families throughout development. If the preschool- or school-age child is a witness to conflict and fighting between the parents, for example, he or she is likely to become distressed and to try to figure out what these events mean for his or her own welfare. The child may think, "This is my fault," or "My mom and dad are going to get a divorce, and what will happen to me?" The child may also try to cope with the distressing situation by intervening in some way. One approach is for the child to try to act as a family peacemaker, working toward decreasing the conflict between the parents (Cummings, Papp, &

Kouros, 2009). If the child "succeeds" as a peacemaker, the usual pattern of distress and comforting will be reversed, with the *child* providing social regulation for the parents' reactivity.

In a second coping pattern, the child may develop active behavior problems that will distract the parents from conflicts with each other as they focus on the problem child. In a third coping strategy, the child may try to avoid the conflict situation altogether (Cummings et al., 2009). Each of these patterns of family interaction can be analyzed in terms of social reactivity and regulation, and when siblings are added to the mix, there are additional possibilities for conflict and coping (Volling, Kolak, & Blandon, 2009). Within the family, children may take on roles that also describe their attempts at coping: the peacemaker, the troublemaker, the entertainer, the withdrawn child, etc., and if one of these roles is already taken, the younger child may need to take on another.

It is important to remember, however, that a coping strategy that succeeds in the short term or in one situation with one set of people may be unadaptive in the long term or in another setting. Thus each of the children's coping strategies observed by Cummings and his associates (2009)—mediating parent conflict, negative emotional outbursts, and detached avoidance, can lead to future problems. In the marital conflict situation, the child is doing the best he or she can, but the child's strategies may or may not be helpful to him or her in the future. Emotional outbursts, for example, can lead to dysregulated emotion and behavior at school or with one's playmates, leading to peer rejection and teacher disapproval.

In studies of marital conflict, parents also differ in how they express their conflict. Some show destructive patterns and use threats, expressions of hostility, and personal insults. Others show more constructive patterns, expressing conflict but also affection, support, humor, and problem solving (Cummings et al., 2009). When parents handle their conflicts constructively, their children are less likely to show distress. Indeed, children might also see how warmth, humor, and problem solving can solve or reduce the negative effects of conflict. Just as it is helpful to recognize, think about, and deal with negative emotion, so it is important to recognize, think about, and deal with social conflict.

Resilience, or the ability to recover from threat or stress, develops out of the child's experience of coping with stressors. When a stressor is too threatening or intense, the child's self-regulation and active coping attempts will not be effective, and the child may withdraw and give up. When children are able to cope with situations, however, they gain strategies for coping with new stressors, and develop the attitude that problems can be overcome through personal effort. With manageable stresses and their repair come expectations of being able to deal with almost any problem. This approach can fail, however, when the child's strategies are applied to situations where the child is not in control. As life progresses, we will also have to deal with severe stresses that we cannot control (job loss, divorce, disease, disability, and death of those close to us). Here, resilience can be found in part through an acceptance of things we cannot control.

REACTIVITY AND REGULATION
IN OLDER CHILDREN AND ADULTS

In older children and adults, negative emotion that is not adequately regulated is associated with mood disorders and can also lead to antisocial behavior. Personality disorders can be related to the exaggerated social emotion of pride in the narcissist and separation anxiety in the borderline personality. Do these patterns develop out of temperament alone? They may for some problems, but many possibilities exist for problems in older children and adults that do not exist for infants. These include concepts and evaluations of the self and others, and habitual ways of dealing with interpersonal problems. A number of mood problems involve ruminating or repeatedly thinking about and reliving events that have distressed us in the past (Beck & Alford, 1988). We would not expect distress in an infant to be accompanied by ruminative thoughts about why negative events have happened and one's role in those events. This requires language and a differentiated view of self and others. The adolescent, on the other hand, can relive situations and think about multiple possibilities for the future.

The basic idea here is that "Pathology can occur at any point in development and it will be different given the capacities at the time it is developed and will be transformed as later developing processes come into place." (Tronick, 2007, pp. 40–41; see also Blatt & Luyten, 2009, and Hyde et al., 2008). We have reviewed a number of temperament influences on the development of problems; these can also be related to changes with development (Rothbart & Posner, 2006). For example, temperament can influence the person's choice of environments, and these may put the person at risk for developing problems. Young children often have little choice over where they live and what they do, but with development the person has increasing control over "niche picking." The older child and adolescent will also have an established and active sense of self, and judgments about the self and others, especially evaluative ones, can serve as additional sources of stress.

Although older children and adults have more possible sources of problems, they also have more capacities for self-regulatory control over thoughts and behavior. They can use effortful control to observe the reactions of self and others, analyze them, and if necessary program different responses to them. This requires a more objective stance toward the self, and a relatively detached platform from which to observe their own and others' actions. Finally actions are practiced that are more in accordance with the person's values. As positive self-change occurs, one can also see oneself in a more positive way. This creates a process where the person creates actions and thinking in line with his or her values, and as those acts and thoughts develop, so does one's positive evaluation of the self (Rothbart, 2009).

Adult aging is also related to how the person recognizes and thinks about the emotions. In a longitudinal study of adults, Labouvie-Vief and her colleagues identified four different patterns in adults' experience and thinking about emotion (LaBouvie-Vief & Marquez, 2004). The first, or *integrated* group of adults, showed generally high positive emotion, low negative emotion, and were well adjusted socially. They were open to information and to ambiguity, and were high in empathy and well-being. Although they experienced positive emotion, they also acknowledged the negative emotions and described them as part of their lives. Their narratives about their own lives frequently included references to distress, disturbance, and repair.

Two other styles were seen as less well integrated. The *complex* group was open to emotions and ideas, complex in thinking about emotions, and tolerant of others and events, but they experienced more negative emotion and were less socially adjusted than the integrated group. These individuals appeared to be devoting themselves "to cope with a core sense of social inadequacy and isolation" (Labouvie-Vief & Marquez, 2004, p. 256) and often were seekers of personal growth. The *self-protective* group was high on positive emotion and saw their social relations as positive, but also showed high conformity, denial and repression of negative emotions, low tolerance of depressive mood, and a striking lack of empathy. The self-protective group differed from the integrated and complex groups in their treatment of negative emotion; in the integrated group, negative emotion was recognized as a part of life; in the complex group, negative emotion was heightened; and in the self-protective group, negative emotion was avoided or denied. In the fourth, the *dysregulated* group, there was both low recognition of emotion and low socioemotional adjustment (Labouvie-Vief & Medler, 2002). I suspect that the fourth group may be further divided into those who are low in recognition of emotion and highly intellectual in coping, and those who are low in recognition of emotion and simplified in their thinking about positive and negative emotions. It would be very interesting to see how temperament might influence the development of these styles.

In Labouvie-Vief's (2008) research on development over the lifespan, the integrated group increased in size from 14% of the 10- to 30-year-olds to 43% of both middle age and older individuals, indicating increases in mature thinking over time. The dysregulated group also decreased from 44% in the young to 30% in the middle age to 26% in the older group (Labouvie-Vief & Medler, 2002). Older adults showed the fewest members in the complex, more negative group (moving from 35 to 47 to 18%), and their percentage increased in the self-protective group, moving from 17 to 26 to 57% (Labouvie-Vief, 2008). Overall, aging has been associated with increased positive emotion and well-being (Carstensen, 1992), and this could result from either more integrated or more self-protective thinking. One other strategy may be to choose social networks to make positive emotion more likely and negative emotion less likely (Carstensen, 1993; Carstensen, Gross, & Fung, 1998), or to simplify one's life so that fewer stressors are experienced (Baltes & Baltes, 1990; Labouvie-Vief, 1999).

To look at the development of reactivity and regulation across the lifespan, we must consider the whole range of capacities of the person at the time a problem develops, including ideas about the self and strategies adapted from the past. Even if a person has escaped early insecurity, problems may develop later, as the older child's self-concept and ideas about others and the world develop (Davis-Kean et al., 2008). Consistencies in self-concept can be a force for stability in problem behavior as well as for more positive behavior: Bates finds that working with 3- to 6-year-olds on conduct problems is often preferable to working with older children. The older children have a more highly developed idea of who they are, and may resist change based on the ideas they have about themselves (Bates, personal communication, 2010). I now turn to studies designed to understand the development of behavior problems and of mood and personality disorders. Again, both the temperament of the child and environmental shaping of the child's experience will contribute to these problems.

INDIVIDUAL DIFFERENCES IN STRESS REACTIVITY

Environmental stressors have been linked to the development of many problems in the developing child and adult. However, both the experience of an event as stressful and the child's coping strategies to it will be influenced by the child's temperament (Boyce & Ellis, 2005; Lengua & Long, 2002). Lengua and her colleagues studied temperament in relation to 8- to 12-year-olds' coping with stressors such as parental divorce (Lengua et al., 1999; Lengua & Long, 2002). Children who were higher in negative emotionality evaluated these events as more negative, suggesting that they were experiencing higher levels of stress. Children high in negative emotionality also tended to use avoidant coping strategies (e.g., avoiding thinking about a subject, avoidant actions). Temperamental positive emotionality, on the other hand, predicted both a lower experience of threat and more active coping. Attention control, a component of temperamental effortful control, also predicted more active coping strategies, including decision making, control strategies, direct problem solving, seeking understanding, and positive restructuring of the event. Temperament thus influences both the meaning of an event to the child and the strategies the child uses to cope with that event.

EXTERNALIZING AND INTERNALIZING PATTERNS

Active, assertive versus avoidant coping leads us back to the externalizing and internalizing patterns of adaptation we have previously identified as early in life as Tronick's (2007) observations of infant coding. These two forms of coping are also linked to adult disorders. In factor-analytic studies, Kreuger and Markon (2006) identified two major dimensions of adult psychopathology that they labeled internalizing and externalizing, which I further discuss in Chapter 10. The reader will recall that internalizing and externalizing factors have been found in some of the earliest research on behavior problems in children. Burt (1937), for example, discovered a more specific factor than that of negative emotionality. One pole of this factor was oriented toward "submissiveness, sorrow, tenderness, and disgust, in a word, towards repressive or inhibitive emotions. [The other pole] predisposes people towards assertive, angry, sociable, and inquisitive behavior, in short, towards active or aggressive conduct" (p. 182).

These two forms of negative emotion and coping differ in their assertiveness and attempts at active control versus inhibition and withdrawal. Anger/irritability and aggression are assertive negative emotions; fear, shyness, and sadness are more nonassertive negative emotions. In the still-face procedure described earlier in this chapter, Tronick (2007) saw both assertive and nonassertive patterns in infant emotion and coping. Internalizing and externalizing problems have also emerged in factor analyses of behavior problems in children (Achenbach & Edelbrock, 1978), and the resulting Child Behavior Checklist is widely used in developmental and child-clinical research. Assertive and nonassertive negative emotion factors have been found in both child and adult temperament and personality (Evans & Rothbart, 2007; Victor et al., 2006).

Externalizing behavior problems are directed outward against others and the environment, and include aggressive and antisocial behavior, delinquency, conduct disorder, and attention-deficit/hyperactivity disorder. Internalizing behavior involves more self-directed mood and body states, including anxiety, depression, social withdrawal, and bodily complaints. Scores on externalizing and internalizing factors are substantially related to each other, and a number of children and adults show both externalizing and internalizing problems (Achenbach & Edelbrock, 1978; Krueger & Markon, 2006).

Why might internalizing (nonassertive coping) and externalizing (assertive coping) problems be found in the same person? One possibility is that both reactions involve defense against threat or loss; they chiefly differ in whether there is active confrontation and assertion (externalizing) or nonassertive withdrawal or inhibition (internalizing). Externalizing reactions are related to surgent temperament tendencies, and involve action against perceived obstacles or threat (Rothbart & Bates, 2006). Internalizing reactions of fear, anxiety, withdrawal, and avoidance are related to low surgency and do not involve confrontation. Internalizing reactions appear to be linked to a judgment (not necessarily a conscious one) that one does not have the power or resources to contend directly with the problem. The person is then likely to withdraw, avoid the threat, inhibit action, or "give up." In externalizing reactions, the person appears to feel some possibility of being effective or in control, and acts in an outward direction.

Depending on the problem and the person's current judgments about whether he or she can actively cope with it, externalizing and internalizing behaviors may thus be shown one after another or in various mixtures. After the loss of a loved one, for example, a person may at first deny the loss, then rage against its having happened. Later, the person appears worn out by the active distress and outward action, and realizes that there is nothing he or she can do about the loss. Over time, the person thus shows denial, anger, sorrow, and depression in a mixture of internalizing and externalizing reactions, and these reactions may alternate over a day's, week's, or month's time. If we view internalizing and externalizing emotions as involving low versus high perceived power over events, we can also better understand why conduct disorders and antisocial behavior (both assertive reactions) are related, as are fear, anxiety, sadness, and depression (nonassertive reactions). We may also think about how a child may be highly assertive in a familiar situation (e.g., the home) while much less assertive in a more threatening and unfamiliar situation (e.g., a new school).

INTERVENTIONS AND PREVENTION

In this section, I describe some of the programs based on ideas of temperament and attention that may be useful for both preventing problems and ameliorating them once they have occurred. I begin by considering the possibility that executive attention can be trained in young children.

Training Attention

At Oregon, we have developed a 5-day attention-training program to test whether executive attention in young children could be strengthened (Rueda, Rothbart, McCandliss, Saccomanno, & Posner, 2005). We examined the effects of this training in children during a period of rapid development of executive attention, presenting the program to 4-year-olds and 6-year-olds. Our computer-based training program was based on methods used by Duane Rumbaugh and David Washburn (1992) to train executive attention in rhesus monkeys for more efficient performance in space flights.

We adapted the monkey exercises to children by making them part of an interesting story. In the first training exercise, a cat on the video screen (called "cat") was moved around the screen with a joystick. Training began as children learned to use the joystick to move the cat to an area of grass, avoiding an area of mud (children were told that the cat likes grass and flowers, but doesn't like mud). Over a series of trials, the area of grass became smaller and the area of mud increased, requiring greater control of the cursor to bring the cat to the grass. Once skill with the cursor was developed, children learned to predict the movement of a duck across a pond. The duck moved either above the water, or below the water, where the children could not see the duck's movement. Children were also given exercises in working memory and practice in resolving cognitive conflict. Children who had five training sessions were then compared to a randomly selected control group that interacted with child-appropriate videos for the same amount of time.

Before and after training, children were given the ANT for children, and EEG brain activity was recorded (Rueda et al., 2005). Children who had received the training showed improvement in the executive attention network in the EEG measures whereas control children did not. For trained 6-year-olds, EEG patterns during the ANT resembled patterns of ACC activation found in adults. In the 4-year-olds, training had a greater influence on ACC locations related to emotional control. The trained children also showed increases on a measure of intelligence (the K-Bit Test: Kaufman & Kaufman, 1990) when compared to control children, suggesting that training had quite general effects on children's cognitive processing (Rueda et al.). Parents did not report changes in children's temperament over the course of the training, but since the CBQ (Rothbart et al., 2001) asks about the child's behavior over the last 6 months, its time scale would not be sensitive to change over such a short period.

Recently a replication and extension of this study was carried out with 5-year-olds in a Spanish preschool (Rueda, Checa, & Santonja, 2008). Several exercises were added to strengthen training and 10 days of attention training were given. As in the United States, the control group interacted with child-appropriate videos for the same amount of time. A follow-up assessment was also given 2 months after training. Both training and control groups showed improvement in intelligence scores and in executive attention as measured by the ANT immediately following training. The training group, however, maintained their improvement over the 2-month follow-up period, whereas the control group did not. Attention training also improved children's performance on tasks requiring emotion regulation and self-control, including delay of reward and children's gambling tests.

The attention-training program has also been adapted to children with autism and children diagnosed with attention-deficit/hyperactivity disorder (Tamm et al., 2008). In addition, other training programs in the schools (e.g., Diamond et al., 2007) have successfully improved self-regulation in young children. In these Tools of the Mind programs (Bodrova & Leong, 2007), children are given concrete aids to help them organize their work (e.g., putting on a pair of lensless eyeglasses to give the children "editor's eyes"). Wearing the glasses encourages careful and disciplined written work. Imaginary play is also important; to play their roles appropriately, children need to both inhibit and activate actions (Bodrova & Leong). In doctor–patient play, for example, the child playing the patient must resist taking the stethoscope away from the child who is playing the doctor. As children's pretend play becomes more complex, children have additional opportunities to practice self-regulation.

Research in both laboratory and school thus indicates that attention is trainable, and Lengua's (2007, 2008) identification of the preschool age as sensitive for the development of effortful control suggests that preschool and kindergarten programs may be especially useful sites for attention-training programs (Posner & Rothbart, 2007a). Programs designed to inform children, parents, and teachers about individual differences in temperament have also had positive effects, and we now turn to two such approaches.

A Temperament Program
for the Elementary School Classroom

A program for school-age children is used to educate children, parents, and teachers about temperament. Sandee McClowry and her associates tested a temperament-based program called INSIGHTS in inner-city New York schools (McClowry, Snow, & Tamis-LeMonda, 2005), where the program led to decreases in children's behavior problems. The INSIGHTS program is offered to first- and second-grade children, their teachers, and parents. In this program, parents and teachers are given information about temperament and encouraged to support the temperamental individuality of their own and other children. They are also taught strategies for preventing and dealing with behavior problems related to temperament. Finally, they are taught positive parenting strategies that are likely to benefit children regardless of temperament.

Adults are taught to recognize the temperament qualities of each child, and to understand that no temperament is ideal for all situations. They are also shown videotapes of children who differ in temperament. The adults take part in discussions and role playing, and are given general information about temperament and take-home assignments. Teachers are also given information on the research studies that provide the foundation for INSIGHTS. Teachers and parents are trained to use their understanding of temperament to gain the compliance of their children. They are also encouraged to recognize and support their children's needs for independence, and to promote responsibility and positive habits in children regardless of their temperament.

In the part of the program designed for school-age children, four puppets are used to personify temperament characteristics. The puppets are Fredrico the Friendly (a surgent puppet), Gregory the Grumpy (an angry and irritable puppet), Hilary the Hard Worker (high in effortful control), and Coretta the Cautious (a fearful puppet). Puppets and children work together to solve daily social dilemmas; the puppets also talk to the children about individual differences in temperament. In solving dilemmas, children gain practice for improving their own interactions with parents, teachers, and friends. Classes are also designed to enhance children's empathy skills, their appreciation of the uniqueness of family members, friends, and teachers, and their use of problem solving to deal with daily problems.

Although the program was used with regular first- and second-grade inner-city classrooms, fully 28% of the children were identified at the beginning of INSIGHTS as showing disruptive (externalizing) behavior problems. Effects of the program were compared with a reading-aloud control group. Both programs led to a decrease in behavior problems, but greater reductions were found for the INSIGHTS group than for the control children. Children in INSIGHTS who had been diagnosed with disruptive problems showed the greatest decreases in problems. The evaluation of the INSIGHTS program suggests the usefulness of including temperament information in child, parent, and teacher training.

Parenting Training and Support: Birth To Three for New Parents

Finally, I would like to present an example of a parent education and support program grounded in temperament that extends from infancy through the preschool years. Birth To Three, a program based on information about temperament and child development, also offers the important addition of the social support of other parents, creating a caring and informed community for parents. The three founders of Birth To Three, Minalee Saks, Sue Kelly, and Andie Fischoff, were involved in our home-based observational study of temperament in the 1970s (Rothbart, 1986). During their home visits, they met parents who were often living far from their families, who were lonely and in need of information and support in raising their children. Kelly and Fischoff, the home observers, and Saks, the mother of one of the infants in the study, decided there was something they could do about the problem. They submitted a grant proposal to the U.S. Department of Health, Education, and Welfare, and with government funding, Birth To Three was born. Birth To Three is now 30 years old, and has served over 80,000 families locally. The program's curriculum is also used in over 800 sites in the United States and in 13 other countries.

Birth To Three offers new parents information on services for young families and the opportunity to join a parent support group. The parenting groups are formed based on the date of a child's birth, so that each group will include a range of socioeconomic status, culture, and education. Three age-graded programs for newborns, infants, and toddlers are available. Infants often attend meetings with their parents, and the older children play in a separate room, providing a real-life laboratory for observing children's temperament. At Birth To Three meetings, parents are offered information about child development. They are also able to discuss this material and any problems that have developed with their own children with a facilitator and other parents. The social support aspect of Birth To Three's program has been very successful, and groups originally based on the infant's date of birth have continued to meet well beyond the first 3 years of the children's lives. Some groups have continued to meet after their children have gone to college and out into the working world.

In the series of 10 Birth To Three meetings for each age group, parents are asked to think about what their children need to learn about the world as they grow up, and how they as parents can guide their children toward appropriate learning. They are also encouraged to think about how much *they as parents* need to learn about child development to respond appropriately to the child. Parents are encouraged to inhibit some of their more automatic responses, especially angry ones, to the behavior of their children. Instead, they are encouraged to reflect on the current problem and their own contributions to it, and to see the situation as offering the possibility for more positive learning. Parents thus become more mindful of their actions, reflecting on what a particular interaction might be actually teaching the child, and realizing that what is taught is often unintended.

Weekly discussions include watching and discussing videos on brain development and caregiver–child interaction. At the end of every session, parents sing to their children, learning songs that will become part of their everyday routine. They are also given take-home assignments, some involving observation of the infant through "Baby Watch." Parent–infant play is encouraged. With the support of University of Oregon psychologists, Birth To Three's curriculum has now been published, allowing hospitals, organizations, and communities to implement the approach (see *birthto3.org*; Rothbart, 2007b). Scientists at Oregon Research Institute are now evaluating video applications of the program. Parenting programs like Birth To Three help to prevent the development of negative parent–child relationships and to promote positive ones. In fact, it is hard for me to look at intervention programs that do not begin until late childhood or adolescence without thinking there must be a way to avoid many, though not all, of these problems from developing in the first place.

SUMMARY

In this chapter I first considered how reactivity and regulation operate in a social situation, using the parent–infant interaction as an example. Social regulation operates with the newborn and is likely to continue through life. In early infancy, the parent compensates for a lack of self-regulation in the child, but over the course of development the child engages in greater self-regulation and may even offer social regulation to parents who are quarreling. Reactivity and social regulation or its lack are seen in family, among friends, and in intimate situations. I also introduced two negative emotion clusters and their related coping mechanisms that are linked to the development of emotional and conduct problems. Finally, I described three programs that have used temperament and attention ideas with newborn, preschool-age and school-age children. In Chapter 10, I offer a review of interactions between temperament and environment in predicting problems.

Temperament, Environment, and Psychopathology

Up until now I have considered individual differences in how we develop, from our early emotional reactivity and activity level to control by fear to effortful control. I have discussed the development of a sense of self and cognitive conceptions of self, and how our idea of self can be threatened in social settings. I have also shown the social adaptations occurring in the home and school, some of which will support future positive adaptations, and some of which will come to cause pain for the self and others. I have considered how problems can develop out of our temperament and our experiences. The very nature of mental and behavioral disturbance will differ with increasing capacities of the older child and adult. As representations develop, they can further add to the development of problems and solutions.

This chapter focuses on how temperament and environment work together to create problem behavior. I have used the word *psychopathology* in the title with some trepidation. Just as the field of physical medicine has been moving in a direction that "medicalizes" conditions previously viewed as within the normal range (Conrad, 2007), there has also been a tendency to "pathologize" temperamental characteristics that do not agree with our cultural image of the ideal child (Carey, 1998). Judging shyness or extremes in infant distress to be pathological conditions are two such examples. Here the term "psychopathology" refers to mental or behavioral problems or disorders, and I review both direct links between temperament and behavior problems, and also the way problems develop in interaction with the child's experience of the social environment.

TEMPERAMENT, PERSONALITY, AND PSYCHOPATHOLOGY

It has been proposed that temperament provides the foundation for psychopathology (Watson, Kotov, & Gamez, 2006), and it has also been proposed that personality provides the building blocks of psychopathology (Markon, Krueger, & Watson, 2005). In our understanding of how problems develop and our definition of personality as including representations of self and others, both views are probably correct. Problems can develop out of unregulated negative emotion and temperament-related behavior as early as infancy. Problems can also develop out of cognitions of the self and others that lead to unregulated negative emotion or behavior in later childhood or adulthood. Temperament provides the initial dispositions toward the development of problems, but the child's experiences and developing understanding of the meaning of events (personality) will strongly influence development, adaptive or maladaptive. This chapter is organized around (1) direct relations between temperament and problem development, and (2) interactions between temperament and environment in promoting problem behavior.

DIRECT RELATIONS BETWEEN TEMPERAMENT AND PROBLEM DEVELOPMENT

During the past decade, research has focused on how the dimensions of temperament are related to the development of disorder. A number of the relations between temperament and problem development can be seen in Figure 10.1. This figure shows links found between temperament in childhood and internalizing and externalizing problems in early adolescence.

Ormel et al. (2005), for example, used the Early Adolescent Temperament Questionnaire-Revised (EATQ-R; Ellis et al., 2004) at ages 10–11 years and predicted the development of behavior problems at 12–14 years. Anger/frustration at the younger age predicted both externalizing and internalizing, whereas fear predicted internalizing and lower externalizing problems. Surgency at the younger age predicted later externalizing problems (aggression and conduct problems) and fewer internalizing problems (fear, sadness, low self-esteem). Affiliativeness predicted both lower externalizing and higher internalizing problems (Ellis et al.). Effortful control appeared to regulate both negative emotion and activity, and protected against both kinds of behavior problems as the children developed.

I now consider each of these temperament dimensions and their relations with the development of problems. These include negative emotionality and its facets of anger, fear and anxiety, surgency/extraversion, affiliative-

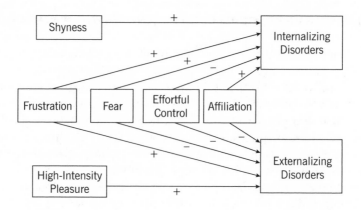

FIGURE 10.1. Temperament in relation to developing behavior problems.

ness, and effortful control; later in the chapter I consider how these dimensions interact with the child's environment in the development of problems.

Negative Emotionality

Temperamental negative emotionality has frequently been linked to the development of later problems and disorders (Waldman, Singh, & Lahey, 2006; see review by Rothbart & Bates, 2006). In factor analysis of personality and disorder measures, negative emotion was linked to both internalizing and externalizing disorders (Markon et al., 2005). Negative reactivity in infancy has also been found to predict internalizing and externalizing problems in adulthood. In the Uppsala longitudinal study, negative emotional reactivity as reported by parents of 10- to 15-month-olds predicted self-reported internalizing and externalizing problems of their children when they were 21 years old (Hagekull & Bohlin, 2008). Negative reactivity predicted both internalizing and externalizing problems, but showed a stronger relationship to internalizing. Links between negative reactivity in infancy and the development of problems in childhood have also been reported. Kagan, Snidman, Zentner, and Peterson (1999), for example, found that highly (negatively) reactive infants at 4 months showed more fearful inhibition at 4 years, and more anxious symptoms at age 7.

Fear and Anger

Within negative emotionality, there are two major pathways to problems: fear and the internalizing emotions, and anger and the externalizing emotions (Rothbart & Bates, 2006). In predicting problems from infant negative emotions, the closest links are found between fear and the internalizing disorders, and anger/irritability and externalizing. Fear also has a negative relation to externalizing, with higher fear often predicting *lower* externalizing, protecting against the development of aggression and conduct problems (see review in Rothbart & Bates). In our research, infants' fearfulness in the laboratory during the first year of life predicted mothers' reports of lower aggression, impulsivity, and activity at age 7 (Rothbart et al., 2000). Fearfulness in infancy also predicted the socializing emotions of guilt, shame, and empathy (Rothbart, Ahadi, et al., 1994). These emotions can also serve to counteract conduct problems. I also noted in Chapter 7 that fear is related to the early development of conscience (Kochanska, 1995), and shyness (social fear) is related to lower aggressive behavior as well as lower prosocial behavior in preschool (Russell, Hart, Robinson, & Olsen, 2003).

The internalizing disorders have been further divided into those that involve fear reactivity to specific cues (e.g., the phobias and panic disorder) and those involving a generalized anxious and depressed disposition to distress (e.g., general distress proneness/dysthymia, major depression, general anxiety disorder and PTSD (Walker, Toufexis, & Davis, 2003; Krueger, 1999; Watson, 2005). In development, fear reactivity is seen as preceding anxiety/depression, with the idea that traumatic experiences may lead to more generalized anxiety or depression, especially for those who are more fearful to begin with (Rosen & Schulkin, 1998). Anxiety and depression are experienced over a much longer period and over a wider range of situations than simple fear to a specific threat, and both anxiety and depression can involve ruminating over pieces of information.

Surgency

Temperamental surgency predicts later problems, with exuberance (surgency) in infancy positively predicting externalizing problems (Martin & Fox, 2006). Surgency is related to the assertiveness of the child's response, and that response may include anger or aggression. In our research, infant surgency predicted children's greater aggressiveness at ages 6–7 years (Rothbart et al., 2000). Hagekull (1994) also found that children's early impulsivity predicted later externalizing, but not internalizing problems. Early activity level predicted later higher externalizing and lower internalizing problems, and negative reactivity predicted both kinds of problems.

Surgency is positively related to anger, aggression, and externalizing problems, but appears to be negatively related to internalizing problems, especially to depressed mood (Caspi, 1995; Tellegen, 1985). The surgent emotions appear to bias the child toward assertive negative emotion and against nonassertive negative emotion. Also, because positive and sociable infants are especially likely to elicit positive reactions in adults, they may be more likely to develop supportive relationships with other adults. Positive relationships with a supportive adult, who need not be the parent, can protect children from developing problems even when they have grown up under considerable adversity and risk (Rutter, 1989; Werner & Smith, 1982).

The positive emotions and sociability can also protect against problems in institutionalized children, where children may be neglected unless they offer pleasure and positive experiences to overworked staff (Werner & Smith, 1982). The more positive child may also develop more active styles of coping. Werner and Smith found links between children's early coping skills and their later adjustment, and in Chapter 6, I noted that positive emotionality is related to both lower appraisal of threat and more active coping in children (Lengua et al., 1999; Lengua & Long, 2002).

Affiliativeness and the Development of Problems

As seen in Figure 10.1, affiliativeness in the EATQ-R was positively related to internalizing problems and *negatively* related to externalizing problems (Ellis et al., 2004). Affiliation puts adolescents at risk for problems like depressed mood, while at the same time protecting against externalizing problems. It is not surprising that affiliative caring about others would help the person inhibit actions likely to hurt others (lower externalizing) but how might affiliativeness contribute to greater internalizing? Depression often develops after the experience of a loss through rejection, abandonment, divorce, desertion, or death (Brown, Bifulco, & Harris, 1987), and those who are more strongly affiliative may simply suffer more from a social loss. If one strongly seeks to be loved, the loss of love and experience of rejection will have more serious effects. Affiliative children and adolescents may also have developed coping strategies that involve others, such as identifying with others' strengths or becoming dependent on others for help, support, and regulation. These coping strategies would make the loss of the other person particularly difficult.

Agency, Communion, and the Personality Disorders

Horowitz (2004) described how personality disorders emerge out of interpersonal relations and temperament. Personality disorders, such as the dependent, avoidant, paranoid, and antisocial disorders, are seen to develop out of personality traits and coping strategies that have been maintained over time. These traits may have been adaptive at first, for example, when the young child's dependency on others yields help and support. When the situation has changed or the trait no longer leads to satisfaction, however, problems may develop. Horowitz's model is organized over two broad dimensions, communion and agency. They are also related to the two issues of autonomy and independence versus closeness with others that I considered earlier in infant development.

In Horowitz's (2004) model, the antisocial or paranoid person is high in agency and low in communion. In avoidant, schizotypal, or schizoid personality disorders, both agency and communion are low, and in borderline disorder and histrionic personality, both agency and communion are high. The dependent and avoidant disorders are linked to low agency and high communion. These tendencies can become goals in themselves. Thus the communion-oriented child may use agency skills to achieve at school in order to please his or her parents. In temperament, the more internalizing emotions and low surgency may predispose toward dependent and avoidant disorders, and the externalizing emotions toward paranoid and antisocial disorders. Exactly how these tendencies will develop will vary from person to person, but they further emphasize that coping is fundamentally social and involves one's orientations to others in ways that can be adaptive or maladaptive. Another exciting area for development involves parents' and teachers' promotion of *autonomy*.

Effortful Control Protects against Problem Development

If problems are more likely to develop in children high in negative emotion or surgency, then we would expect the child's self-regulative capacities, including effortful control, to help protect against problems. Higher effortful control, in fact, predicts fewer problems in development, although it is more strongly related to protecting against externalizing problems (Eisenberg et al., 1998; Lengua, 2003; Morris et al., 2002; review by Muris & Ollendick, 2005). Effortful control also protects against the effects of early negative emotionality on later problems (Eisenberg et al., 1996; Rothbart & Bates, 2006). Effortful control supports children's use of more positive alternatives to problem behavior, such as compliance, empathy, and social competence (Eisenberg et al., 2003; Kochanska, 1997). When a child can inhibit tendencies toward anger and avoidance, he or she can instead focus on the needs of others and on repairing current problems.

Effortful control also contributes to children's school readiness and success, and to their social skills at school (Blair & Razza, 2007; Checa, Rodriguez-Bailon, & Rueda, 2008; Rueda, Checa, & Santonja, 2008; Valiente, Lemery-Chalfant, Swanson, & Reiser, 2008). Finally, effortful control contributes to children's positive adjustment and active coping (Lengua, 2002;

Lengua & Long, 2002; review by Eisenberg, Fabes, Guthrie, & Reiser, 2000). Although active coping is usually seen as a positive reaction to bad situations, we need to remember that this may not be the case in highly dangerous environments (Tolan & Grant, 2009). Active coping in response to urban violence, for example, contributes to increased externalizing problems (Rosario et al., 2003), whereas the avoidant coping that is linked to poorer outcomes in relatively safe environments is associated with more positive outcomes in dangerous ones. Tolan and Grant conclude that "Adopting a more realistic . . . view that 'there is little one can do to change things' may serve individuals better when facing great stress than to insistently attempt to change circumstances beyond their control or to consider a given event's occurrence and impact as one's personal responsibility" (p. 67).

Because effortful control is so important to development, Lengua and her colleagues have studied factors that might influence its development. In both preschool-age children and 8- to 12-year-olds, she found that environmental factors, including family income, parent education, neighborhood, negative life events, family conflict, maternal depression, and quality of parenting, were related to lower effortful control in children. Although environmental influences did not predict growth in effortful control between 8 and 12 years (Lengua, 2006, 2008; Lengua, Bush, Long, Trancik, & Kovacs, 2008), environmental factors were both related to the child's current level of effortful control, *and* predicted increases in effortful control over the preschool years (Lengua, 2007; Lengua, Honorado, & Bush, 2007). Mothers' appropriate setting of limits and support of their child's autonomy also predicted increases in effortful control over this time. These findings suggest that effortful control may be particularly sensitive to parenting and environmental influences during the preschool years, and we know that this is also a time when some of the greatest increases in effortful control are taking place (Rothbart & Rueda, 2005).

INTERACTIONS BETWEEN TEMPERAMENT
AND PARENTING IN DEVELOPMENT
OF BEHAVIOR PROBLEMS

Jack Bates and I wrote reviews for the *Handbook of Child Psychology* in 1998 and again in 2006 (Rothbart & Bates, 2006). Jack wrote the sections on development of adjustment in children, and one of the processes he was especially interested in was how temperament and environment might interact with each other, that is, how the effect of one factor (e.g., high vs. low negative emotionality) might be dependent on the characteristics of the other (e.g., good vs. poor parenting) in the development of problems. In our 1998 review there were very few examples of interaction. In our review of temperament and adjustment in 2006, however, a substantial number of interactions were found (Rothbart & Bates, 2006). The effect of one influence, such as poor parenting, on the child's behavior often depended on the temperament of the child: children who were high in negative emotionality were more strongly affected by poor parenting in the development of problems. Both temperament and environmental factors thus contribute to problems in children's coping, and each can heighten or diminish the effects of the other.

Interactions are difficult to detect, requiring replications and large samples of subjects. They are important, however, because they allow us to get away from a view of *either* temperament *or* environment being responsible for the development of problems. Instead, they let us understand that a given situation may present more challenges to one child than another, based on temperament. In addition, the effects of temperament on the development of problems can be tempered or moderated by good parenting.

In the next section, I consider temperament–environment interactions as they relate to the development of externalizing and internalizing problems. This section should be considered along with the gene–environment interactions discussed in Chapter 3. In those studies, the genes stand in for temperament, and it is possible to look at the outcomes for a child with a given genetic background depending on that child's experiences in development. I now begin with effects on externalizing problems.

Externalizing Problems

In general, poor-quality parenting (parent hostility, marital conflict) and low positive parenting seem to intensify externalizing problems for children who are already at temperamental risk by being high in negative emotionality (Calkins & Fox, 2002; Morris et al., 2002; Tschann, Kaiser, Chesney, Alkon, & Boyce, 1996). When children are less prone to the negative emotions, the quality of parenting does not appear to influence the development of externalizing problems (Belsky, Hsieh, & Crnic, 1998; Stoolmiller, 2001; Wills, Sandy, Yaeger, & Shinar, 2001).

At the same time, however, children who are negative and unregulated may themselves contribute to poor parenting. For example, parents of children with conduct problems are more likely to reject or punish their children. However, when boys with conduct problems were observed interacting with their own and with other mothers, *both* the biological and non-biological mothers directed more commands and negative responses toward the boys with conduct problems (Anderson, Lytton, & Romney, 1986). These findings suggest that the children were at least to some extent driving the adults' behavior.

How might children's temperament affect adult–child interaction? Lee and Bates (1985) observed mothers' interactions with 2-year-olds in their homes when the mothers were trying to control their child's troublesome behavior. More distress-prone children approached trouble more often, and they tended to resist their mother's attempts to control them. Their mothers were also more likely to use aversive discipline. These interactions resembled the coercive cycle of parent–child interaction described in socially aggressive boys and their mothers (Patterson, 1979, 1980). Coercive cycles are seen when child and parent alternate in using pain to control the other, increasing levels of hostility and aggression with each cycle. Children's aversive behavior can encourage their mothers to use aversive discipline, and the mother may ultimately withdraw from the interaction, leading to the development of coercive relationships and to children's problems with aggression and lack of self-regulation (Lee & Bates).

Parents and their biological children also share in their genetic endowment, and they may also share dispositions to assertive negative emotion. If aggressive children's parents are also more aggressive, they may try to control their children's behavior by inflicting pain, further contributing to coercive cycles. The child's problem behavior can thus lead to poorer parenting, which in turn leads to greater problems in regulation. Lengua (2006; Lengua & Kovacs, 2005) found that over time, irritability in the child predicted greater rejection and inconsistent discipline from parents, which in turn predicted greater irritability in the child.

Internalizing Problems

There appear to be different parent influences on the development of children's inhibited (internalizing) behavior than on externalizing (Rothbart & Bates, 2006). Arcus (2001) found that highly reactive younger infants were less likely to show fearful inhibition at 14 months if their mothers had been high in setting limits or if they had interfering siblings. She suggests that firm mothers and intrusive siblings present more challenges to the fearful infant's self-regulatory abilities than would a more accommodating environment. Belsky et al. (1998) found that infants high in negative emotion were less inhibited at 3 years if their fathers were more negative and less positive; fathers had no influence on infants who were low in temperamental negativity. In the Uppsala study, infants who were high in negative emotion tended to show greater internalizing problems as adults, but those distress-prone children who had been in day care showed fewer problems than those who had not (Hagekull & Bohlin, 2008). No effects of day care were found for children who were low in negative emotion. Chess and Thomas (1984) also reported that withdrawing children developed best when parents provided repeated and firm, but not overwhelming, challenges to their children.

Thus moderately challenging situations appear to reduce the likelihood of inhibition and internalizing. Both setting limits, without hostility, for more aggressive children and providing graded challenges for more fearful children appear to be helpful approaches for parents. Parents may also ask themselves, "What is my child learning in this interaction?" The child may be learning that aggression works or that an appeal to parents leads to their assistance whenever there is a problem. By changing their own attitudes and behavior, the parent who asks this question may be able to repair some of these outcomes in the future.

Effortful Control and Parenting

Although negative emotionality heightens the effects of poor parenting on externalizing, effortful control appears to protect or buffer the child against poor parenting. Morris and his colleagues found that children rated by their mothers as high in effortful control showed less effect of mothers' hostility on their externalizing problems in school (Morris et al., 2002). Rubin, Burgess, Dwyer, and Hastings (2003) found that when children's parenting was poor, children's 2-year-old self-regulation predicted lower externalizing problems at age 4; when parenting was good, children's earlier self-regulation was not related to their development of problems.

Can parenting compensate for deficiencies in children's effortful control? There is some evidence that it can. For highly impulsive adolescents, higher parent control and support are associated with lower antisocial behavior (Stice & Gonzales, 1998). Parent management may also lessen the likelihood that children's low self-control will lead to problems. However, high levels of parent control may not be ideal for all children: High maternal control with highly manageable children has been linked to children's development of greater externalizing behavior (Bates, Pettit, Dodge, & Ridge, 1998).

Effortful Control and Resiliency

How do we account for resiliency in children who have grown up in adverse environments, but do not seem to have developed problems (Garmezy, 1974; Masten, 2001; Werner & Smith, 1982)? Children's effortful control may be particularly important in the development of resiliency. Gardner, Dishion, and Connell (2008), for example, found that effortful control protected against the effects of belonging to delinquent or deviant peer groups in young people (see also Goodnight, Bates, Newman, Dodge, & Pettit, 2006). Lengua and Long (2002) found that when children were low in self-regulation, family stress led to greater internalizing problems than when the children were high in self-regulation. Effortful control also promotes prosocial behavior, even when parenting is not ideal. Parents' negative emotion, for example, is associated with greater sympathy in the child, but only when the child is high in effortful control (Valiente et al., 2004).

Can there be too much self-regulation? I believe the answer is yes. When fear or effortful control is used to develop rigid and inflexible responses that protect the child from information or experience, the Blocks' concept of *ego control* comes into play. Jack and Jeanne Block found that a moderate amount of ego control is related to adjustment (Block & Block, 1980), but that low or high levels of ego control were related to problems. They also studied *ego resiliency*, the ability to flexibly change the amount of control used in challenging versus playful situations. Higher levels of resiliency are related to adjustment, and also to flexible and adaptive responses to challenge and change. In the Blocks' view, one can never have too much ego resiliency, although even high resiliency can support problems. In Woody Allen's 1983 movie *Zelig*, the title character was so flexible in adapting to and conforming with others that there seemed to be no core of consistency in his behavior at all.

Affiliativeness, Parenting, and Problems

Agreeableness or affiliativeness (involvement with and caring about others) can also protect against the development of problems when parenting is poor. For children low in agreeableness, parents' angry discipline was more strongly related to behavior problems than when children were highly agreeable (Prinzie, Onghena, & Hellinckx, 2003). Highly agreeable children also showed lower externalizing whether discipline was angry or not. In our research on early adolescence and behavior problems (Ellis et al., 2004), affiliativeness protected against externalizing problems, but put children at risk for developing internalizing problems.

When both fear and affiliativeness are very low, the *callous–unemotional* trait may also be observed (see review in Rothbart & Bates, 2006). Callous–unemotional behavior in children is similar to psychopathic behavior in adults (Glenn et al., 2007), and it involves manipulation of others as well as a lack of empathy, anxiety, and guilt. It appears to depend more on low affiliativeness and low fear than on impulsivity or effortful control. In research on parenting and the callous–unemotional trait, children who were *low* in callous–unemotionality were more affected by poor parenting, but the quality of parenting did not influence outcomes for children high on callous–unemotionality (Wooten et al., 1997).

Until now, we have found that a child's temperamental disposition toward problems (e.g., high negative emotionality) appears to be intensified by poor parenting. For callous–unemotionality, however, there was a different outcome: When children were *low* on the callous–unemotional scale and therefore at lower temperamental risk of problems, poorer parenting was related to the development of conduct problems. Children who were highly callous and unemotional and therefore at higher temperamental risk, were less affected by parenting as measured in this study, suggesting that for some children, parents may have difficulty in preventing the development of problems. This is an area where future work will be important in understanding the roots of callous–unemotional behavior.

Gender Influences

With the exception of higher activity level in male infants (Eaton, 1994), sex differences have rarely been found in infant assessments of temperament, but more boys than girls develop behavior problems in childhood. In addition, the problems that develop tend to differ for girls and boys. Antisocial behavior and attention-deficit/hyperactivity disorder are generally found at higher rates for boys than for girls (Eagly & Steffen, 1986), whereas girls are more likely to develop depression in early adolescence or later (Zahn-Waxler, Cole, & Barrett, 1991). In a meta-analysis of gender findings from over 200 studies of 3- to 13-year-olds, large gender differences were found on temperamental effortful control, with girls showing greater effortful control (Else-Quest, Hyde, Goldsmith, & Van Hulle, 2006). In this review, boys also showed higher surgency than girls. These differences are in keeping with the finding of aggression and conduct problems in boys. Surgency would support assertive negative emotion, and boys may also lack the effortful control capacities that would protect against the development of problems.

The picture for gender differences in the development of depression is more complex. By the age of 13, children's capacities for representing the self, tendencies to self-appraisal and rumination, as well as pubertal changes, would be added to any early temperamental vulnerabilities. In a model developed by Hyde and her colleagues (2008), girls are more prone to depression in several ways. They have more depressive cognitive styles, negative body representations, and negative effects of early puberty. These factors, in interaction with negative life events, increase the likelihood of depression in early adolescence for girls.

Block and Gjerde (1990) predicted depressive mood at age 18 from children's 3- to 4-year-old and their later 7-year-old behavior. Since depressive mood is usually linked to low self-esteem, they were surprised to find that preschool girls' *higher* self-worth, attentiveness, verbal fluency, and appropriate emotional behavior predicted higher depressive mood at age 18. At age 7, girls who would later become depressed had developed close and genuine relationships, but were also shy and liked to be alone. Boys' depressive mood at age 18, on the other hand, was predicted by their having short-lived relationships and not admitting negative feelings at 3–4 years, and by their stretching limits and trying to be the center of attention at age 7. Thus higher early regulation in girls and lower regulation in boys predicted depressive mood at age 18 (Gjerde, Block, & Block, 1988). Peer rejection may have influenced boys' development of aggression here, whereas a more highly socialized girl may be more sensitive to not living up to the cultural standard.

Positive correlations have also been found between conduct disorder and depression for preadolescent boys, but not for girls (Edelbrock & Achenbach, 1980; Puig-Antich, 1982). Patterson and Capaldi (1990) identified rejection by peers as a central influence on fourth-grade boys' depressed mood. Unregulated behavior in the boys may have led to peer rejection, which in turn was related to depressive mood. For girls, Zahn-Waxler et al. (1991) noted a vulnerability to depression in highly socialized (and presumably affiliative) girls, who might be especially saddened by social loss. Differences in boys' and girls' development of depression suggest that there are multiple pathways to similar outcomes.

The importance of the significance or meaning of an event in the development of depression has been stressed by Brown et al. (1987), Beck (1983), and others. In their models, the loss of a significant other, a job, a role, a belief, health, achievement status, and so on, and the stress related to that loss can lead to depression. For depression to occur, however, the loss needs to be highly significant in the person's view of the world. If social relations are seen as less important than job achievement and there are social losses, one may be less affected by social loss than the person for whom social relations are highly prized. Brown's model also includes general vulnerabilities to depression like low self-esteem and low social support (Brown et al.), as well as failure in achieving outside goals or relationships (Nietzel & Harris, 1990). This theory supports "vulnerability matching" in the development of depression (Hammen, 2001). As girls become more involved in careers, they may be put at a double risk of depression, having both traditional social and newer achievement-related vulnerabilities.

ATTENTION AND PSYCHOPATHOLOGY

Michael Posner has identified three attention networks, each with its own functions and brain organization (Posner & Peterson, 1990; Posner & Rothbart, 2007b). These networks are the (1) alerting, (2) orienting, and (3) executive attention networks. Individual differences in the executive attention that supports effortful control are central to children's adaptive development (Posner & Rothbart, 2007a) and help to prevent the development of psychopathology. We have also reviewed research relating attention to other disorders, and a few examples are given here (Rothbart & Posner, 2006). Attention-deficit/hyperactivity disorder (ADHD) appears to involve a deficit in alerting (Halperin & Schulz, 2006) as well as a deficit in executive attention (Johnson et al., 2008). Infants and toddlers who are higher in temperamental activity level and anger and lower in effortful control (executive functioning) are more likely to develop ADHD (Auerbach et al., 2008; Willcutt, Doyle, Nigg, Faraone, & Pennington, 2005). In keeping with their greater anger problems, children with ADHD also show general problems with emotion regulation (Pliszka, Carlson, & Swanson, 1999).

Individual differences in orienting, on the other hand, appear to be involved in anxiety disorders. Anxious individuals show difficulty orienting away from a negative target (Derryberry & Reed, 1994; Fox, Russo, Bowles, & Dutton, 2001). Autism is also related to deficits in orienting (Landry & Bryson, 2004), and schizophrenia has been associated with both deficits in orienting (Early, Posner, Reiman, & Raichle, 1989) and deficits in executive attention (Wang et al., 2005). Alexithymia, the inability to identify and communicate emotions, is also related to low effortful control (Gu et al., 2008).

We have worked with clinical researchers to identify temperament dimensions related to borderline personality disorder (Posner et al., 2002). Borderline personality disorder involves great fluctuations in emotion and difficulties in interpersonal relations. Borderline patients were compared to a control group of nondisordered individuals who had been matched on temperament dimensions. An executive attention deficit in the borderline patients was found on the ANT in comparison with controls (Posner et al.). Borderline patients also showed less activation of executive attention brain areas, particularly the ACC, when negative emotion was elicited and motor inhibition was required. Borderline patients with higher effortful control and more efficient performance on the ANT also responded more positively to therapy (Silbersweig et al., 2007).

Recent research has also linked rejection sensitivity to the borderline diagnosis. When high rejection sensitivity is combined with low executive control, borderline problems are more likely to develop (Ayduk et al., 2008). As we combine temperament and personality measures, measures of attention, and imaging studies, we will be better able to understand how disorders develop and how they may be treated. In an *Annual Review* paper, we (Posner & Rothbart, 2007b) propose a general model for psychology that links research in each of these areas.

SUMMARY

Both children's behavior problems and adult disorders are organized on internalizing and externalizing dimensions. These forms of disorder are in turn related to the more assertive and nonassertive emotions that are part of temperament. Temperament differences in interaction with parent behavior and other environmental influences are linked to the development of problems, and effortful control is important in preventing their development as well as correcting them after they have occurred. This is an area where much future research is to be expected. In our 1998 review (Rothbart & Bates, 1998), Jack Bates found very little evidence for interactions in problem development. By 2006, he found many interactions (Rothbart & Bates, 2006). Although these studies typically investigate only two influences on the development of problems, in the future we will be able to be much more specific about the temperament dimensions and the aspects of the environment that are important to development.

CHAPTER 11

Some Final Observations

At the turn of the 20th century, Milicent Shinn was the first woman to receive a doctorate at the University of California at Berkeley, and her doctoral thesis was based on extensive notes she had made on the development of her niece, Ruth. These notes were made in Ruth's home "on a fruit ranch, in the neighborhood of San Francisco Bay" (Shinn, 1909, p. 5). For a student of temperament, reading Shinn's notes offers great pleasure. In addition, her research allows us to reflect on what we have learned about temperament.

I begin by examining some of Shinn's (1909) notes on Ruth's development, followed by observations by Charles Darwin (1877) of his oldest son, William Erasmus. Darwin's observations of his son provide a strong contrast in temperament to the descriptions of Shinn's niece. I then revisit a number of the questions about temperament posed in the introduction to this book. I also consider human development more generally, placing the study of temperament and personality within more general influences on development. Finally, I discuss research directions for the future and consider the value of temperament diversity for our individual and social lives.

But first, let me introduce Ruth. From Shinn's notes, Ruth was a very positive infant from early in life. At 2 months, she smiled at faces; at 3 months, she often sat propped up among her cushions, playing with a rattle and happily vocalizing. During the fourth month, she displayed "the most vivacious delight, with smiles and movements, cooing and crowing" (1909, p. 238). Although much of Ruth's positive display was social, she showed "similar jubilant behavior when she lay by herself on bed or floor, kicking, crowing, smiling and murmuring, delighted if paid attention to, and happy if not" (p. 238). Ruth also showed little fear, suffering

> scarcely at all from timidity. With strangers, she was as a rule happy and sociable, and ready to respond with great gayety to advances toward a frolic. In the ninth and tenth months, she suffered a little from timidity to strangers, and she had a few frights from severe falls and other causes, but on the whole her absence of fear either of persons or things, was noticeable. She was not easily startled, and novel sights and sounds excited a pleasant interest instead of fear. (p. 244)

Ruth *did* object, however, when her urge to movement and activity was held in check. She objected to being restrained and disliked being dressed. Early in Ruth's development of language, she took up the word *caught* (pronounced without the *t*) to indicate that she was being held against her will. Even so, she recovered quickly from frustration and distress:

> Notes occur from time to time of crying over refusals or deprecations; hurts too were sometimes loudly lamented. But in the main, it continued true that the child threw off disagreeable feelings readily and took nothing very hard . . . would let a thing be taken forcibly from her hand with little protest, and was easily diverted. (Shinn, 1909, p. 244)

In her lack of anger and fear and her rapid recovery from distress (soothability), Ruth showed low negative emotionality and high soothability. She also showed signs of high surgency in her motor activity and positive emotion: "At three months, she liked to be tossed in her father's arms and during the fourth month, would crow and smile when she was tossed in the air, slid down one's knees, or otherwise tumbled about" (Shinn, 1909, p. 202).

In Ruth's development, high surgency and sociability did not, however, include high affiliative tendencies. Although Ruth was gregarious, she did not like to be held or to sit on anyone's lap. Once she could walk, she almost never asked to be held or carried. Because she recovered so quickly from negative emotion, Ruth also rarely needed to be consoled and appeared to see others chiefly as a source of excitement. Shinn's observations support the idea that a child can be surgent without showing strong early signs of affiliation.

Ruth showed little dependency on others and Shinn was curious about whether a need for others might ever be shown. She found it when Ruth woke from sleep and called for her mother. Ruth had considerable difficulty falling asleep, gave up her second nap quickly, and when she woke up from a nap, would often be in a state of distress. Her mother would soothe her at these times. She also began to show signs of dependency after waking, and these were specifically directed toward her mother. If her mother was not there when she woke up, Ruth would cry for her. "In the third as in the second year, the feeling of peculiar dependence on her mother seemed connected with the time of waking, rather than going to sleep" (Shinn, 1909, p. 89). These observations led Shinn to propose "the roots of the emotional relation between mother and child are struck mainly in the association of her with the vaguely but intensely susceptible states that border on sleep" (p. 291). Another possibility, however, is that dependency and related affiliation may develop from caregiver soothing, however it occurs.

Affiliation is also related to empathy. Ruth showed little empathy, and her first evidence of it was to a book describing a baby waking up in distress:

> A book had been given her in which was a little picture story of a baby who waked up and cried in her mother's absence and was cleverly tended by a clever dog. Instead of being pleased, she found it deeply pathetic, put up her lip and nearly cried over it—a striking sensibility, as she was hardly at all susceptible to imaginative sympathy. Hearing me tell her mother of it, she almost cried again. (Shinn, 1909, p. 290)

Shinn's observations raise important questions about the development of empathy in children who are rarely distressed and show little need to be soothed. Could children's moments of vulnerability provide an opportunity for learning empathy? For more exuberant, less negatively reactive children, might it be as important for the parent to be available when the child is in a needy state, as to reinforce the child for being good? Recall that Kochanska's (1995) more unfearful children were likely to develop conscience if an attachment had formed with the parent. In our studies (Rothbart, Ahadi, et al., 1994), childhood fear predicted later empathy, guilt, and shame. These findings suggest that, in addition to providing the negative affect that can support conscience, distress proneness and feelings of vulnerability may serve as a "sounding board," reflecting others' distress and supporting the desire to help them.

Ruth also expressed what might be called nonangry aggression. She did this by carrying out actions that were likely to be physically hurtful but delivered without angry intent. In Shinn's (1909) descriptions of Ruth:

> Slapping and striking, however, was from the twelfth month, a common action of this roguish roughness. At intervals during the whole of the second

and third year, the child would, when taken in arms, slap merrily at our faces, snatch at our hair, etc.; by the end of the nineteenth month, she would strike with a stick . . . and on into the fourth year. I have notes of her striking people merely because she found a convenient stick in her hand. . . . In the thirty-fourth month, she slapped her kitten sometimes, without discernable motive. I find but a single note of her ever striking in anger; this was when her grandmother held her still to be wiped, when she was in romping spirits after her bath (thirty-fifth month). (p. 394)

Because researchers can code the facial expressions and body movements of infants and young children, it would be possible to observe whether a given aggressive act is performed with the anger expression or without it. Anger-free aggression is clearly different from the child's "reactive aggression" to a hurt or slight. It may also broaden our view of "instrumental aggression," defined as goal-directed action, as when the child snatches the toy of another child. This action can take place without anger. In Ruth's case, however, the only goal seems to be carrying out the action of hitting when prompted by the presence of a stick. It might be called stimulation seeking aggression, although it probably will require a better name. It is likely related to her temperamental surgency combined with lack of fear.

There are so many other interesting observations in Shinn's notes that a long list of research questions could be generated from Shinn's (1909) observations alone. For example, Ruth, like our older more surgent son, required relatively intense soothing methods when she (rarely) became highly distressed. She was also not very much interested in the sound of words, in their meter or rhythm. She showed only a little distress from teething, a relative insensitivity to pain, and a relative insensitivity to cuddling and the "tender" emotions.

Given our approach to individual differences, we might expect that notes taken on other children would reveal considerable temperament differences from Ruth. Here, we can look in on some of Darwin's observations of his firstborn son, William Erasmus (Doddy). First, his observations on Doddy's anger:

It was difficult to decide at how early an age anger was felt. . . . When nearly four months old, and perhaps much earlier, there could be no doubt, from the manner in which the blood gushed into his whole face and scalp, that he could easily be got into a violent passion. A small cause sufficed; thus, when a little over seven months old, he screamed with rage because a lemon slipped away and he could not seize it with his hands. . . . When eleven months old, if a wrong plaything was given him, he would push it away and beat it. (as cited in Kessen, 1965, p. 121)

Doddy, in contrast to Ruth, showed a disposition toward anger, and he often combined it with physical action against an offensive object. He also showed definite fear reactions: "Before the present one [Doddy] was 4½ months old, I had been accustomed to make close to him many strange and loud noises, which were all taken as excellent jokes, but at this period I one day made a loud snoring noise which I had never done before; he instantly looked grave and then burst out crying" (as cited in Kessen, 1965, p. 121). Darwin took Doddy to the Zoological Gardens when the child was 26 months old. There, Doddy "enjoyed looking at all the animals which were like those that he knew, such as deer, antelopes, etc., and all the birds, even the ostriches, but was much alarmed at the various larger animals in cages. He often said afterwards that he wished to go again, but not to see the 'beasts in houses'" (p. 122).

In contrast to the relative lack of empathy in Ruth, empathy was seen in Doddy quite early in life. It "was clearly shown at 6 months and 11 days by his melancholy face, with the corners of his mouth well depressed, when his nurse pretended to cry" (as cited in Kessen, 1965, p. 125). Doddy also showed evidence of the "moral sense" as early as 13 months; when

> it became easy to work with his feelings and make him do whatever was wanted. At 2 years and 3 months old, he gave his last bit of gingerbread to his little sister, and then cried out with high self approbation, "Oh kind Doddy, kind Doddy." As the child was educated solely by working on his good feeling, he soon became as truthful, open, and tender as anyone could desire. (p. 126)

Although I could go on at much greater length on these observations and their relation to temperament, I will stop here to consider some of the more general issues discussed in this book, to suggest how we might place the study of temperament within a wider scientific framework, and to think about topics for future research and scholarship.

GENERAL QUESTIONS ON TEMPERAMENT

In the Introduction, I posed a number of important questions:

What are the basic dimensions of temperament?
How do they relate to human biology?
How does temperament provide the building blocks for social and personality development?
When and how do changes in temperament occur?

How does the balance between different temperament dimensions change with development?

How does temperament affect children's coping with and adaptations to challenge?

How do the child's constructions of self affect children's emotional life and their ability to regulate the emotions?

How does temperament affect adjustment and the development of psychopathology?

Can temperament-related interventions lead to change?

In the following sections, I summarize some of the answers to these questions.

Dimensions of Temperament

In Chapter 2, I identified a set of temperament dimensions that have emerged from questionnaire research and have been related to the biology of the organism. These include fear, frustration, surgency, affiliation, perceptual sensitivity, and effortful control. The structure of adult personality traits in the Big Five model and FFM of personality maps quite directly onto these temperament dimensions, suggesting that much of personality may develop from the biologically based core of temperament. The basic dimensions of temperament are also related to the development of behavior problems and disorders of regulation, with similarities between temperament and the structure of disorders in both childhood and adulthood.

Temperament and Experience

Temperamental dispositions are played out in the child's specific experiences in the world. If a temperament-based reaction is not elicited in a given situation (if there is no press for the reaction), the reaction will not occur and will not be represented in the child's memory or in future expectations about that situation. However, when temperament-based reactions *are* elicited, they will likely lead to coping attempts. A given coping strategy may or may not be successful, and the reaction and consequences of the coping will provide the child with further evaluative information. We may think about this information as constituting the "meaning" of situations, persons, and objects that will be carried forward to future events and generalized to similar situations. Representations and coping strategies may differ, depending on the child's temperament, the child's history of experience, and the constraints of the particular situation. Early temperament reactions themselves give meaning to objects and events, and because circumstances differ from one situation to another, an individual child will not represent every situation in the same way. As the child develops, he or she carries a host of meaning structures that have developed out of specific experiences. The child may also choose situations that are unlikely to trigger negative emotions, or be moved to a situation with less press for the reaction.

The Cognitive Level of Personality

With development, the toddler and preschool-age child also come to adopt cognitions about the self and others, and these further support the child's specific expectations, hopes, and anxieties. Self-protective strategies can now be developed for maintaining the person's constructions and view of the self in what I have called the defensive stance, and these strategies will also be influenced by temperament reactions. Temperamental dispositions are thus transformed into the cognitive levels of personality, providing conceptual levels of meaning that can operate simultaneously with emotional and behavioral reactions. Different levels of meaning may also not agree. Consider the person whose life's dream is to go into auto sales but who is temperamentally shy. This person may experience distress due to conflict between different levels of functioning, cognitive and behavioral. In adults' judgments of their own behavior, one might say, "I couldn't have hurt her; I'm a kind person" or "I just wasn't myself."

The Development of Temperament

There is continued interplay between reactivity and self-regulation in development. Self-regulation increases over time, and the self-regulatory strategies applied are likely to differ from one situation to another and from one relationship to another. In early development, the child shows skills at self-soothing and begins to develop behavior patterns that will elicit care from others. As self-regulatory aspects of fear develop, inhibiting approach, impulsive action and the expression of emotion may also result. In the toddler period and beyond, the development of effortful control allows more flexible regulation of emotions, action, and thought. Mechanisms of effortful control will ultimately allow us to observe our emotions, actions, and thoughts, and to deliberately act in ways that can change our habitual actions and our view of ourselves.

The temperament dispositions of early infancy are chiefly reactive, involving negative emotions, orienting, positive emotion, and as motor systems develop, surgency. In general, self-regulatory capacities are added to reactive ones with development, but the child's self-soothing is a notable self-regulatory exception in infancy. As inhibitory aspects of fear develop, children show a balance between the impulse to act and the tendency to hesitate or withdraw from a given situation. As effortful control develops during the preschool years, children can choose among options, inhibit a desired action or emotion, and activate actions that the child might not otherwise have chosen.

Temperament, Adaptation, and Change

Temperament plays an important role in the development of competence and social skills, and is related to the child's development of language (Dixon & Shore, 1997; Dixon & Smith, 2000) and developing cognitions about the self and the world. Although temperament itself may be relatively resistant to change, we are able to influence its expression through a choice of environment and through cognitive change in our views of the self and the world. We can also approach emotions and value-laden thoughts less seriously, letting them arise and fall within experience, and identifying less with them. When anxiety and self-defensiveness is reduced we can also become more open to the positive emotions and to feelings of affiliation with others, adopting more of an open stance. Temperament systems give us the tools for achieving greater freedom from cognitive and emotion-based limitations, and experiencing more positive lives.

TEMPERAMENT AND THE DISCIPLINES

Before addressing future research directions, I would like to consider temperament within a broader scientific framework, thinking about research questions that cut across different levels of social, psychological, and biological analysis. One of the great developmental thinkers of the past half century is the British psychologist Robert Hinde, who offers a frameworks for thinking about organisms and the environment. In Hinde's (1998) view:

> Environment not only impinges on, but also is created by, the individual at each stage in development. Individuals respond selectively to the environment, assign meanings to it, change it, and are changed by it. So far as psychological development is concerned, the most important part of that environment is constituted by other persons. Individuals interact with others, form relationships with them, and participate in groups. . . . The rub is that these aspects of behavior have become the subject matter of different disciplines—physiology, individual psychology, social psychology, sociology, anthropology, political science, and economics, among others. (p. 166)

Research at each level makes important contributions to our understanding, and a full understanding of development requires making connections between different levels (Hinde, 1998; Figure 11.1). One level of the framework can influence a quite distant level, and influence goes in both directions. Thus poverty in a family, affected by a downturn in the economy, influences the nutrition of the child and thereby affects the child's behavior and the parent–child and teacher–child interactions that support the child's relationships. An economic downturn with the threat or actu-

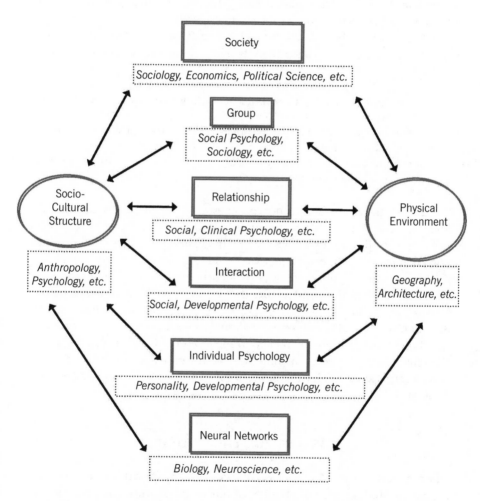

FIGURE 11.1. An adaptation of Hinde's (1998) framework for study in the human sciences. The levels of influence are listed within solid rectangles and circles; below, in dashed rectangles, are areas of study related to these influences.

ality of unemployment also increases stress levels in the parent, which in turn influence the parent's relationship to the child and the child's personality. Society is affected if children grown to adulthood are less prepared to perform work roles than previous generations. Each level can thus influence and be influenced by the others. Throughout his analysis, Hinde emphasizes the power of relationships in the home, the workplace, and the social world. In relationships, each partner contributes to the experience of the other and to the constructions one comes to hold about the self. As these experiences become consolidated, each partner has developed expectations about what the partner could (or should) do next.

Each level is also related to what Hinde (1998) calls the sociocultural structure, that is, the norms, values, beliefs, and institutional roles of a culture:

> At the individual level, these influences involve behavioral, cognitive, and affective processes, mediated (once a given stage of development is passed) by the meanings attributed to events and situations. Thus each level, including that of the individual, is to be seen not as an entity but as involving processes of continuous creation, change, or degradation through the dialectical relations within and between levels. (p. 168)

Different explanatory concepts apply at different levels of analysis, and each contributes to a better understanding of development. Conflicts between societies, for example, may be understood in terms of the history and interactions between complex communities (Niebuhr, 1932), whereas conflicts between siblings may be related to competition for the parent's attention and affection, and involve the child's views of the self and the sibling. Sibling conflicts exist at the level of the person-to-person relationship, although they are also influenced by family, societal, and sociocultural values. Temperament is chiefly related to the levels of biology, psychology, and the relationship. However, as noted in the Introduction, the temperament of a nation's leader can have important influences both within and between societies.

ISSUES FOR THE FUTURE

In an article written for the *Merrill–Palmer Quarterly's* 50th anniversary, I argued for making several changes in our research and theory that might improve our understanding of temperament (Rothbart, 2004). The first of these is the pressing need for development of a common language. Temperament dimensions are frequently given different labels in different laboratories, even though the definitions of the dimensions are very similar, and measures of the differently named dimensions are substantially intercorrelated (Goldsmith, Rieser-Danner, & Briggs, 1991). If future temperament research and reviews were to use a common language, progress could occur at a much greater speed and outside observers of the field would be less likely to view the field as confused and difficult to understand.

A second need is to make greater connections between temperament, personality, and development of the whole child:

> How do we get from initial temperament tendencies to the self-related emotions and cognitions?
>
> How do openness and effortful control interact in the course of development?
>
> How do temperament tendencies toward fear and anger/frustration, in interaction with parenting, influence development of disordered regulation and the internalizing and externalizing disorders?
>
> When personality changes, how will it affect temperament?

A third need is for longitudinal studies using multiple measures of both temperament and personality. Longitudinal research has already contributed greatly to our understanding of the development of temperament, and now we can add an investigation of the contribution of both genes and environment to developmental outcomes.

We need to be able to measure temperament in terms of both broad higher-order variables and more narrowly defined dimensions so that we can study how temperament dimensions interact with each other and environmental events in development. We have already learned that fear and anger tendencies tend to set up different routes or trajectories for the development of behavior problems, and that fear can inhibit the expression of anger. Another important research question is how social and nonsocial temperament reactions such as general fear and social fear (shyness) can be differentiated at different ages. Developmental transitions are very important, as in the development and consolidation of models of the self. When, for example, is social fear (shyness) first differentiated from fear of objects? What are the effects of cognitive models of the self on the development of social and nonsocial fear? Aksan and Kochanska (2004) have distinguished between joy toward objects and toward people in infancy, and studying similarities and differences between surgency and affiliation will also contribute to a better understanding of social and personality development.

Hinde's (1998) framework allows us to pose many additional research questions. For example, cross-cultural studies of shyness have identified links between shyness and the values of a culture. How, in addition, does culture influence the development of warm intimate relationships, leadership qualities, and political values? Studies of genetic contributions to development will also allow us to investigate interactions between genes, environment, and sociocultural values on temperament and personality outcomes.

We will probably always need more research on the components of temperament:

How does a broader temperament dimension like surgency or effortful control break down into component processes, and how are these related to individual biology?

What are the links between social fear (shyness), nonsocial fear, and cognition at different points in development?

When and how does surgent temperament diverge into its relatively socialized and unsocialized trajectories?

How do the child's structures of meaning, especially cognitions about the self and others, affect the expression of temperament, and how does temperament affect children's structures of meaning?

How is both broad and differentiated temperament related to genetic structure, and how do environmental events interact with the effects of genes to predict outcomes?

The neurosciences will continue to make contributions to our understanding of individual differences in temperament. As temperament is increasingly linked to brain structure and function, our understanding of both temperament and neuroscience will be enriched.

Research is also needed to identify discontinuities as well as continuities in temperament development. For example:

How is temperament expressed differently from one situation to another for an individual child?

Do some temperament dimensions vary more across situations than others?

How does our own variability in different situations affect how we see ourselves?

How does the cognitive self affect our behavior, and what happens when there is conflict between who the child thinks he or she is and what he or she thinks, feels, or does?

What influences people to ignore basic moral injunctions such as the Golden Rule (Pfaff, 2007)?

How do different cultures socialize temperament and how is this related to cultural values?

What happens when a child's temperament conflicts with the cultural ideal, the requirements of a school or a specific job?

Do caregiver–child "issues" differ in different cultures?

How do temperamental differences contribute to family interaction?

We also continue to need more direct observational research. This work has been done by the students of parent–infant interaction, and we have seen it done by Sander (1962, 1969) as described in Chapter 4 and Shinn (1909) and Darwin (1877 cited in Kessen, 1965) in this chapter. Observation gives us a deeper understanding of temperament in development, and generates important hypotheses for research. Crockenberg and Leerkes (2003) have also proposed more small-sample research, in which observations of parent–child interaction are combined with parent interviews, studies of parent relationships with each other, and with the child. This smaller-scale research can then lead to identification of patterns to be further tested in large samples of families.

Finally, there is a very pressing need for more reviews in the area of temperament and individual differences. I began this book with doubts that the rapidly expanding research literature on temperament and related issues could be synthesized. Having completed the book, I am convinced that keeping up with progress in the field is far beyond what any single author can do. I have been amazed at the number and high quality of recent contributions to our understanding of temperament, and regret not being able to be more comprehensive in this book. We need a greater number of reviews, including reviews that cut across the levels of analysis described above. Reviews are needed both within and across the usual levels of study, examining influences that are both adjacent to and distant from the levels on Hinde's (1998) developmental model. Current reviews in the biological and cognitive sciences can serve as models for this important project, and an upcoming book, *Handbook of Temperament* (Zentner & Shiner, in press) will contribute to this effort.

THE VALUE OF TEMPERAMENT DIVERSITY

How can we respect individual differences in the child's temperament, while at the same time fostering and supporting our children's growth?

What kinds of experiences can improve the future of young children, and how do they vary as a function of the child's temperament? How can we use our political will to make sure that children's environments will be favorable ones? The answers to these questions clearly involve different levels within Hinde's (1998) hierarchy. At base, however, they require us to see temperament variability in a more positive way, reflecting the possibilities that exist for each child and for society, if we make sure that the best environments for all our children are realized.

There is much discussion about the value of different kinds of diversity: the diversity of species, the diversity of cultures, and the diversity of ethnicity, race, gender, and sexual orientation, among others. These discussions are important, but to date they say little about the value of diversity in temperament. Temperamental diversity allows for both variations in social experiences and the possibility of effective cooperation in work settings. Thomas and Chess' (1977) idea of "goodness of fit" can be extended to allow for individual contributions toward a common goal in a larger group. We would hope that we could both value the temperament diversity that can contribute to our social goals, while at the same time not being fearful of the ways in which others differ from us.

In the infant, we see temperament in all of its diversity. Fortunately, this is also a time in life when it is especially easy to love and value the child just as he or she is (Welwood, 2006). As the child grows, valuing temperament diversity can allow us to maintain our love of the child, and to accept the responsibility for providing the opportunities and challenges that will bring out the best in each person. In this view, the future is seen not so much in terms of who the child is expected to become, but in terms of who the child is and how he or she is developing.

Finally, one of the major arguments of this book has been that we all share each of the temperament processes, although to a greater or lesser degree. These tendencies involve both reactivity and self-regulation, and they function in social settings and with social groups. Although one way of looking at temperament emphasizes differences between us and others, another way allows us to see ourselves in others and others in ourselves through the psychological processes we all share. Welwood (2006) argues that the second time in life when it is especially easy to love and value another person is as he or she lies dying. If we could extend our appreciation of differences and similarities beginning with childhood and continuing through the life cycle, we would be able to better appreciate who we all are.

References

Achenbach, T. M., & Edelbrock, C. S. (1978). The classification of child psychopathology: A review and analysis of empirical efforts. *Psychological Bulletin, 85,* 1275–1301.

Adamec, R. E. (1990). Amygdala kindling and anxiety in the rat. *NeuroReport, 1,* 3–4.

Adler, A. (1946). *The practice and theory of individual psychology.* London: Routledge & Kegan Paul.

Ahadi, S. A., Rothbart, M. K., & Ye, R. (1993). Children's temperament in the U.S. and China: Similarities and differences. *European Journal of Personality, 7,* 359–378.

Ainsworth, M. D. S. (1973). The development of infant–mother interaction. In B. M. Caldwell, & H. N. Ricciuti (Eds.), *Review of child development research* (Vol. 3, pp. 1–94). Chicago: University of Chicago Press.

Ainsworth, M. D. S., Blehar, M. C., Waters, E., & Wall, S. (1978). *Patterns of attachment: A psychological study of the Strange Situation.* Hillsdale, NJ: Erlbaum.

Aksan, N., & Kochanska, G. (2004). Links between systems of inhibition from infancy to preschool years. *Child Development, 75,* 1477–1490.

Aksan, N., & Kochanska, G. (2005). Conscience in childhood: Old questions, new answers. *Developmental Psychology, 41,* 506–516.

Allik, J., Laidra, K., Realo, A., & Pullmann, H. (2004). Personality development from 12 to 18 years of age: Changes in mean levels and structure of traits. *European Journal of Personality, 18,* 445–462.

Allman, J. M., Hakeem, A., Erwin, J. M., Nimchinsky, E., & Hof, P. (2001). The anterior cingulate cortex: The evolution of an interface between emotion and cognition. In A. R. Damasio, A. Harrington, J. Kagan, B. S. McEwen, S. H. Moss, et al. (Eds.), Unity of knowledge: The convergence of natural and human science. *Annals of the New York Academy of Sciences, 935,* 107–117.

Allman, J. M., Watson K. K., Tetreault N. A., & Hakeem A. Y. (2005). Intuition and autism: A possible role for Von Economo neurons. *Trends in Cognitive Science, 9*(8), 367–373.

Allport, G. W. (1937). *Personality: A psychological interpretation.* New York: Holt.

Allport, G. W. (1961). *Pattern and growth in personality.* New York: Holt, Rinehart & Winston.

Amsterdam, B. K. (1972). Mirror self-image reactions before age two. *Developmental Psychobiology, 5,* 297–305.

Anders, T., Goodlin-Jones, B., & Sadeh, A. (2000). Sleep disorders. In C. H. Zeanah (Ed.), *Handbook of infant memtal health, 2nd edition* (pp. 326–338). New York: Guilford Press.

Anderson, K., Lytton, H., & Romney, D. M. (1986). Mothers' interactions with normal and conduct-disordered boys: Who affects whom? *Developmental Psychology, 22,* 604–609.

Anscombe, G. E. M. (1958). Modern moral philosophy. *Philosophy 33*(124), 1–33.

Arcus, D. (2001). Inhibited and uninhibited children: Biology in the social context. In T. Wachs & D. Kohnstamm (Eds.), *Temperament in context* (pp. 43–60). Hillsdale, NJ: Erlbaum.

Asendorpf, J. B. (1989). Shyness as a final common pathway for two different kinds of inhibition. *Journal of Personality and Social Psychology, 57,* 481–492.

Asendorpf, J. B. (1991). Development of inhibited children's coping with unfamiliarity. *Child Development, 62,* 1460–1474.

Asendorpf, J. B. (1993). Social inhibition: A general-developmental perspective. In H. C. Traue & J. W. Pennebaker (Eds.), *Emotion inhibition and health* (pp. 80–99). Ashland, OH: Hogrefe & Huber.

Asendorpf, J. B., Borkenau, P., Ostendorf, F., & van Aken, M. A. G. (2001). Carving personality description at its joints: Confirmation of three replicable personality prototypes for both children and adults. *European Journal of Personality, 15,* 169–198.

Asendorpf, J. B., Denissen, J. J. A., & van Aken, M. A. G. (2008). Inhibited and aggressive preschool children at 23 years of age: Personality and social transitions into adulthood. *Developmental Psychology, 44,* 997–1011.

Asendorpf, J. B., & Nunner-Winkler, G. (1992). Children's moral motive strength and temperamental inhibition reduce their immoral behavior in real moral conflicts. *Child Development, 63*(5), 1223–1235.

Asendorpf, J. B., & van Aken, M. A. G. (1991). Correlates of the temporal consistency of personality patterns in childhood. *Journal of Personality, 59,* 689–703.

Assor, A., Roth, G., & Deci, E. L. (2004). The emotional costs of parents' conditional regard: A Self-Determination Theory analysis. *Journal of Personality, 77,* 47–88.

Auerbach, J. G., Berger, A., Atzaba-Poria, N., Arbelle, S., Cypin, N., Friedman, A., et al. (2008). Temperament at 7, 12, and 25 months in children at familial risk for ADHD. *Infant and Child Development, 17*(4), 321–338.

Auerbach, J. G., Faroy, M., Ebstein, R., Kahana, M., & Levine, J. (2001). The association of the dopamine D4 receptor gene (DRD4) and the serotonin transporter promotor gene (5-HTTLPR) with temperament in 12-month-old infants. *Journal of Child Psychology Psychiatry and Allied Disciplines, 42*, 777–783.

Auerbach, J. G., Geller, V., Lezer, S., Shinwell, E., Belmaker, R. H., Levine, J., et al. (1999). Dopamine D4 receptor (D4DR) and serotonin transporter promoter (5-HTTLPR) polymorphisms in the determination of temperament in 2-month-old infants. *Molecular Psychiatry, 4*(4), 369–373.

Ausubel, D. P. (1996). *Ego development and psychopathology.* New Brunswick, NJ: Transaction.

Ausubel, D. P., & Sullivan, E. V. (1970). *Theory and problems of child development* (2nd ed.). New York: Grune & Stratton.

Ausubel, D. P., Sullivan, E. V., & Ives, S. W. (1980). *Theory and problems of child development* (3rd ed.). New York: Grune & Stratton.

Ayduk, O., Mendoza-Denton, R., Mischel, W., & Downey, G. (2000). Regulating the interpersonal self: Strategic self-regulation for coping with rejection sensitivity. *Journal of Personality and Social Psychology, 79*(5), 776–792.

Ayduk, O., Zayas, V., Downey, G., Cole, A. B., Shoda, Y., & Mischel, W. (2008). Rejection sensitivity and executive control: Joint predictors of borderline personality features. *Journal of Research in Personality, 42*(1), 151–168.

Ayers, T., Sandler, I. N., West, S. G., & Roosa, M. W. (1996). A dispositional and situational assessment of children's coping: Testing alternative models of coping. *Journal of Personality, 64*, 923–958.

Bakeman, R., & Brown, J. V. (1980). Early interaction: Consequences for social and mental development at three years. *Child Development, 51*, 437–447.

Bakermans-Kranenburg, M. J., & van IJzendoorn, M. H. (2006). Gene–environment interaction of the dopamine D4 receptor (DRD4) and observed maternal insensitivity predicting externalizing behavior in preschoolers. *Developmental Psychobiology, 48*(5), 406–409.

Bakermans-Kranenburg, M. J., van IJzendoorn, M. H., & Juffer, F. (2003). Less is more: Meta-analyses of sensitivity and attachment interventions in early childhood. *Psychological Bulletin, 129*(2), 195–215.

Bakermans-Kranenburg, M. J., van IJzendoorn, M. H., Pijlman, F. T. A., Mesman, J., & Juffer, F. (2008). Experimental evidence for differential susceptibility: Dopamine D4 Receptor Polymorphism (DRD4 VNTR) moderates intervention effects on toddlers externalizing behavior in a randomized controlled trial. *Developmental Psychology, 44*, 293–300.

Baltes, P. B., & Baltes, M. M. (1990). Psychological perspectives on successful aging: The model of selective optimization with compensation. In P. B. Baltes & M. M. Baltes (Eds.), *Successful aging: Perspectives from the behavioral sciences* (pp. 1–34). New York: Cambridge University Press.

Balzac, H. (1995). *Eugenie Grandet.* Lonfon: Penguin Books. (Original work published 1833)

Bandura, A. (1986). *Social foundations of thought and action: A social cognitive theory.* New York: Prentice-Hall.

Banks, M. R., & Banks, W. A. (2002). The effects of animal-assisted therapy on loneliness in an elderly population in long-term care facilities. *Journals of Gerontology Series A: Biological Sciences and Medical Science,* 57, M428–M432.

Baron-Cohen, S., Tager-Flusberg, H., & Cohen, D. J. (Eds.) (2000). *Understanding other minds. Perspectives from autism and developmental cognitive neuroscience* (2nd ed.). London: Oxford University Press.

Barrett, K. C., & Morgan, G. A. (1995). Continuities and discontinuities in mastery motivation during infancy and toddlerhood: A conceptualization and review. In R. H. MacTurk & G. A. Morgan (Eds.), *Mastery motivation: Origins, conceptualizations, and applications* (pp. 57–93). Norwood, NJ: Ablex.

Barry, R. A., Kochanska, G., & Philibert, R. A. (2008). GXE interaction in the organization of attachment: Mothers' responsiveness as a moderator of children's genotypes. *Journal of Child Psychology and Psychiatry, 49*(12), 1313–1320.

Bates, J. E. (1987). Temperament in infancy. In J. D. Osofsky (Ed.), *Handbook of infant development* (2nd ed., pp. 1101–1149). New York: Wiley.

Bates, J. E. (1989a). Applications of temperament concepts. In G. A. Kohnstamm, J. E. Bates, & M. K. Rothbart (Eds.), *Temperament in childhood* (pp. 321–355). Chichester, UK: Wiley.

Bates, J. E. (1989b). Concepts and measures of temperament. In G. A. Kohnstamm, J. E. Bates, & M. K. Rothbart (Eds.), *Temperament in childhood* (pp. 3–26). Chichester, UK: Wiley.

Bates, J. E. (1994). Parents as scientific observers of their children's development. In S. L. Friedman & H. C. Haywood (Eds.), *Developmental follow-up: Concepts, domains and methods* (pp. 197–216). New York: Academic Press.

Bates, J. E., Freeland, C. A. B., & Lounsbury, M. L. (1979). Measurement of infant difficultness. *Child Development, 5,* 794–803.

Bates, J. E., & Pettit, G. S. (2007). Temperament, parenting and socialization. In J. E. Grusec & P. D. Hastings (Eds.), *Handbook of socialization* (pp. 153–177). New York: Guilford Press.

Bates, J. E., Pettit, G. S., Dodge, K. A., & Ridge, B. (1998). Interaction of temperamental resistance to control and restrictive parenting in the development of externalizing behavior. *Developmental Psychology, 34*(5), 982–995.

Bates, J. E., Schermerhorn, A. C., & Goodnight, J. A. (2010). Temperament and personality through the lifespan. In R. M. Lerner, M. E. Lamb, & A. M. Freund (Eds.), *The handbook of life-span development: Vol. 2. Social and emotional development.* New York: Wiley.

Bates, J. E., Viken, R. J., Alexander, D. B., Beyers, J., & Stockton, L. (2002). Sleep and adjustment in preschool children: Sleep diary reports by mothers relate to behavior reports by teachers. *Child Development, 73*(1), 62–74.

Bates, J. E., & Wachs, T. D. (1994). *Temperament: Individual differences at the interface of biology and behavior.* Washington, DC: American Psychological Association Press.

Baumrind, D. (1967). Child care practices anteceding three patterns of preschool behavior. *Genetic Psychology Monographs, 75*(1), 43–88.

Bayley, N., & Schaefer, E. S. (1963). Maternal behavior, child behavior, and their intercorrelations from infancy through adolescence. *Monographs of the Society for Research in Child Development, 28*(3, Whole No. 87), 1–127.

Beauchaine, T. P. (2001). Vagal tone, development, and Gray's motivational theory: Toward an integrated model of autonomic nervous system functioning in psychopathology. *Development and Psychopathology, 13,* 183–214.

Beck, A. T. (1967). *Depression: Clinical, experimental, and theoretical aspects.* New York: Harper & Row.

Beck, A. T. (1983). Cognitive therapy of depression: New perspectives. In P. J. Clayton & J. E. Barnett (Eds.), *Treatment of depression: Old controversies and new approaches* (pp. 265–290). New York: Raven Press.

Beck, A. T., & Alford, B. A. (2009). *Depression: Causes and treatment.* Philadelphia: University of Pennsylvania Press.

Beebe, B. (2003). Brief mother–infant treatment: Psychoanalytically informed video feedback. *Infant Mental Health Journal, 24,* 24–52.

Beebe, B., Jaffe, J., Lachmann, F., Feldstein, S., Crown, C., & Jasnow, M. (2000). Systems models in development and psychoanalysis: The case of vocal rhythm coordination and attachment. *Infant Mental Health Journal, 21*(1–2), 99–122.

Bell, R. Q. (1968). A reinterpretation of the direction of effects in studies of socialization. *Psychological Review, 75,* 81–95.

Bell, R. Q. (1974). Contributions of human infants to caregiving and social interaction. In M. Lewis & L. A. Rosenblum (Eds.), *The effect of the infant on its caregiver* (pp. 1–20). New York: Wiley.

Bell, R. Q. (1989). *Neonatal behavior predictors of security of attachment* (No. 12). Sapporo, Japan: Hokkaido University.

Bell, R. Q., Weller, G. M., & Waldrop, M. (1971). Newborn and preschooler: Organization of behavior and relations between periods. *Monographs of the Society for Research in Child Development, 2*(1–2, Whole No. 142).

Belsky, J., Friedman, S. L., & Hsieh, K-H. (2001). Testing a core emotion-regulation prediction: Does early attentional persistence moderate the effect of infant negative emotionality on later development? *Child Development, 72*(1), 123–133.

Belsky, J., Hsieh, K., & Crnic, K. (1998). Mothering, fathering, and infant negativity as antecedents of boys' externalizing problems and inhibition at age 3: Differential susceptibility to rearing influence? *Development and Psychopathology, 10,* 301–319.

Benedict, R. (1947). *The chrysanthemum and the sword.* London: Secker & Warburg.

Benes, F. M. (1999). Alterations of neural circuitry within layer II of anterior cingulate cortex in schizophrenia. *Journal of Psychiatric Research, 33*(6), 511–512.

Bennett, M., & Sani, F. (2004). *The development of the social self.* New York: Psychology Press.

Bergman, P., & Escalona, S. (1949). Unusual sensitivities in very young children. *Psychoanalytic Study of the Child, 3–4,* 333–352.

Berlyne, D. E. (1971). *Aesthetics and psychobiology.* New York: Appleton-Century.

Biederman, J., Rosenbaum, J. F., Hirshfeld, D. R., Faraone, S. V., Bolduc, E. A., Gersten, M., et al. (1990). Psychiatric correlates of behavioral inhibition in young children of parents with and without psychiatric disorders. *Archives of General Psychiatry, 47*(1), 21–26.

Bigelow, A. E., & Birch, S. (1999). The effects of contingency in previous interactions on infants' preference for social partners. *Infant Behavior and Development, 22,* 367–382.

Birns, B. (1965). Individual differences in human neonates' responses to stimulation. *Child Development, 36,* 249–256.

Birns, B., Barten, S., & Bridger, W. (1969). Individual differences in temperamental characteristics of infants. *Transactions of the New York Academy of Sciences, 31,* 1071–1082.

Black, J. E., & Greenough, W. T. (1991). Developmental approaches to the memory processes. In J. L. Martinez Jr., & R. P. Kesner (Eds.), *Learning and memory: A biological view* (2nd ed., pp. 61–91). San Diego, CA: Academic Press.

Blair, C., & Razza, R. A. (2007). Relating effortful control, executive function, and false belief understanding to emerging math and literacy ability in kindergarten. *Child Development, 78,* 647–663.

Blair, R. J. R., Jones, L., Clark, F., & Smith, M. (1997). The psychopath: A lack of responsiveness to distress cues? *Physiology, 34,* 192–198.

Blanchard, D. C., & Takahashi, S. N. (1988). No change in intermale aggression after amygdala lesions which reduce freezing. *Physiology and Behavior, 42*(6), 613–616.

Blasi, G., Mattay, G. S., Bertolino, A., Elvevåg, B., Callicott, J. H., Das, S., et al. (2005). Effect of cCatechol-O-Methyltransferase val 158 met genotype on attentional control. *Journal of Neuroscience, 25*(20), 5038–5045.

Blatt S. J., & Luyten, P. (2009). A structural–developmental psychodynamic approach to psychopathology: Two polarities of experience across the life span. *Development and Psychopathology, 21*(3), 793–814.

Block, J. (1971). *The Q-sort method in personality assessment and psychiatric research.* Springfield, IL: Thomas.

Block, J. (1995). Overly positive self-evaluations and personality: Negative implications for mental health. *Journal of Personality and Social Psychology, 6*(6), 1152–1162.

Block, J. (1996). Some jangly remarks on Baumeister and Heatherton. *Psychological Inquiry, 7,* 28–32.

Block, J., & Gjerde, P. F. (1990). Depressive symptomatology in late adolescence: A longitudinal perspective on personality antecedents. In J. E. Rolf, A. Masten, D. Cicchetti, K. Neuchterlein, & S. Weintraub (Eds.), *Risk and protective factors in the development of psychopathology* (pp. 334–360). New York: Cambridge University Press.

Block, J., Gjerde, P. F., & Block, J. H. (1991). Personality antecedents of depressive tendencies in 18-year-olds: A prospective study. *Journal of Personality and Social Psychology, 60,* 726–738.

Block, J. H. (2002). *Personality as an affect-processing system.* Mahwah, NJ: Erlbaum.

Block, J. H., & Block, J. (1980). The role of ego-control and ego-resiliency in the organization of behavior. In W. A. Collins (Ed.), *Minnesota symposium on child psychology* (Vol. 13, pp. 39–101). Hillsdale, NJ: Erlbaum.

Bodrova, E., & Leong, D. (2006). *Tools of the mind: The Vygotskian approach to early childhood education* (2nd ed.). Columbus, OH: Merrill/Prentice-Hall.

Bohlin, G., & Hagekull, B. (2009). Socio-emotional development: From infancy to young adulthood. *Scandinavian Journal of Psychology, 50*, 592–601.

Boivin, M., Hymel, S., & Bukowski, W. M. (1995). The roles of social withdrawal, peer rejection, and victimization by peers in predicting loneliness and depressed mood in childhood. *Development and Psychopathology, 7*, 765–785.

Bolger, N. (1990). Coping as a personality process: A prospective study. *Journal of Personality and Social Psychology, 59*, 525–537.

Bornstein, M. H., Tal, J., & Tamis-LeMonda, C. S. (1991). Parenting in cross-cultural perspective: The United States, France, and Japan. In M. H. Bornstein (Ed.), *Cultural approaches to parenting* (pp. 69–90). Hillsdale, NJ: Erlbaum.

Bornstein, M. H., Toda, S., Azuma, H., Tamis-LeMonda, C. S., & Ogino, M. (1990). Mother and infant activity and interaction in Japan and in the United States: II. A comparative microanalysis of naturalistic exchanges focused on the organization of infant attention. *International Journal of Behavioral Development, 13*, 289–308.

Botvinick, M., Cohen, J. D., & Carter, C. S. (2004). Conflict monitoring and anterior cingulate cortex: An update. *Trends in Cognitive Sciences, 8*, 539–546.

Botvinick, M. M., Braver, T. S., Barch, D. M., Carter, C. S., & Cohen, J. D. (2001). Conflict monitoring and cognitive control. *Psychological Review, 108*(3), 624–652.

Bowlby, J. (1969). *Attachment and loss: Vol. 1. Attachment*. New York: Basic Books.

Bowlby, J. (1973). *Attachment and loss: Vol. 2. Separation*. New York: Basic Books.

Bowlby, J. (1977). The making and breaking of affectional bonds: I. Aetiology and psychopathology in the light of attachment theory. *British Journal of Psychiatry, 130*, 201–210.

Bowlby, J. (1982). Attachment and loss: Retrospect and prospect. *American Journal of Orthopsychiatry, 52*(4), 664–678.

Boyce, W. T., & Ellis, B. J. (2005). Biological sensitivity to context: I. An evolutionary–developmental theory of the origins and functions of stress reactivity. *Development and Psychopathology, 17*, 271–301.

Bramlett, R. K., Scott, P., & Rowell, R. K. (2000). A comparison of temperament and social skills in predicting academic performance in first graders. *Special Services in the Schools, 16*(1–2), 147–158.

Brazelton, T. B., & Cramer, B. (1990). *The earliest relationship*. New York: Addison Wesley.

Brazelton, T. B., Koslowski, B., & Main, M. (1974). The origins of reciprocity: The early mother–infant interaction. In M. Lewis & L. Rosenblum (Eds.), *The effect of the infant on its caregiver* (pp. 49–76). New York: Wiley.

Brazelton, T. B., & Nugent, J. K. (1995). *The neonatal behavioural assessment scale* (3rd ed.). London: MacKeith Press.

Brazelton, T. B., Nugent, J. K., & Lester, B. M. (1987). Neonatal behavioral assessment scale. In J. D. Osofsky (Ed.), *Handbook of infant development* (pp. 780–817). New York: Wiley.

Bretherton, I. (1985). Attachment theory: Retrospect and prospect. In I. Bretherton & E. Waters (Eds.), Growing points of attachment theory and research. *Monographs of the Society for Research in Child Development, 50*(1–2, Serial No. 209), 3–35.

Bridges, K. (1931). *Social and emotional development of the pre-school child.* London: Kegan Paul, Trench, Trubner.

Bronson, M. B. (2000). *Self-regulation in early childhood: Nature and nurture.* New York: Guilford Press.

Brookings, J. B., Zemara, M. J., & Hochstetlerb, G. M. (2002). An interpersonal circumplex/five-factor analysis of the Rejecion Sensitivity Questionnaire. *Personality and Individual Differences, 34,* 439–461.

Brown, G. W., Bifulco, A., & Harris, T. O. (1987). Life events, vulnerability, and onset of depression: Some refinements. *British Journal of Psychiatry, 150,* 30–42.

Brown, J. R., Ye, H., Bronson, R. T., Dikkes, P., & Greenberg, M. E. (1996). A defect in nurturing in mice lacking the immediate early gene fosb. *Cell, 86*(2), 297–309.

Brown, K. W., Ryan, R. M., & Creswall, J. D. (2007). Mindfulness: Theoretical foundations and evidence for salutary effects. *Psychological Inquiry, 18,* 211–237.

Brownell, C. A., & Kopp, C. B. (2007). Transitions in toddler socioemotional development: Behavior, understanding, relationships. In C. A. Brownell & C. B. Kopp (Eds.), *Socioemotional development in the toddler years: Transitions and transformations* (pp. 1–42). New York: Guilford Press.

Budaev, S. V. (1997). The statistical analysis of behavioural latency measures. *ISCP Newsletter, 14*(1), 1–4.

Burgess, K. B., Marshall, P. J., Rubin, K. H., & Fox, N. A. (2003). Infant attachment and temperament as predictors of subsequent externalizing problems and cardiac physiology. *Journal of Child Psychology and Psychiatry and Allied Disciplines, 44*(6), 819–831.

Burt, C. L. (1937). The analysis of temperament. *British Journal of Medical Psychology, 17,* 158–188.

Burt, C. L. (1938). *The young delinquent.* London: University of London Press.

Burt, S. A., McGue, M., Krueger, R. F., & Iacono, W. G. (2005). Sources of covariation among the child-externalizing disorders: Informant effects and the shared environment. *Psychological Medicine, 35*(8), 1133–1144.

Burton, R. (1921). *The anatomy of melancholy.* Oxford, UK: Oxford Press.

Bush, G., Luu, P., & Posner, M. I. (2000). Cognitive and emotional influences in anterior cingulate cortex. *Trends in Cognitive Sciences, 4,* 215–222.

Buss, A. H. (1986). A theory of shyness. In W. H. Jones, J. M. Cheek, & S. R. Briggs (Eds.), *Shyness: Perspectives on research and treatment* (pp. 39–46). New York: Plenum Press.

Buss, A. H., & Plomin, R. (1975). *A temperament theory of personality development.* New York: Wiley.

Buss, A. H., & Plomin, R. (1984). *Temperament: Early developing personality traits*. Hillsdale, NJ: Erlbaum.

Butler, R. A. (1954). Curiosity in monkeys. *Scientific American, 190*(2), 70–75.

Butler, R. A. (1957). The effect of deprivation of visual incentives on visual exploration motivation in monkeys. *Journal of Comparative and Physiological Psychology, 50*, 177–179.

Cacioppo, J. T., & Berntson, G. G. (1994). Relationship between attitudes and evaluative space: A critical review, with emphasis on the separability of positive and negative substrates. *Psychological Bulletin, 115*(3), 401–423.

Calder, A. J., Lawrence, A. D., & Young, A. W. (2001). Neuropsychology of fear and loathing. *Nature Reviews Neuroscience, 2*(5), 352–363.

Calkins, S. D., & Fox, N. A. (1992). The relations among infant temperament, security of attachment, and behavioral inhibition at twenty-four months. *Child Development, 63*, 1456–1472.

Calkins, S. D., & Fox, N. A. (2002). Self-regulatory processes in early personality development: A multilevel approach to the study of childhood social withdrawal and aggression. *Development and Psychopathology, 14*, 477–498.

Calkins, S. D., Fox, N. A., & Marshall, T. R. (1996). Behavioral and psychological antecedents of inhibition in infancy. *Child Development, 67*, 523–540.

Calkins, S. D., & Williford, A. (2003, April). *Anger regulation in infancy: Correlates and consequences*. Paper presented at the Biennial Meeting of the Society for Research in Child Development, Tampa, Florida.

Campos, J. J., Barrett, K. C., Lamb, M. E., Goldsmith, H. H., & Stenberg, C. (1983). Socioemotional development. In P. H. Mussen, M. M. Haith, & J. J. Campos (Eds.), *Handbook of child psychology* (Vol. 2, pp. 783–915). New York: Wiley.

Canli, T. (Ed.). (2006). *Biology of personality and individual differences*. New York: Guilford Press.

Canli, T., Zhao, Z., Desmond, J. E., Kang, E., Gross, J., & Gabrieli, J. D. E. (2001). An fMRI study of personality influences on brain reactivity to emotional stimuli. *Behavioral Neuroscience, 115*(1), 33–42.

Carey, W. B. (1994). Specific uses of temperament data in pediatric behavioral interventions. In W. B. Carey & S. C. McDevitt (Eds.), *Prevention and early intervention: Individual differences as risk factors for the mental health of children: A festschrift for Stella Chess and Alexander Thomas* (pp. 215–225). Philadelphia: Brunner/Mazel.

Carey, W. B. (1998). Temperament and behavior problems in the classroom. *School Psychology Review, 27*(4), 522–534.

Carey, W. B., & McDevitt, S. C. (1978). Revision of the infant temperament questionnaire. *Pediatrics, 61*(5), 735–739.

Carlson, S. M. (2005). Developmentally sensitive measures of executive function in preschool children. *Developmental Neuropsychology, 28*, 595–616.

Carlson, S. M., & Moses, L. J. (2001). Individual differences in inhibitory control and children's theory of mind. *Child Development, 72*, 1032–1053.

Carskadon, M. A. (Ed.). (2002). *Adolescent sleep patterns: Biological, social, and psychological influences*. New York: Cambridge University Press.

Carstensen, L. L. (1992). Social and emotional patterns in adulthood: Support for socioemotional selectivity theory. *Psychology and Aging, 7,* 331–338.

Carstensen, L. L. (1993). Motivation for social contact across the life span: A theory of socioemotional selectivity. In J. E. Jacobs (Ed.), *Nebraska symposium on motivation: 1992. Developmental perspectives on motivation* (Vol. 40, pp. 209–254). Lincoln: University of Nebraska Press.

Carstensen, L. L., Gross, J., & Fung, H. (1997). The social context of emotion. In M. P. Lawton & K. W. Schaie (Eds.), *Annual review of geriatrics and gerontology* (pp. 325–352). New York: Springer.

Carstensen, L. L., Pasupathi, M., Mayr, U., & Nesselroade, J. R. (2000). Emotional experience in everyday life across the adult life span. *Journal of Personality and Social Psychology, 79,* 644—655.

Carter, C. S. (1986). The reproductive and adrenal systems. In M. G. H. Coles, E. Donchin, & S. W. Porges (Eds.), *Psychophysiology* (pp. 172–182). New York: Guilford Press.

Case, R. (1991). Stages in the development of the young child's first sense of self. *Developmental Review, 11,* 210–230.

Caspi, A. (1995). Temperamental origins of child and adolescent behavior problems: From age three to age fifteen. *Child Development, 66,* 55–66.

Caspi, A., Elder, G. H., & Bem, D. J. (1988). Moving away from the world: Life-course patterns of shy children. *Developmental Psychology, 24*(6), 824–831.

Caspi, A., Harrington, H., Milne, B., Amen, J. W., Theodore, R. F., & Moffitt, T. E. (2003). Children's behavioral styles at age 3 are linked to their adult personality traits at age 26. *Journal of Personality, 71*(4), 494–513.

Caspi, A., Henry, B., McGee, R. O., Moffitt, T. E., & Silva, P. A. (1995). Temperamental origins of child and adolescent behavior problems: From age three to age fifteen. *Child Development, 66,* 55–68.

Caspi, A., McClay, J., Moffitt, T., Mill, J., Martin, J., Craig, I. W., et al. (2002). Role of genotype in the cycle of violence in maltreated children. *Science, 297*(5582), 851–854.

Caspi, A., & Shiner, R. L. (2006). Personality development. In W. Damon & R. Lerner (Series Eds.) & N. Eisenberg (Vol. Ed.), *Handbook of child psychology: Vol. 3. Social, emotional, and personality development* (6th ed., pp. 300–365). New York: Wiley.

Caspi, A., & Silva, P. A. (1995). Temperamental qualities at age three predict personality traits in young adulthood: Longitudinal evidence from a birth cohort. *Child Development, 66,* 486–498.

Cattell, R. B. (1933). Temperament tests I: Temperament. *British Journal of Psychology, 23,* 308–329.

Cattell, R. B. (1957). *Personality and motivation structure and measurement.* Yonkers, NY: World Book.

Cattell, R. B. (1963). Theory of fluid and crystallized intelligence: A critical experiment. *Journal of Educational Psychology, 54*(1), 1–22.

Cattell, R. B. (1973). *Personality and mood by questionnaire.* Oxford, UK: Jossey-Bass.

Caudill, W. D., & Weinstein, H. (1969). Maternal care and infant behavior in Japan and America. *Psychiatry, 32,* 12–43.

Chamove, A. S., Eysenck, H. J., & Harlow, H. F. (1972). Personality in monkeys: Factor analysis of rhesus social behaviour. *Quarterly Journal of Experimental Psychology, 24,* 496–504.

Champoux, M., Bennett, A., Shannon, C., Higley, L. D., Lesch, K. P., & Suomi, S. J. (2002). Serotonin transporter gene polymorphism, differential early rearing, and behavior in rhesus monkey neonates. *Molecular Psychiatry, 7*(10), 1058–1063.

Checa, P., Rodriguez-Bailon, R., & Rueda, M. R. (2008). Neurocognitive and temperamental systems of self-regulation and early adolescents' social and academic outcomes. *Mind, Brain, and Education, 2*(4), 177–187.

Chen, X., Cen, G., Li, D., & He, Y. (2005). Social functioning and adjustment in Chinese children: The imprint of historical time. *Child Development, 76,* 182–195.

Chen, X., He, Y., & Li, D. (2004). Self-perceptions of social competence and self-worth in Chinese children: Relations with social and school performance. *Social Development, 13*(4), 570–589.

Chen, X., Rubin, K. H., & Li, Z. (1995). Social functioning and adjustment in Chinese children: A longitudinal study. *Developmental Psychology, 31,* 531–539.

Chen, X., Rubin, K. H., & Sun, Y. (1992). Social reputation and peer relationships in Chinese and Canadian children: A cross-cultural study. *Child Development, 63,* 1336–1343.

Chess, S., & Thomas, A. (1984). *Origins and evolution of behavior disorders: Infancy to early adult life.* New York: Brunner/Mazel.

Chess, S., & Thomas, A. (1986). *Temperament in clinical practice.* New York: Guilford Press.

Chess, S., & Thomas, A. (1990). The New York Longitudinal Study (NYLS): The young adult periods. *Canadian Journal of Psychiatry, 35*(6), 557–561.

Chess, S., Thomas, A., & Birch, H. G. (1985). *Your child is a person.* New York: Penguin Books.

Chisholm, J. (1978). Swaddling, cradleboards, and the development of children. *Early Human Development, 2*(3), 255–275.

Church, J. (1961). *Language and the discovery of reality.* New York: Vintage Books.

Clarke, A., & Boinski, S. (1995). Temperament in nonhuman primates. *American Journal of Primatology, 37*(2), 103–125.

Clohessy, A. B., Posner, M. I., & Rothbart, M. K. (2001). Development of the functional field. *Acta Psychologica, 106,* 51–68.

Cloninger, C. R. (1986). A unified biosocial theory of personality and its role in the development of anxiety states. *Psychiatric Developments, 4*(3), 167–226.

Cloninger, C. R. (1987). A systematic method for clinical description and classification of personality variants. *Archives of General Psychiatry, 44,* 573–588.

Cohen, N. J., Lojkasek, M., Muir, E., Muir, R., & Parker, C. J. (2002). Six month follow-up of two mother–infant psychotherapies: Convergence of therapeutic outcomes. *Infant Mental Health Journal, 23,* 361–380.

Compas, B. E. (1987). Coping with stress during childhood and adolescence. *Psychological Bulletin, 101,* 393–403.

Compas, B. E., Connor-Smith, J. K., Salzman, H., Thomsen, A. H., & Wadsworth, M. E. (2001). Coping with stress during childhood and adolescence: Problems, progress, and potential in theory and research. *Psychological Bulletin, 68*, 901–916.

Conner, B. (2007). *Unplugged play: No batteries. No plugs. Pure fun.* New York: Workman.

Connor-Smith, J. K., & Flachsbart, C. (2007). Relations between personality and coping. *Journal of Personality and Social Psychology, 93*, 1080–1107.

Conrad, P. (2007). *The medicalization of society: On the transformation of human conditions into treatable disorders.* Baltimore: Johns Hopkins Press.

Cooley, C. H. (1902). *Human nature and social order.* New York: Scribners.

Corbetta, M., Kincade, J. M., & Shulman, G. L. (2002). Neural systems for visual orienting and their relationships to spatial working memory. *Journal of Cognitive Neuroscience, 14*(3), 508–523.

Costa, P. T., & McCrae, R. R. (1992a). The five-factor model of personality and its relevance to personality disorders. *Journal of Personality Disorders, 6*(4), 343–359.

Costa, P. T., & McCrae, R. R. (1992b). *Revised NEO Personality Inventory* (NEO-PI-R). Odessa, FL: Psychological Assessment Resources.

Costa, P. T., Jr., & McCrae, R. R. (1994). Stability and change in personality from adolescence through adulthood. In C. F. Halverson Jr., G. A. Kohnstamm, & R. P. Martin (Eds.), *The developing structure of temperament and personality from infancy to adulthood* (pp. 139–150). Hillsdale, NJ: Erlbaum.

Costa, P. T., Jr., & McCrae, R. R (2001). A theoretical context for adult temperament. In T. D. Wachs & G. A. Kohnstamm (Eds.), *Temperament in context* (pp. 1–21). Hillsdale, NJ: Erlbaum.

Costello, E. J., Angold, A., Burns, B. J., Stangl, D. K., Tweed, D. L., Erkanli, A., et al. (1996). The Great Smoky Mountains Study of youth: Goals, design, methods, and the prevalence of DSM-III-R disorders. *Archives of General Psychiatry, 53*, 1129–1136.

Cramer, P. (2006). *Protecting the self: Defense mechanisms in action.* New York: Guilford Press.

Crockenberg, S. B. (2003). Rescuing the baby from the bathwater: How gender and temperament (may) influence how child care affects child development. *Child Development, 74*, 1038.

Crockenberg, S. B., & Leerkes, E. (2000). Infant social and emotional development in family context. In C. H. Zeanah Jr. (Ed.), *Handbook of infant mental health* (2nd ed., pp. 60–90). New York: Guilford Press.

Crockenberg, S. B., & Acredolo, C. (1983). Infant temperament ratings: A function of infants, or mothers, or both? *Infant Behavior and Development, 6*, 61–72.

Crockenberg, S. B., & Leerkes, E. M. (2003). Negative infant emotionality and the development of family relationships in infancy and early childhood. In A. C. Crouter & A. Booth (Eds.), *Children's influence on family dynamics: The neglected side of family relationships* (pp. 57–78). Mahwah, NJ: Erlbaum.

Crockenberg, S. B., & Smith, P. (1982). Antecedents of mother–infant interaction and infant irritability in the first three months of life. *Infant Behavior and Development*, 5, 105–119.

Culpeper, N., & London, W. R. (Trans.). (1657). *Galen's art of physic*. London: Peter Cole.

Cummings, E. M., Papp, L. M., & Kouros, C. D. (2009). Regulatory processes in children's coping with exposure to mental conflict. In S. L. Olson & A. J. Sameroff (Eds.), *Biopsychosocial regulatory processes in the development of childhood behavior problems* (pp. 212–237). New York: Cambridge University Press.

Damon, W., & Hart, D. (1982). The development of self-understanding from infancy through adolescence. *Child Development*, 53, 841–864.

Darwin, C. (1877). *A biographical sketch of an infant. Mind II*. (Reprinted from *The child*, pp. 286–294, by W. Kessen, Ed., 1965, New York: Wiley)

Davidson, R. J. (2003). Affective neuroscience and psychophysiology: Toward a synthesis. *Psychophysiology*, 40, 655–665.

Davidson, R. J., Putnam, K. M., & Larson, C. L. (2000). Dysfunction in the neural circuitry of emotion regulation—a possible prelude to violence. *Science*, 289(5479), 591–594.

Davis, M. (1998). Are different parts of the external amygdala involved in fear versus anxiety? *Biological Psychiatry*, 44, 1239–1247.

Davis, M., Hitchcock, J. M., & Rosen, J. B. (1987). Anxiety and the amygdala: Pharmacological and anatomical analysis of the fear-potentiated startle paradigm. In G. Bower (Ed.), *The psychology of learning and motivation: Advances in research and theory* (Vol. 21, pp. 263–305). San Diego, CA: Academic Press.

Davis-Kean, P. E., Huesmann, L. R., Jager, J., Collins, W. A., Bates, J. E., & Lansford, J. E. (2008). Changes in the relation of self-efficacy beliefs and behaviors across development. *Child Development*, 79(5), 1257–1269.

Deary, I. J. (1996). A (latent) Big Five personality model in 1915? A reanalysis of Webb's data. *Journal of Personality and Social Psychology*, 71(5), 992–1005.

de Beauvoir, S. (1958). *Memoirs of a dutiful daughter* (J. Kirkup, Trans.). Paris: Gallimard.

Decety, J., & Jackson, P. L. (2004). The functional architecture of human empathy. *Behavioral and Cognitive Neuroscience Reviews*, 3(2), 71–100.

Declerck, C. H., Boone, C., & De Brabander, B. (2006). On feeling in control: A biological theory for individual differences in control perception. *Brain and Cognition*, 62(2), 143–176.

De Fruyt, F., Bartels, M., Van Leeuwen, K. G., De Clercq, B., Decuyper, M., & Mervielde, I. (2006). Five types of personality continuity in childhood and adolescence. *Journal of Personality and Social Psychology*, 91, 538–552.

Depue, R. A., & Collins, P. F. (1999). Neurobiology of the structure of personality: Dopamine, facilitation of incentive motivation, and extraversion. *Behavioral and Brain Sciences*, 22(3), 491–569.

Depue, R. A., & Iacono, W. G. (1989). Neurobehavioral aspects of affective disorders. In M. R. Rosenzweig & L. Y. Porter (Eds.), *Annual review of psychology* (Vol. 40, pp. 457–492). Palo Alto, CA: Annual Reviews.

Depue, R. A., & M. F. Lenzenweger. (2006). A multidimensional neurobehavioral model of personality disturbance. In R. F. Kreuger & J. L. Tackett (Eds.), *Personality and psychopathology* (pp. 210–261). New York: Guilford Press.

Derryberry, D., & Reed, M. A. (1994). Temperament and attention: Orienting toward and away from positive and negative signals. *Journal of Personality and Social Psychology, 66*, 1128–1139.

Derryberry, D., & Reed, M. A. (1996). Regulatory processes and the development of cognitive representations. *Development and Psychopathology, 8*, 215–234.

Derryberry, D., & Reed, M. A. (2002). Anxiety-related attentional biases and their regulation by attentional control. *Journal of Abnormal Psychology, 111*, 225–236.

Derryberry, D., & Rothbart, M. K. (1988). Arousal, affect, and attention as components of temperament. *Journal of Personality and Social Psychology, 55*(6), 958–966.

Dettling, A. C., Gunnar, M. R., & Donzella, B. (1999). Cortisol levels of young children in full-day childcare centers: Relations with age and temperament. *Psychoneuroendocrinology, 24*, 519–536.

Dettling, A. C., Parker, S. W., Lane, S., Sebanc, A., & Gunnar, M. R. (2000). Quality of care and temperament determine changes in cortisol concentrations over the day for young children in childcare. *Psychoneuroendocrinology, 25*(8), 819–836.

De Waal, F. (2001). *The ape and the sushi master: Cultural reflections of a primatologist.* New York: Basic Books.

Diamond, A., Barnett, S., Thomas, J., & Munro, S. (2007). Preschool program improves cognitive control. *Science, 318*, 1387–1388.

Diamond, S. (1957). *Personality and temperament.* New York: McGraw-Hill.

Diamond, S. (1974). *The roots of psychology: A sourcebook in the history of ideas.* New York: Basic Books.

DiBiase, R., & Lewis, M. (1997). The relation between temperament and embarrassment. *Cognition and Emotion, 11*(3), 259–271.

Dienstbier, R. A. (1984). The role of emotion in moral socialization. In C. E. Izard, J. Kagan, & R. B. Zajonc (Eds.), *Emotions, cognition, and behavior* (pp. 484–514). New York: Cambridge University Press.

Digman, J. M. (1972). High school academic achievement as seen in the context of a longitudinal study of personality. *Proceedings of the Annual Convention of the American Psychological Association, 7*(Pt. 1), 19–20.

Digman, J. M. (1989). Five robust trait dimensions: Development, stability, and utility. *Journal of Personality, 57*(2), 195–214.

Digman, J. M. (1990). Personality structure: Emergence of the five-factor model. *Annual Review of Psychology, 41*, 417–440.

Digman, J. M. (1996). The curious history of the five-factor model. In J. S. Wiggins (Ed.), *The five-factor model of personality: Theoretical perspectives* (pp. 1–20). New York: Guilford Press.

Digman, J. M., & Inouye, J. (1986). Further specification of the five robust factors of personality. *Journal of Personality and Social Psychology, 50*, 116–123.

Digman, J. M., & Shmelyov, A. G. (1996). The structure of temperament and personality in Russian children. *Journal of Personality and Social Psychology, 71*(2), 341–351.

Digman, J. M., & Takemoto-Chock, N. K. (1981). Factors in the natural language of personality: Re-analysis, comparison, and interpretation of six major studies. *Multivariate Behavioral Research, 16,* 149–170.

Ding, Y. C., Chi, H. C., Grady, D. L., Morishima, A., Kidd, J. R., Kidd, K. K., et al. (2002). Evidence of positive selection acting at the human dopamine receptor D4 gene locus. *Proceedings of the National Academy of Sciences of the United States of America, 99,* 309–314.

Diorio, J., & Meaney, M. J. (2007). Maternal programming of defensive responses through sustained effects on gene expression. *Journal of Psychiatry and Neuroscience, 32*(4), 275–284.

Dishion, T., & Patterson, G. R. (2006). The development and ecology of antisocial behavior in children and adolescents. In D. Cicchetti & D. J. Cohen (Eds.), *Developmental psychopathology: Vol. 3. Risk, disorder, and adaptation* (2nd ed., pp. 503–541). Hoboken, NJ: Wiley.

Dixon, W., & Shore, C. (1997). Temperamental predictors of linguistic style during multiword acquisition. *Infant Behavior and Development, 20,* 99–103.

Dixon, W. E., & Smith, P. H. (2000). Links between temperament and language acquisition. *Merrill-Palmer Quarterly, 46,* 417–440.

Dodge, K. A., & Coie, J. D. (1987). Social-information-processing factors in reactive and proactive aggression in children's peer groups. *Journal of Personality and Social Psychology, 53*(6), 1146–1158.

Downey, G., & Feldman, S. I. (1996). Implications of rejection sensitivity for intimate relationships. *Journal of Personality and Social Psychology, 70,* 1327–1343.

Drevets, W. C., & Raichle, M. E. (1998). Reciprocal suppression of regional cerebral blood flow during emotional versus higher cognitive processes: Implications for interactions between emotion and cognition. *Cognition and Emotion, 12*(3), 353–385.

Duncan, J., Seitz, R. J., Kolodny, J., Bor, D., Herzog, H., Ahmed, A., et al. (2000). A neural basis for general intelligence. *Science, 289*(5478), 457–460.

Dweck, C. S. (2000). *Self-theories: Their role in motivation, personality, and development.* Philadelphia: Taylor and Francis/Psychology Press.

Dweck, C. S. (2008). Can personality be changed? The role of beliefs in personality and change. *Current Directions in Psychological Science, 17*(6), 391–394.

Eagly, A. H., & Steffen, V. J. (1986). Gender and aggressive behavior: A meta-analytic review of the social psychological literature. *Psychological Bulletin, 100,* 309–330.

Early, T. S., Posner, M. I., Reiman, E. M., & Raichle, M. E. (1989). Hyperactivity of the left striatopallidal projection. Part II: Phenomenology and thought disorder. *Psychiatric Developments, 2,* 109–121.

Eaton, D. K., Kann, L., Kinchen, L., Shanklin, S., Ross, J., Hawkins, J., et al. (2008). Youth risk behavior surveillance—United States, 2007. *Centers for Disease Control and Prevention (CDC) Morbidity and Mortality Surveillance Summary, 57,* 1–131.

Eaton, W. O. (1994). Temperament, development, and the five-factor model: Lessons from activity level. In C. F. Halverson Jr., G. A. Kohnstamm, & R. P. Martin (Eds.), *The developing structure of temperament and personality from infancy to adulthood* (pp. 173–187). Hillsdale, NJ: Erlbaum.

Ebstein, R. P., Levine, J., Geller, V., Auerbach, J., Gritsenko, I., & Belmaker, R. H. (1998). Dopamine D4 receptor and serotonin transporter promoter in the determination of neonatal temperament. *Molecular Psychiatry, 3*(3), 238–246.

Edelbrock, C., & Achenbach, T. M. (1980). A typology of child behavior profile patterns: Distribution and correlates for disturbed children aged 6–16. *Journal of Abnormal Child Psychology, 8*(4), 441–470.

Edwards, C. P. (1995). Parenting toddlers. In M. Bornstein (Ed.), *Handbook of parenting, Vol. 1: Children and parenting* (pp. 41–64). Mahwah, NJ: Erlbaum.

Edwards, C. P., & Liu, W. (2002). Parenting toddlers. In M. C. Bornstein (Ed.), *Handbook of parenting, Vol. 1. Children and parenting* (2nd ed., pp. 45–72). Mahwah, NJ: Erlbaum.

Eigsti, I.-M., Zayas, V., Mischel, W., Shoda, Y., Ayduk, O., Dadlani, M. B., et al. (2006). Predicting cognitive control from preschool to late adolescence and young adulthood. *Psychological Science, 17*(6), 478–484.

Eisenberg, N., Fabes, R. A., Bernzweig, J., Karbon, M., Poulin, R., & Hanish, L. (1993). The relations of emotionality and regulation to preschoolers' social skills and sociometric status. *Child Development, 64*(5), 1418–1438.

Eisenberg, N., Fabes, R. A., Guthrie, I. K., Murphy, B. C., Poulin, R., & Shepard, W. (1996). The relations of regulation and emotionality to problem behavior in elementary school children. *Development and Psychopathology, 8,* 141–162.

Eisenberg, N., Fabes, R. A., Guthrie, I. K., & Reiser, M. (2000). Dispositional emotionality and regulation: Their role in predicting quality of social functioning. *Journal of Personality and Social Psychology, 78,* 136–157.

Eisenberg, N., Fabes, R. A., Shepard, S. A., Murphy, B. C., Guthrie, I. K., Jones, S., et al. (1997). Contemporaneous and longitudinal prediction of children's social functioning from regulation and emotionality. *Child Development, 68*(4), 642–664.

Eisenberg, N., Fabes, R. A., & Spinrad, T. L. (2006). Prosocial development. In N. Eisenberg (Vol. Ed.), W. Damon & R. M. Lerner (Series Ed.), *Handbook of child psychology: Social, emotional, and personality development* (Vol. 3, pp. 646–718). New York: Wiley.

Eisenberg, N., Smith, C. L., Sadovsky, A., & Spinrad, T. L. (2004). Effortful control: Relations with emotion regulation, adjustment, and socialization in childhood. In R. F. Baumeister & K. D. Vohs (Eds.), *Handbook of self-regulation: Research, theory, and applications* (pp. 259–282). New York: Guilford Press.

Eisenberg, N., Spinrad, T. L., & Sadovsky, A. (2006). Empathy-related responding in children. In M. Killen & J. Smetana (Eds.), *Handbook of moral development* (pp. 517–549). Mahwah, NJ: Erlbaum.

Eisenberg, N., Valiente, C., Fabes, R. A., Smith, C. L., Reiser, M., Shepard, S. A., et al. (2003). The relations of effortful control and ego control to children's resiliency and social functioning. *Developmental Psychology, 39,* 761–776.

Eisenberger, N. I., Lieberman, M. D., & Williams, K. D. (2003). Does rejection hurt? An fMRI study of social exclusion. *Science, 302*(5643), 290–292.

Ekman, P., Sorenson, E. R., & Friesen, W. V. (1969). Pan-cultural elements in facial displays of emotion. *Science, 164*(875), 86–88.

Ellis, L. K., Rothbart, M. K., & Posner, M. I. (2004). Individual differences in executive attention predict self-regulation and adolescent psychosocial behaviors. *Annals of the New York Academy of Sciences, 1021*, 337–340.

Else-Quest, N. M., Hyde, J. S., Goldsmith, H. H., & Van Hulle, C. (2006). Gender differences in temperament: A meta-analysis. *Psychological Bulletin, 132*, 33–72.

El-Sheikh, M., Kouros, C. D., Erath, S., Cummings, E. M., Keller, P., & Staton, L. (2009). Marital conflict and children's externalizing behavior: Interactions between parasympathetic and sympathetic nervous system activity. *Monographs of the Society for Research in Child Development, 74*(1), vii, 1–79.

Emde, R. N. (1983). The prerepresentational self and its affective core. *Psychoanalytic Study of the Child, 38*, 165–192.

Emde, R. N., Gaensbauer, T. J., & Harmon, R. J. (1976). *Emotional expression in infancy: A biobehavioral study*. New York: International Universities Press.

Epstein, S. (1984). The stability of behavior across time and situations. In R. A. Zucker, J. Aronoff, & A. I. Rabin (Eds.), *Personality and the prediction of behavior* (pp. 209–268). Orlando, FL: Academic Press.

Erez, A., & Isen, A. M. (2002). The influence of positive affect on the components of expectancy motivation. *Journal of Applied Psychology, 87*(6), 1055–1067.

Escalona, S. K. (1968). *The roots of individuality: Normal patterns of development in infancy*. Chicago: Aldine.

Evans, D., & Rothbart, M. K. (2007). Developing a model for adult temperament. *Journal of Research in Personality, 41*, 868–888.

Eysenck, H. J. (1947). *Dimensions of personality*. London: Routledge & Kegan Paul.

Eysenck, H. J. (1957). *The dynamics of anxiety and hysteria*. London: Routledge & Kegan Paul.

Eysenck, H. J. (1967). *The biological basis of personality*. Springfield, IL: Thomas.

Eysenck, H. J., & Eysenck, M. W. (1985). *Personality and individual differences: A natural science approach*. New York: Plenum.

Fabes, R., & Eisenberg, N. (1997). Regulatory control and adults' stress-related responses to daily life events. *Journal of Personality and Social Psychology, 73*, 1107–1117.

Fabes, R., Poulin, R., Eisenberg, N., & Madden-Derdich, D. (2002). The coping with children's negative emotions scale (CCNES): Psychometric properties and relations with children's emotional competence. *Marriage and Family Review, 34*, 285–310.

Fan, J., Fossella, J., Sommer, T., Wu, Y., & Posner, M. I. (2003). Mapping the genetic variation of executive attention onto brain activity. *Proceedings of the National Academy of Sciences of the United States of America, 100*(12), 7406–7411.

Felitti, V. J., Anda, R. F., Nordenberg, D., Williamson, D. F., Spitz, A. M., Edwards, V., et al. (1998). The relationship of adult health status to childhood abuse and household dysfunction. *American Journal of Preventive Medicine, 14*(4), 245–258.

Fernald, A., & Kuhl, P. (1987). Acoustic determinants of infant preference for motherese speech. *Infant Behavior and Development, 10*(33), 279–293.

Fernández-Duque, D., & Black, S. E. (2006). Attentional networks in normal aging and Alzheimer's disease. *Neuropsychology, 20*(2), 133–143.

Field, T. M. (1977). Effects of early separation, interactive deficits, and experimental manipulations on infant–mother face-to-face interaction. *Child Development, 48,* 763–771.

Field, T. M. (1981). Infant gaze aversion and heart rate during face-to-face interactions. *Infant Behavior and Development, 4,* 307–315.

Field, T. M. (2007). *The amazing infant.* London: Blackwell.

Fivush, R., & Reese, E. (1991, July). *Parental styles for talking about the past.* Paper presented at the International Conference on Memory in Lancaster, UK.

Flavell, H. (1963). *The developmental psychology of Jean Piaget.* New York: Van Nostrand.

Fogel, A. (1992). Co-regulation, perception and action. *Human Movement Science, 11,* 505–523.

Foley, D., Ancoli-Israel, S., Britz, P., & Walsh, J. (2004). Sleep disturbances and chronic disease in older adults: Results of the 2003 National Sleep Foundation Sleep in America Survey. *Journal of Psychosomatic Research, 56*(5), 497–502.

Forkman, B., Furuhaug, I. L., & Jensen, P. (1995). Personality, coping patterns, and aggression in piglets. *Applied Animal Behaviour Science, 45*(1–2), 31–42.

Fossella, J., Posner, M. I., Fan, J., Swanson, J. M., & Pfaff, D. W. (2002). Attentional phenotypes for the analysis of higher mental function. *Scientific World Journal, 2*(Cited April 1, 2002), 217–223.

Fox, E., Russo, R., Bowles, R. J., & Dutton, K. (2001). Do threatening stimuli draw or hold visual attention in sub-clinical anxiety? *Journal of Experimental Psychology: General, 130,* 681–700.

Fox, M. D., Snyder, A. Z., Vincent, J. L., Corbetta, M., Van Essen, D. C., & Raichle, M. E. (2005). The human brain is intrinsically organized into dynamic, anticorrelated functional networks. *Proceedings of the National Academy of Sciences of the United States of America, 102*(27), 9673–9678.

Fox, N. A., Calkins, S. D., & Bell, M. A. (1994). Neural plasticity and development in the first two years of life: Evidence from cognitive and socioemotional domains of research. *Development and Psychopathology, 6,* 677–696.

Fraiberg, S. (1977). *Insights from the blind.* New York: Basic Books.

Fraiberg, S. (1980). *Clinical studies in infant mental health: The first year of life.* New York: Basic Books.

French, J. M. (1993). Assessment of donkey temperament and the influence of home environment. *Applied Animal Behaviour Science, 36*(2–3), 249–257.

Frick, P. J., Cornell, A. H., Bodin, S. D., Dane, H. E., Barry, C. E., & Loney, B. R. (2003). Callous–unemotional traits and developmental pathways to severe conduct problems. *Developmental Psychology, 39,* 246–260.

Frick, P. J., & Dickens, C. (2006). Current perspectives on conduct disorder. *Current Psychiatry Reports, 8*(1), 59–72.

Friedman, E., Katcher, A. H., Lynch, J. J., & Thomas, S. A. (1980). Animal companions and one-year survival of patients after discharge from a coronary care unit. *Public Health Reports, 95*(4), 307–312.

Fries, M. E. (1954). Some hypotheses on the role of the congenital activity type in personality development. *International Journal of Psycho-Analysis, 35*, 206–207.

Fries, M. E., & Woolf, P. J. (1953). Some hypotheses on the role of the congenital activity type in personality development. *Psychoanalytic Study of the Child, 8*, 48–62.

Gale, R. F. (1974). *Who are you? The psychology of being yourself.* New York: Prentice-Hall.

Gallese, V. (2001). The "shared manifold" hypothesis: From mirror neurons to empathy. *Journal of Consciousness Studies, 8*, 33–50.

Ganiban, J. M., Saudino, K. S., Ulbricht, J., Neiderhiser, J. M., & Reiss, D. (2008). Stability and change in temperament during adolescence. *Journal of Personality and Social Psychology, 95*, 222–236.

Gardner, T. W., Dishion, T. J., & Connell, A. M. (2008). Adolescent self-regulation as resilience: Resistance to antisocial behavior within the deviant peer context. *Journal of Abnormal Child Psychology, 36*(2), 273–284.

Garmezy, N. (1974). The study of competence in children at risk for severe psychopathology. In E. J. Anthony & C. J. Kopernik (Eds.), *The child in his family* (pp. 77–89). New York: Wiley.

Garmezy, N., & Masten, M. S. (1986). Stress, competence, and resilience: Common frontiers for therapist and psychopathologist. *Behavioral Therapy, 17*, 500–521.

Garnet, J. C. M. (1918). General ability, cleverness and purpose. *British Journal of Psychology, 9*, 345–366.

Gartstein, M. A., & Rothbart, M. K. (2003). Studying infant temperament via the revised Infant Behavior Questionnaire. *Infant Behavior and Development, 26*(1), 64–86.

Gerardi-Caulton, G. (2000). Sensitivity to spatial conflict and the development of self-regulation in children 24–36 months of age. *Developmental Science, 3*(4), 397–404.

Gest, S. D. (1997). Behavioral inhibition: Stability and associations with adaptation from childhood to early adulthood. *Journal of Personality and Social Psychology, 72*(2), 467–475.

Ghera, M. M., Hane, A. A., Malesa, E. E., & Fox, N. A. (2006). The role of infant soothability in the relation between infant negativity and maternal sensitivity. *Infant Behavior and Development, 29*(2), 289–293.

Gilliom, M., & Shaw, D. S. (2004). Codevelopment of externalizing and internalizing problems in early childhood. *Development and Psychopathology, 16*(2), 313–333.

Gjerde, P. F., Block, J., & Block, J. H. (1988). Depressive symptoms and personality during late adolescence: Gender differences in the externalization–internalization of symptom expression. *Journal of Abnormal Psychology, 86*, 475–486.

Glenn, A. L., Raine, A., Venables, P. H., & Mednick, S. A. (2007). Early temperamental and psychophysiological precursors of adult psychopathic personality. *Journal of Abnormal Psychology, 116*(3), 508–518.

Gogol, N. V. (1965). *The overcoat and other tales of good and evil.* New York: Norton. (Original work published 1842)

Gold, K. C., & Maple, T. L. (1994). Personality assessment in the gorilla and its utility as a management tool. *Zoo Biology, 13*(5), 509–522.

Goldberg, L. R. (1990). An alternative "description of personality": The Big-Five factor structure. *Journal of Personality and Social Psychology, 59,* 1216–1229.

Goldberg, L. R. (1993). The structure of phenotypic personality traits. *American Psychologist, 48,* 26–34.

Goldberg, S., & Lewis, M. (1969). Play behavior in the year-old infant: Early sex differences. *Child Development, 40*(1), 21–31.

Goldman-Rakic, P. S. (1988). Topography of cognition: Parallel distributed networks in primate association cortex. *Annual Review of Neuroscience, 11,* 137–156.

Goldsmith, H., Rieser-Danner, L., & Briggs, S. (1991). Evaluating convergent and discriminant validity of temperament questionnaires for preschoolers, toddlers, and infants. *Developmental Psychology, 27*(4), 566–579.

Goldsmith, H. H., Buss, K. A., & Lemery, K. S. (1996). Toddler and childhood temperament: Expanded content, stronger genetic evidence, new evidence for the importance of environment. *Developmental Psychology, 33,* 891–905.

Goldsmith, H. H., & Campos, J. J. (1986). Fundamental issues in the study of early temperament: The Denver twin temperament study. In M. H. Lamb & A. Brown (Eds.), *Advances in developmental psychology* (pp. 231–283). Hillsdale, NJ: Erlbaum.

Goldsmith, H. H., & Rieser-Danner, L. (1986). Variation among temperament theories and validation studies of temperament assessment. In G. A. Kohnstamm (Ed.), *Temperament discussed: Temperament and development in infancy and childhood* (pp. 1–9). Lisse, The Netherlands: Swets & Zeitlinger.

Goldsmith, H. H., & Rothbart, M. K. (1990). *The Laboratory Temperament Assessment Battery (LabTAB): Prelocomotor and locomotor versions.* Technical Manual, Department of Psychology, University of Wisconsin, Madison.

Goldsmith, H. H., & Rothbart, M. K. (1991). Contemporary instruments for assessing early temperament by questionnaire and in the laboratory. In A. Angleitner & J. Strelau (Eds.), *Explorations in temperament: International perspectives on theory and measurement* (pp. 249–272). New York: Plenum Press.

Goleman, D. P. (1995). *Emotional intelligence: Why it can matter more than IQ for character, health and lifelong achievement.* New York: Bantam Books.

Gonzalez, C., Fuentes, L. J., Carranza, J. A., & Estevez, A. F. (2001). Temperament and attention in the self-regulation of 7-year-old children. *Personality and Individual Differences, 30,* 931–946.

Goodenough, W. H. (1981). *Culture, language, and society.* Menlo Park, CA: Benjamin.

Goodnight, J. A., Bates, J. E., Newman, J. P., Dodge, K. A., & Pettit, G. W. (2006). The interactive influences of friend deviance and disinhibition on the development of externalizing behavior during middle adolescence. *Journal of Abnormal Child Psychology, 34*(5), 573–583.

Gorsuch, R. L. (1983). *Factor analysis*. Hillsdale, NJ: Erlbaum.

Gosling, S. D., & John, O. P. (1999). Personality dimensions in nonhuman animals: A cross-species review. *Current Directions in Psychological Science, 8*(3), 69–75.

Gray, J. (1980). *Ivan Pavlov*. New York: Viking.

Gray, J. A. (1978). The neuropsychology of anxiety. *British Journal of Psychology, 69*, 417–434.

Gray, J. A. (1979). A neuropsychological theory of anxiety. In C. E. Izard (Ed.), *Emotions in personality and psychopathology*. New York: Oxford University Press.

Gray, J. A. (1982). *The neuropsychology of anxiety: An enquiry into the functions of the septo-hippocampal system*. London: Oxford University Press.

Gray, J. A., & McNaughton, N. (1996). *The neuropsychology of anxiety: Reprise*. Paper presented at the Nebraska Symposium on Motivation: Vol. 38. Perspectives on anxiety, panic, and fear, Lincoln, NB.

Greene, D., & Lepper, M. R. (1974). Effects of extrinsic rewards on children's subsequent intrinsic interest. *Child Development, 45*, 1141–1145.

Greenspan, S. I. (1995). *The challenging child*. New York: Da Capo Press.

Gu, X., Liu, X., Guise, K. G., Fossella, J., Wang, K., Fan, J., et al. (2008). Alexithymic trait and voluntary control in healthy adults. *PLoS ONE, 3*(11), [online] e3702. doi:10.1371/journal.pone.0003702

Guerin, D. W., & Gottfried, A. W. (1994). Developmental stability and change in parent reports of temperament: A ten-year longitudinal investigation from infancy through preadolescence. *Merrill–Palmer Quarterly, 40*(3), 334–355.

Guerin, D. W., Gottfried, A. W., Oliver, P. H., & Thomas, C. W. (2003). *Temperament: Infancy through adolescence*. New York: Kluwer Academic/Plenum.

Guidano, V. F. (1987). *Complexity of the self: A developmental approach to psychopathology and therapy*. New York: Guilford Press.

Gunnar, M. R. (1994). Psychoendocrine studies of temperament and stress in early childhood: Expanding current models. In J. E. Bates & T. D. Wachs (Eds.), *Temperament: Individual differences at the interface of biology and behavior* (pp. 175–198). Washington, DC: American Psychological Association.

Gunnar, M. R. (2004). Psychoendocrine studies of temperament and stress in early childhood: Expanding current models. In J. E. Bates & T. D. Wachs (Eds.), *Temperament: Individual differences at the interface of biology and behavior* (pp. 175–198). Washington, DC: American Psychological Association.

Gunnar, M. R., & Cheatham, C. L. (2003). Brain and behavior interface: Stress and the developing brain. *Journal of Infant Mental Health, 24*, 195–211.

Gunnar, M. R., & Quevedo, K. (2007). The neurobiology of stress and development. *Annual Review of Psychology, 58*, 145–173.

Gunnar, M. R., & Vazquez, D. (2006). Stress neurobiology and developmental psychopathology. In D. Cicchetti & D. Cohen (Eds.), *Developmental psychopathology: Vol. 2. Developmental neuroscience* (2nd ed., pp. 533–577). New York: Wiley.

Guthrie, I. K., Eisenberg, N., Fabes, R. A., Murphy, B. C., Holmgren, R., Mazsk, P., et al. (1997). The relations of regulation and emotionality to children's situational empathy-related responding. *Motivation and Emotion, 21,* 87–108.

Haden, C. A., Ornstein, P. A., Eckerman, C. O., & Didow, S. M. (2001). Mother–child conversational interactions as events unfold: Linkages to subsequent remembering. *Child Development 72,* 1016–1031.

Hagekull, B. (1994). Infant temperament and early childhood functioning: Possible relations to the five-factor model. In C. F. Halverson, G. A. Kohnstamm, & R. P. Martin (Eds.), *The developing structure of temperament and personality from infancy to adulthood* (pp. 227–240). Hillsdale, NJ: Erlbaum.

Hagekull, B., & Bohlin, G. (2008, October). *Predictions from childhood temperament to social–emotional functioning in early adulthood.* Presented at the 17th meeting of the Occasional Temperament Conference in San Rafael, CA.

Hagekull, B., & Bohlin, G. (1995). Day care quality, family and child characteristics, and socioemotional development. *Early Childhood Research Quarterly, 10,* 505–526.

Haith, M. M., Hazan, C., & Goodman, G. S. (1988). Expectation and anticipation of dynamic visual events by 3.5-month-old babies. *Child Development, 59,* 467–479.

Halperin, J. M., & Schulz, K. P. (2006). Revisiting the role of the prefrontal cortex in the pathophysiology of attention-deficit/hyperactivity disorder (ADHD). *Psychological Bulletin, 132*(4), 560–581.

Halverson, C. F., Jr., Kohnstamm, G. A., & Martin, R. P. (1994). *The developing structure of temperament and personality from infancy to adulthood.* Hillsdale, NJ: Erlbaum.

Hammen, C. (2001). Vulnerability to depression in adulthood. In R. Ingram & J. Price (Eds.), *Handbook of vulnerability to psychopathology: Risk across the lifespan* (pp. 226–257). New York: Guilford Press.

Hariri, A. R. (2009). The neurology of individual differences in complex behavioral traits. *Annual Review of Neuroscience, 32,* 225–247.

Hariri, A. R., Mattay, V. S., Tessitore, A., Fera, F., & Weinberger, D. R. (2003). Neocortical modulation of the amygdala response to fearful stimuli. *Biological Psychiatry, 53*(6), 494–501.

Harkness, S., & Super, C. M. (1983). The cultural construction of child development: A framework for the socialization of affect. *Ethos, 11*(4), 221–231.

Harman, C., Rothbart, M. K., & Posner, M. I. (1997). Distress and attention interactions in early infancy. *Motivation and Emotion, 21,* 27–43.

Harter, S. (1980). The development of competence motivation in the mastery of cognitive and physical skills: Is there still a place for joy? In C. H. Nadeau (Ed.), *Psychology of motor behavior and sport* (pp. 3–20). Champaign, IL: Human Kinetics.

Harter, S. (1983). Developmental perspectives on the self-system. In P. H. Mussen (Ed.), *Handbook of child psychology: Vol. 4. Socialization, personality, and social development* (pp. 275–386). New York: Wiley.

Harter, S. (1998). The development of self-representations. In W. Damon (Series Ed.)

& Nancy Eisenberg (Vol. Ed.), *Handbook of child psychology: Vol. 3. Social, emotional, and personality development* (5th ed., pp. 553–617). New York: Wiley.

Harter, S. (2006). The self. In N. Eisenberg (Ed.), *Handbook of child psychology: Vol. 3. Social, emotional, and personality development* (6th ed., pp. 505–570). Hoboken, NJ: Wiley.

Hartman, C., Hox, J., Mellenbergh, G. J., Boyle, M. H., Offord, D. R., Racine, Y., et al. (2001). DSM-IV internal construct validity: When a taxonomy meets data. *Journal of Child Psychology and Psychiatry, 42*, 817–836.

Hasher, L., & Zachs, R. T. (1979). Automatic and effortful processes in memory. *Journal of Experimental Psychology: General, 108*(3), 356–388.

Havill, V. L., Allen, K., Halverson, C. F., & Kohnstamm, G. A. (1994). Parents use of Big Five categories in their natural language descriptions of children. In C. F. Halverson, G. A. Kohnstamm, & R. P. Martin (Eds.), *The developing structure of temperament and personality for infancy to adulthood* (pp. 371–386). Hillsdale, NJ: Erlbaum.

Hegvik, R. L., McDevitt, S. C., & Carey, W. B. (1982). The middle childhood temperament questionnaire. *Developmental and Behavioral Pediatrics, 3*, 197–200.

Henderson, N. D. (1982). Human behavior genetics. *Annual Review of Psychology, 33*, 403–440.

Hermans, H. J. M., & Kempen, H. J. G. (1998). Moving cultures: The perilous problems of cultural dichotomies in a globalizing society. *American Psychologist, 53*, 1111–1120.

Heymans, G., & Wiersma, E. D. (1906). Beiträge zur speziellen psychologie auf Grund einer Messenuntersuchungung. *Zeitschrift fur Psychologie, 42*, 81–127, 258–301.

Higgins, E. T. (1991). Development of self-regulatory and self-evaluative processes: Costs, benefits, and tradeoffs. In M. R. Gunnar & L. A. Sroufe (Eds.), *Self processes and development: The Minnesota symposia on child psychology* (Vol. 23, pp. 125–165). Hillsdale, NJ: Erlbaum.

Hinde, R. A. (1997). *Relationships: A dialectical perspective*. Psychology Press: Erlbaum, Taylor & Francis.

Hinde, R. A. (1998). Integrating across levels of complexity. In D. M. Hann, L. C. Huffman, I. I. Lederhendler, & D. Meineke (Eds.), *Advancing research on developmental plasticity* (pp. 165–173). Bethesda, MD: National Institute of Mental Health, NIH.

Hoff-Ginsberg, E. (1991). Mother–child conversation in different social classes and communicative settings. *Child Development, 62*(4), 782–796.

Hoffman, M. L. (1975). Developmental synthesis of affect and cognition and its implications for altruistic motivation. *Developmental Psychology, 11*, 607–622.

Hoffman, M. L. (1979). Development of moral thought, feeling, and behavior. *American Psychologist, 34*(10), 958–966.

Hoffman, M. L. (1983). Affective and cognitive processes in moral internalization. In E. T. Higgins, D. Ruble, & W. Hartup (Eds.), *Social cognition and social development: A sociocultural perspective* (pp. 236–274). New York: Cambridge University Press.

Hoffman, M. L. (2000). *Empathy and moral development: Implications for caring and justice.* New York: Cambridge University Press.

Homiak, M. (2007, winter). *Moral character.* In E. N. Zalta (Ed.), Stanford Encyclopedia of Philosophy web site. Retrieved December, 2008, from *plato.stanford.edu/archives/win2007/entries/moral-character*

Honzik, M. P. (1965). Prediction of behavior from birth to maturity. Review of Birth to Maturity, by J. Kagan & H. Moss. *Merrill–Palmer Quarterly, 11,* 77–88.

Horn, J. L., & Cattell, R. B. (1966). Refinement and test of the theory of fluid and crystallized general intelligence. *Journal of Educational Psychology, 57*(5), 253–270.

Horney, K. (1939). *The neurotic personality of our time.* New York: Norton.

Horney, K. (1945). *Our inner conflicts.* New York: Norton.

Horney, K. (1950). *Neurosis and human growth.* New York: Norton.

Howard, J. W. & Rothbart, M. (1980). Social categorization and memory for in-group and out-group behavior. *Journal of Personality and Social Psychology, 38*(2), 301–310.

Hwang, J. Y. (2002). *Development of a temperament self-report measure for young children.* Doctoral dissertation, University of Oregon (Pub. No. AAT 3072589).

Hwang, J. Y., & Rothbart, M. K. (2003). Behavior genetics studies of infant temperament: Findings vary across parent-report instruments. *Infant Behavior and Development, 26*(1), 112–114.

Hyde, J. S., Mezulis, A. H., & Abramson, L. Y. (2008). The ABCs of depression: Integrating affective, biological, and cognitive models to explain the emergence of the gender difference in depression. *Psychological Review, 115*(2), 291–313.

Hyson, M. (2008). *Enthusiastic and engaged learners: Approaches to learning in the early childhood classroom.* New York: Teachers College Press.

Insel, T. R. (2003). Is social attachment an addictive disorder? *Physiology and Behavior, 79*(3), 351–357.

Ito, T. A., & Cacioppo, J. T. (2005). Variations on a human universal: Individual differences in positivity offset and negativity bias. *Cognition and Emotion, 19,* 1–26.

Izard, C. E. (1991). *The psychology of emotions.* New York: Plenum Press.

Izard, C. E. (1993). Four systems for emotion activation: Cognitive and noncognitive processes. *Psychological Review, 100,* 68–90.

Jackson, P. W. (2002). *John Dewey and the philospher's task.* New York: Teacher's College Press.

Jaffe, J., Beebe, B., Feldstein, S., Crown, C. L., & Jasnow, M. (2001). Rhythms of Dialogue in Infancy. *Monographs of the Society for Research in Child Development,* Series 264, *66*(2), 1–132.

Jahromi, L. B., Putnam, S. P., & Stifter, C. A. (2004). Maternal regulation of infant reactivity from 2 to 6 months. *Developmental Psychology, 40*(4), 477–487.

John, O. P., & Srivastava, S. (1999). The Big Five trait taxonomy: History, measurement, and theoretical perspectives. In L. A. Pervin & O. P. John (Eds.), *Handbook of personality: Theory and research* (2nd ed., pp. 102–138). New York: Guilford Press.

Johnson, K. A., Robertson, I. H., Barry, E., Mulligan, A., Daibhis, A., Daly, M., et al. (2008). Impaired conflict resolution and alerting in children with ADHD: Evidence from the attention network task (ANT). *Journal of Child Psychology and Psychiatry, 49*(12), 1339–1347.

Johnson, M. H., Posner, M. I., & Rothbart, M. K. (1991). Components of visual orienting in early infancy: Contingency learning, anticipatory looking, and disengaging. *Journal of Cognitive Neuroscience, 3*, 335–344.

Johnson, M. H., Posner, M. I., & Rothbart, M. K. (1994). Facilitation of saccades toward a covertly attended location in early infancy. *Psychological Science, 5*, 90–93.

Jones, L. B., Rothbart, M. K., & Posner, M. I. (2003). Development of executive attention in preschool children. *Developmental Science, 6*(5), 498–504.

Jones, S., Eisenberg, N., Fabes, R. A., & MacKinnon, D. P. (2002). Parents' reactions to elementary school children's negative emotions: Relations to social and emotional functioning at school. *Merrill-Palmer Quarterly, 48*(2), 133–159.

Jones, W. H., Cavert, C., & Indart, M. (1983). *Impressions of shyness.* Paper presented at the annual meeting of the American Psychological Association, Anaheim, CA.

Jones, W. H., & Carpenter, B. N. (1986). Shyness, social behavior, and relationships. In W. H. Jones, J. M. Cheek, & S. R. Briggs (Eds.), *Shyness: Perspectives on research and treatment* (pp. 227–238). New York: Plenum.

Jung, C. G. (1923). *Psychological types or the psychology of individuation.* New York: Harcourt Brace.

Jung, C. G. (1928). *Contributions to analytic psychology.* London: Routledge & Kegan Paul.

Kagan, J. (1984). *The nature of the child.* New York: Basic Books.

Kagan, J. (1994). *Galen's prophecy: Temperament in human nature.* New York: Basic Books.

Kagan, J. (1997). Temperament and the reactions to unfamiliarity. *Child Development, 68*(1), 139–143.

Kagan, J. (1998). Biology and the child. In W. Damon & N. Eisenberg (Eds.), *Handbook of child psychology: Vol. 3. Social, emotional and personality development* (5th ed., pp. 177–235). New York: Wiley.

Kagan, J., & Fox, N. A. (2006). Biology, culture, and temperamental biases. In W. Damon & N. Eisenberg (Eds.), *Handbook of child psychology: Vol. 3. Social, emotional, and personality development* (6th ed., pp. 167–225). Hoboken, NJ: Wiley.

Kagan, J., & Moss, H. A. (1962). *Birth to maturity.* New York: Wiley.

Kagan, J., Reznick, J. S., & Snidman, N. (1988). Biological bases of childhood shyness. *Science, 240*(4849), 167–171.

Kagan, J., & Snidman, N. (1999). Early childhood predictors of adult anxiety disorders. *Biological Psychiatry, 46*(11), 1536–1541.

Kagan, J., Snidman, N., & Arcus, D. (1998). Childhood derivatives of high and low reactivity in infancy. *Child Development, 69*(6), 1483–1493.

Kagan, J., Snidman, N., Zentner, M., & Peterson, E. (1999). Infant temperament and anxious symptoms in school age children. *Development and psychopathology, 11*(2), 209–224.

Kagan, S. L., Moore, E., & Bredekamp, S. (Eds.). (1995, June). *Reconsidering children's early development and learning: Toward common views and vocabulary. Goal 1: Technical Planning Group Report 95-03*. Washington, DC: National Education Goals Panel.

Kanske, P. (2008). *Exploring executive attention in emotion: ERP and fMRI evidence. MPI series in human cognitive and brain sciences: Vol. 106*. [Dissertation]. Leipzig, Germany: Max Planck Institute for Human Cognitive and Brain Sciences, University of Leipzig.

Kaufman, A., & Kaufman, N. (1990). *Kaufman brief intelligence test*. Circle Pines, MN: American Guidance Service.

Keily, M. K., Lofthouse, N., Bates, J. W., Dodge, K. A., & Pettit, G. S. (2003). Differential risks of covarying and pure components in mother and teacher reports of externalizing and internalizing behavior across ages 5 to 14. *Journal of Abnormal Child Psychology, 31*, 267–283.

Keogh, B. K. (1989). Applying temperament research to school. In G. A. Kohnstamm, J. Bates, & M. K. Rothbart (Eds.), *Temperament in childhood* (pp. 437–450). Chichester, UK: Wiley.

Keogh, B. K. (2003). *Temperament in the classroom*. Baltimore: Brookes.

Kerr, M. (2001). Culture as a context for temperament: Suggestions from the life courses of shy Swedes and Americans. In T. D. Wachs & G. A. Kohnstamm (Eds.), *Temperament in context* (pp. 139–152). Mahwah, NJ: Erlbaum.

Kerr, M., Lambert, W. W., & Bem, D. J. (1996). Life course sequelae of childhood shyness in Sweden: Comparison with the United States. *Developmental Psychology, 32*, 1100–1105.

Kerr, M., & Stattin, H. (2000). What parents know, how they know it, and several forms of adolescent adjustment: Further evidence for a reinterpretation of monitoring. *Developmental Psychology, 36*, 366–380.

Kessen, W. (1965). *The child*. New York: Wiley.

Kieras, J. E., Tobin, R. M., Graziano, W. G., & Rothbart, M. K. (2005). You can't always get what you want: Effortful control and children's responses to undesirable gifts. *Psychological Science, 16*(5), 391–396.

Kim-Goodwin, Y. S. (2003). Postpartum beliefs and practices among non-Western cultures. *MCN: The American Journal of Maternal/Child Nursing, 28*, 74–78.

King, J. E., & Figueredo, A. J. (1997). The five-factor model plus dominance in chimpanzee personality. *Journal of Research in Personality, 31*(2), 257–271.

Kochanska, G. (1991). Socialization and temperament in the development of guilt and conscience. *Child Development, 62*, 1379–1392.

Kochanska, G. (1993). Toward a synthesis of parental socialization and child temperament in early development of conscience. *Child Development, 64*, 325–347.

Kochanska, G. (1995). Children's temperament, mothers' discipline, and security of attachment: Multiple pathways to emerging internalizations. *Child Development, 66*, 597–615.

Kochanska, G. (1997). Multiple pathways to conscience for children with different temperaments: From toddlerhood to age 5. *Developmental Psychology, 33*, 228–240.

Kochanska, G., & Aksan, N. (2007). Conscience in childhood: Past, present, and future. In G. W. Ladd (Ed.), *Appraising the human developmental sciences: Essays in honor of Merrill–Palmer Quarterly* (pp. 238–249). Detroit, MI: Wayne State University Press.

Kochanska, G., Aksan, N., & Joy, M. E. (2007). Children's fearfulness as a moderator of parenting in early socialization: Two longitudinal studies. *Developmental Psychology, 43*(1), 222–237.

Kochanska, G., DeVet, K., Goldman, M., Murray, K. T., & Putnam, S. P. (1993). Maternal reports of conscience development and temperament in young children. *Child Development, 65*(3), 852–868.

Kochanska, G., Gross, J. N., Lin, M-H., & Nichols, K. E. (2002). Guilt in young children: Development, determinants, and relations with a broader system of standards. *Child Development, 73*(2), 461–482.

Kochanska, G., Murray, K. T., & Coy, K. C. (1997). Inhibitory control as a contributor to conscience in childhood: From toddler to early school age. *Child Development, 68*, 263–277.

Kochanska, G., Murray, K. T., & Harlan, E. T. (2000). Effortful control in early childhood: Continuity and change, antecedents, and implications for social development. *Developmental Psychology, 36*(2), 220–232.

Kochanska, G., Murray, K. T., Jacques, T. Y., Koenig, A. L., & Vandegeest, K. A. (1996). Inhibitory control in young children and its role in emerging internalization. *Child Development, 67*, 490–507.

Kochanska, G.. Philibert, R. A., & Barry, R. A. (2009). Interplay of genes and early mother–child relationship in the development of self-regulation from toddler to preschool. *Journal of Child Psychology and Psychiatry, 50*(11), 1331–1338

Kochanska, G., Tjebkes, T. L., & Forman, D. R. (1998). Children's emerging regulation of conduct: Restraint, compliance, and internalization from infancy to the second year. *Child Development, 69*, 1378–1389.

Kohlberg, L. (1969). Stage and sequence: The cognitive-developmental approach to socialization. In D. A. Goslin (Ed.), *Handbook of socialization theory and research* (pp. 347–480). Chicago: Rand McNally.

Kohlberg, L. (1976). Moral stages and moralization: The cognitive-developmental approach. In T. Lickona (Ed.), *Moral development and behavior: Theory, research, and social issues* (pp. 31–53). New York: Holt, Rinehart and Winston.

Kohnstamm, G. A. (1989). Temperament in childhood: Cross-cultural and sex differences. In G. A. Kohnstamm, J. E. Bates, & M. K. Rothbart (Eds.), *Temperament in childhood* (pp. 483–508). Chichester, UK: Wiley.

Kohnstamm, G. A., Bates, J. E., & Rothbart, M. K. (Eds.). (1989). *Temperament in childhood*. Chichester, UK: Wiley.

Kohnstamm, G. A., Halverson, C. F. J., Mervielde, I., & Havill, V. L. (Eds.). (1998). *Parental descriptions of child personality: Developmental antecedents of the Big Five?* Mahwah, NJ: Erlbaum.

Komsi, N., Raikkonen, K., Pesonen, A., Heinonen, K., Keskivaara, A., & Strandberg, T. E. (2006). Continuity of temperament from infancy to childhood. *Infant Behavior and Development, 29*, 494–508.

Konner, M. (2002). *The tangled wing: Biological constraints on the human spirit* (2nd ed). New York: Holt.

Kopp, C. B. (1989). Regulation of distress and negative emotions: A developmental view. *Developmental Psychology, 25*, 343–354.

Kopp, C. B. (1992). Emotional distress and control in young children. In N. Eisenberg & R. A. Fabes (Eds.), *Emotion and its regulation in early development. New directions for child development: No. 55. The Jossey-Bass education series* (pp. 41–56). San Francisco: Jossey-Bass.

Kopp, C. B. (2009). Emotion-focused coping in young children: Self and self-regulatory processes. In E. A. Skinner & M. J. Zimmer-Gembeck (Eds.), *Coping and the development of regulation. New directions for child and adolescent development* (pp. 33–46). San Francisco: Jossey-Bass.

Korn, S. J., & Gannon, S. (1983). Temperament, cultural variation, and behavior disorder in preschool children. *Child Psychiatry and Human Development, 12*(4), 203–212.

Korner, A. F. (1964). Some hypotheses regarding the significance of individual differences at birth for later development. *Psychoanalytic Study of the Child, 19*, 58–72.

Korner, A. F. (1972). State as a variable, as obstacle and as mediator of stimulation in infant research. *Merrill–Palmer Quarterly, 18*, 77–94.

Korner, A. F., Zeanah, C. H., Linden, J., Kraemer, H. C., Kerkowitz, R. I., & Agras, W. S. (1985). Relation between neonatal and later activity and temperament. *Child Development, 56*, 38–42.

Kramer, P. D. (1993). *Listening to Prozac*. New York: Viking.

Kremen, A. M., & Block, J. (1998). The roots of ego control in young adulthood: Links with parenting in early childhood. *Journal of Personality and Social Psychology, 75*, 1062–1075.

Krueger, R. F. (1999). The structure of common mental disorders. *Archives of General Psychiatry, 56*, 921–926.

Krueger, R. F., & Markon, K. E. (2006). Reinterpreting comorbidity: A model based approach to understanding and classifying psychopathology. *Annual Review of Clinical Psychology, 2*, 111–133.

Krueger, R. F., & Johnson, W. (2008). Behavioral genetics and personality. In L. Q. Pervin, O. P. John, & R. W. Robins (Eds.), *Handbook of personality: Theory and research* (3rd ed., pp. 287–310). New York: Guilford Press.

Krueger, R. F., South, S., Johnson, W., & Iacono, W. (2008). The heritability of personality is not always 50%: Gene–environment interactions and correlations between personality and parenting. *Journal of Personality, 76*, 1485–1522.

Kubzansky, L. D., Martin, L. T., & Buka, S. L. (2004). Early manifestations of personality and adult emotional functioning. *Emotion, 4*(4), 364–377.

Labouvie-Vief, G., (2008). Dynamic integration theory: Emotion, cognition, and equilibrium in later life. In V. Bengtson, M. Silverstein, N. Putney, & D. Gans (Eds.), *Handbook of theories of aging* (pp. 253–267). New York: Springer.

Labouvie-Vief, G., & Marquez, M. G. (2004). Dynamic integration: Affect optimization and differentiation in development. In D. Y. Dai & R. J. Sternberg (Eds.),

Motivation, emotion and cognition: Integrative perspectives on intellectual functioning and development (pp. 237–272). Mahwah, NJ: Erlbaum.

Labouvie-Vief, G., & Medler, M. (2002). Affect optimization and affect complexity: Modes and styles of regulation in adulthood. *Psychology and Aging, 17,* 571–587.

Ladygina-Kots, N. N. (2002). *Infant ape and human child (instincts, emotions, play, habits).* New York: Oxford University Press. (Original work published 1935 by the Museum Darwinianum, Moscow)

Landry, R., & Bryson, S. (2004). Impaired disengagement of attention in young children with autism. *Journal of Child Psychology and Psychiatry, 45*(6), 1115–1122.

Larson, S. K., DiPietro, J. A., & Porges, S. M. (1987, April). *Neonatal and NBAS performance are related to development across at 15 months.* Paper presented at the Society for Research in Child Development, Baltimore, MD.

Lawrence, A. D., & Calder, A. J. (2004). Homologizing human emotions. In D. Evans & P. Cruse (Eds.), *Emotion, evolution, and rationality* (pp. 15–47). Oxford, UK: Oxford University Press.

Lawrence, A. D., Calder, A. J., McGowan, S. W., & Grasby, P. M. (2002). Selective disruption of the recognition of facial expressions of anger. *Neuroreport, 13*(6), 881–884.

Leary, M. R. (2004). *The curse of the self: Self-awareness, egotism, and the quality of human life.* New York: Oxford University Press.

LeDoux, J. E. (1987). Emotion. In F. Plum (Ed.), *Handbook of physiology. Section 1: The nervous system: Vol. V. Higher functions of the brain, Part 1* (pp. 419–460). Bethesda, MD: American Physiological Society.

LeDoux, J. E. (1989). Cognitive-emotional interactions in the brain. *Cognition and Emotion, 3,* 267–289.

LeDoux, J. E. (1996). *The emotional brain: The mysterious underpinnings of emotional life.* New York: Simon & Schuster.

Lee, C. L., & Bates, J. E. (1985). Mother–child interaction at age two and perceived difficult temperament. *Child Development, 56,* 1314–1325.

Leerkes, E. M., & Crockenberg, S. C. (2002). The development of maternal self-efficacy and its impact on maternal behavior. *Infancy, 3*(2), 227.

Leerkes, E. M., & Crockenberg, S. C. (2006). Antecedents of mothers' emotional and cognitive responses to infant distress: The role of family, mother, and infant characteristics. *Infant Mental Health Journal, 27*(4), 405.

Lemery, K. S., Essex, M., & Smider, N. (2002). Revealing the relationship between temperament and behavior problem symptoms by eliminating measurement confounding: Expert ratings and factor analyses. *Child Development, 73,* 867–882.

Lemery, K. S., Goldsmith, H. H., Klinnert, M. D., & Mrazek, D. A. (1999). Developmental models of infant and childhood temperament. *Developmental Psychology, 35,* 189–204.

Lengua, L. J. (2002). The contribution of emotionality and self-regulation to the understanding of children's response to multiple risk. *Child Development, 73,* 144–161.

Lengua, L. J. (2003). Associations among emotionality, self-regulation, adjustment problems and positive adjustment in middle childhood. *Journal of Applied Developmental Psychology, 24,* 595–618.

Lengua, L. J. (2006). Growth in temperament and parenting as predictors of adjustment during children's transition to adolescence. *Developmental Psychology, 42,* 819–832.

Lengua, L. J. (2007, April). *Family disruptions and parenting as predictors of the development of executive functioning.* Paper presented at the Biennial Meeting for the Society for Research on Child Development, Boston, MA.

Lengua, L. J. (2008, October). *Effortful control in the context of socioeconomic and psychosocial risk.* Invited paper for the symposium: New Directions in Psychological Science and their Implications for Dissemination. Paper presented at the American Psychological Association's fourth annual Science Leadership Conference *Designing the Future: Innovations in Knowledge Dissemination for Psychological Science,* Tempe, AZ.

Lengua, L. J., Bush, N., Long, A. C., Trancik, A. M., & Kovacs, E. A. (2008). Effortful control as a moderator of the relation between contextual risk and growth in adjustment problems. *Development and Psychopathology, 20,* 509–528.

Lengua, L. J., Honorado, E., & Bush, N. (2007). Cumulative risk and parenting as predictors of effortful control and social competence in preschool children. *Journal of Applied Developmental Psychology, 28,* 40–55.

Lengua, L. J., & Kovacs, E. A. (2005). Bidirectional associations between temperament and parenting in the prediction of adjustment problems in middle childhood. *Journal of Applied Developmental Psychology, 26,* 21–38.

Lengua, L. J., & Long, A. C. (2002). The role of emotionality and self-regulation in the appraisal-coping process: Tests of direct and moderating effects. *Journal of Applied Developmental Psychology, 23,* 471–493.

Lengua, L. J., Sandler, I. N., West, S. G., Wolchik, S. A., & Curran, P. J. (1999). Emotionality and self-regulation, threat appraisal, and coping in children of divorce. *Development and Psychopathology, 11*(1), 15–37.

Lepper, M. R., & Greene, D. (1975). Turning play into work: Effects of adult surveillance and extrinsic rewards on children's intrinsic motivation. *Journal of Personality and Social Psychology, 31,* 479–486.

Lesch, K. P. (2003). Neuroticism and serotonin: A developmental genetic perspective. In R. Plomin, J. C. DeFries, I. W. Craig, & P. McGuffin (Eds.), *Behavioral genetics in the postgenomic era* (pp. 389–423). Washington, DC: American Psychological Association.

Levine, S., Haltmeyer, G. C., Karas, G. G., & Denenberg, V. H. (1967). Physiological and behavioral effects of infantile stimulation. *Physiology and Behavior, 2,* 55–59.

Lewis, M., & Brookes, J. (1978). Self-knowledge and emotional development. In M. Lewis & L. A. Rosenblum (Eds.), *The genesis of behavior: Vol. 1. The development of affect* (pp. 205–226). New York: Plenum.

Lewis, M., & Ramsay, D. S. (1997). Stress reactivity and self-recognition. *Child Development, 68,* 621–629.

Lewis, M., & Ramsay, D. S. (2004). Development of self-recognition, personal pronoun use, and pretend play during the 2nd year. *Child Development, 75*(6), 1821–1831.

Lewis, M., Sullivan, M. W., Stanger, C., & Weiss, M. (1989). Self-development and self-conscious emotions. *Child Development, 60*(1), 146–156.

Lewkowicz, D. J., & Turkewitz, G. (1981). Intersensory interaction in newborns: Modification of visual preferences following exposure to sound. *Child Development, 52,* 827–832.

Lillard, A. S. (2005). *Montessori: The science behind the genius.* New York: Oxford University Press.

Lindsay, S. R. (2000). *Handbook of applied dog behavior and training. Vol. 1: Adaptation and learning.* Ames: Iowa State University.

Lindsay, S. R. (2005). *Handbook of applied dog behavior and training. Vol. 3: Procedures and protocols.* Oxford, UK: Blackwell.

Linn, P., & Horowitz, L. F. (1983). The relationship between infant individual differences and mother–infant interaction during the neonatal period. *Infant Behavior and Development, 6,* 415–427.

Loehlin, J. C. (1992). *Genes and environment in personality development.* New York: Sage.

Low, B. (2002). *NFB kids: Portrayals of children by the National Film Board of Canada, 1939–1989.* Waterloo: Wilfred Laurier University Press.

Luu, P., Collins, P., & Tucker, D. M. (2000). Mood, personality, and self-monitoring: Negative affect and emotionality in relation to frontal lobe mechanisms of error monitoring. *Journal of Experimental Psychology: General, 129,* 43–60.

Lynam, D. R., Caspi, A., Moffitt, T., Wilkstron, P. H., Loeber, R., & Novak, S. (2000). The interaction between impulsivity and neighborhood context on offending: The effects of impulsivity are stronger in poorer neighborhoods. *Journal of Abnormal Psychology, 109,* 563–574.

Maccoby, E., & Martin, J. (1983). Socialization in the context of the family: Parent–child interaction. In E. M. Hetherington (Ed.), *Handbook of child psychology: Socialization, personality, and social development* (Vol. 4, pp. 1–101). New York: Wiley.

Mahler, M. S. (1967). On human symbiosis and the vicissitudes of individuation. *Journal of the American Psychoanalytic Association, 15*(4), 740.

Malphurs, J. E., Field, T. M., Larraine, C., Pickens, J., Pelaez-Nogueras, M., Yando, R., et al. (1996). Altering withdrawn and intrusive interaction behaviors of depressed mothers. *Infant Mental Health Journal, 17*(2), 152–160.

Markon, K. E., & Krueger, R. F. (2006). Information-theoretic latent distribution modeling: Distinguishing discrete and continuous latent variable models. *Psychological Methods, 11,* 228–243.

Markon, K. E., Krueger, R. F., & Watson, D. (2005). Delineating the structure of normal and abnormal personality: An integrative hierarchical approach. *Journal of Personality and Social Psychology, 88,* 139–157.

Markus, H. R., & Kitayama, S. (1991). Culture and self: Implications for cognition, emotion, and motivation. *Psychological Review, 98,* 224–253.

Marsh, A. A., Finger, E. C., Mitchell, D. G. V., Reid, M. E., Sims, C., Kosson, D. S., et al., (2008). Reduced amygdala response to fearful expressions in children and adolescents with callous–unemotional traits and disruptive behavior disorders. *American Journal of Psychiatry, 165*(6), 712–720.

Martin, J. (2010). *Neuroanatomy text and atlas* (4th ed.). New York: McGraw-Hill Medical.

Martin, J. N., & Fox, N. A. (2006). Temperament. In K. McCartney & D. Phillips (Eds.), *Blackwell handbook of early childhood development* (pp. 126–146). Malden, MA: Blackwell.

Martin, R. P., Drew, K. D., Gaddis, L. R.; & Moseley, M. (1988). Prediction of elementary school achievement from preschool temperament: Three studies. *School Psychology Review, 17*(1), 125–137.

Martin, R. P. (1989). Activity level, distractibility, and persistence: Critical characteristics in early schooling. In G. A. Kohnstamm, J. E. Bates, & M. K. Rothbart (Eds.), *Temperament in childhood* (pp. 451–461). Chichester, UK: Wiley.

Martin, R. P., Wisenbaker, J., & Huttunen, M. (1994). The factor structure of instruments based on the Chess–Thomas model of temperament: Implications for the Big Five model. In C. F. Halverson, G. A. Kohnstamm, & R. P. Martin (Eds.), *The developing structure of temperament and personality from infancy to adulthood* (pp. 157–172). Hillsdale, NJ: Erlbaum.

Mascolo, M. F. (2004). The coactive construction of selves in cultures. *New Directions for Child and Adolescent Development, 104*, 79–90.

Masten, A. S. (2001). Ordinary magic: Resilience processes in development. *American Psychologist, 56*, 227–238.

Matthews, G., Zeidner, M., & Roberts, R. D. (2002). *Emotional intelligence: Science and myth*. Cambridge, MA: MIT Press.

Matheny, A. P., Jr., Riese, M. L., & Wilson, R. S. (1985). Rudiments of infant temperament: Newborn to nine months. *Developmental Psychology, 21*, 486–494.

McCall, R. B. (1990). Infancy research: Individual differences. *Merrill–Palmer Quarterly, 36*(1), 141–157.

McClowry, S. G., Hegvik, R., & Teglasi, H. (1993). An examination of the construct validity of the middle childhood temperament questionnaire. *Merrill–Palmer Quarterly, 39*, 279–293.

McClowry, S. G., Snow, D. L., & Tamis-LeMonda, C. S. (2005). An evaluation of the effects of INSIGHTS on the behavior of inner city primary school children. *Journal of Primary Prevention, 26*(6), 567–584.

McCrae, R. R. (2001). Trait psychology and culture: Exploring intercultural comparisons. *Journal of Personality, 69*(6), 819–846.

McCrae, R. R., & Costa, P. T., Jr. (1987). Validation of the five-factor model of personality across instruments and observers. *Journal of Personality and Social Psychology, 52*, 81–90.

McCrae, R. R., Costa, P. T., Jr., Ostendorf, F., Angleitner, A., Hrebíčková, M., Avia, M. D., et al. (2000). Nature over nurture: Temperament, personality, and life span development. *Journal of Personality and Social Psychology, 78*(1), 173–186.

McCrae, R. R., & John, O. P. (1992). An introduction to the five-factor model and its applications. *Journal of Personality, 60*, 175–215.

McEwen, B. S. (2007). Physiology and neurobiology of stress and adaptation: Central role of the brain. *Physiological Review, 87,* 873–904.

McGaugh, J. L. (2003). *Memory and emotion: The making of lasting memories.* New York: Columbia University Press.

Mead, G. H. (1934). *Mind, self and society.* Chicago: University of Chicago Press.

Mead, M. (1949). *Male and female.* New York: William Morrow.

Meaney, M. J. (2001). Maternal care, gene expression, and the transmission of individual differences in stress reactivity across generations. *Annual Review of Neuroscience, 24,* 1161–1192.

Meier, C. A. (1989). *Healing dream and ritual: Ancient incubation and modern psychotherapy.* Einsiedeln, Switzerland: Daimon Verlag.

Meili, R., & Meili-Dworetzki, G. (1972). *Grundlagen individueller Personlichkeitsunterscheide.* Bern, Switzerland: Huber.

Messer, D. J. (1995). Mastery motivation: Past, present and future. In R. H. MacTurk & G. A. Morgan (Eds.), *Mastery motivation: Origins, conceptualizations, and applications. Advances in applied developmental psychology* (Vol. 12, pp. 293–316). Norwood, NJ: Ablex.

Mezulis, A. H., Hyde, J. S., & Abramson, L. Y. (2006). The developmental origins of cognitive vulnerability to depression: Temperament, parenting, and negative life events. *Developmental Psychology, 42,* 1012–1025.

Mischel, W. (1968). *Personality and assessment.* New York: Wiley.

Mischel, W. (1983). Delay of gratification as process and as person variable in development. In D. Magnusson & V. P. Allen (Eds.), *Human development: An interactional perspective* (pp. 149–165). New York: Academic Press.

Mischel, W., & Ayduk, O. (2004). Willpower in a cognitive-affective processing system: The dynamics of delay of gratification. In R. F. Baumeister & K. D. Vohs (Eds.), *Handbook of self-regulation: Research, theory, and applications* (pp. 99–129). New York: Guilford Press.

Mischel, W., Shoda, Y., & Rodriguez, M. L. (1989). Delay of gratification in children. *Science, 244*(4907), 933–938.

Mogg, K., Bradley, B. P., & Williams, R. (1995). Attentional bias in anxiety and depression: The role of awareness. *British Journal of Clinical Psychology, 34*(1), 17–36.

Monks of New Skete (1991). *The art of raising a puppy.* Boston: Little, Brown.

Morgan, G. A., Harmon, R. J., & Maslin-Cole, C. A. (1990). Mastery motivation: Definition and measurement. *Early Education and Development, 1,* 318–339.

Morris, A. S., Silk, J. S., Steinberg, L., Sessa, F. M., Avenoli, S., & Essex, M. J. (2002). Temperamental vulnerabilities and negative parenting as interaction predictors of child adjustment. *Journal of Marriage and Family, 64,* 461–471.

Muris, P., & Ollendick, T. H. (2005). The role of temperament in the etiology of child psychopathology. *Clinical Child and Family Psychology Review, 8*(4), 271–289.

Murphy, B. C., Shepard, S., Eisenberg, N., Fabes, R. A., & Guthrie, I. K. (1999). Contemporaneous and longitudinal relations of young adolescents' dispositional sympathy to their emotionality, regulation, and social functioning. *Journal of Early Adolescence, 29,* 66–97.

Murphy, L. B. (1962). *The widening world of childhood*. New York: Basic Books.

Murphy, L. B., & Moriarty, A. (1976). *Vulnerability, coping, and growth from infancy to adolescence*. New Haven, CT: Yale University Press.

Nagin, D., & Tremblay, R. (2005). What has been learned from group-based trajectory modeling? Examples from physical aggression and other problem behaviors. *Annals of the American Academy of Political and Social Science, 602*, 82–117.

Nebylitsyn, V. D. (1972a). *Fundamental properties of the human nervous system*. New York: Plenum.

Nebylitsyn, V. D. (1972b). The problem of general and partial properties of the nervous system. In V. D. Nebylitsyn & J. A. Gray (Eds.), *Biological bases of individual behavior* (pp. 400–417). New York: Academic Press.

Needham, J. (1973). *Chinese science*. Cambridge, MA: MIT Press.

Neilon, P. (1948). Shirley's babies after 15 years: A personality study. *Journal of Genetic Psychology 73*, 175–186.

Nelson, K. (2007). *Young minds in social worlds: Experience, meaning, and memory*. Cambridge, MA: Harvard University Press.

Nelson, R. J., & Young, K. A. (1998). Behavior in mice with targeted disruption of single genes. *Neuroscience and Biobehavioral Reviews, 22*(3), 453–462.

Niebuhr, R. (1932). *Moral man and immoral society*. New York: Scribner's Sons.

Nietzel, M. T., & Harris, M. J. (1990). Relationship of dependency and achievement/autonomy to depression. *Clinical Psychology Review, 10*, 279–297.

Nigg, J. T., Martel, M. M., Nikolas, M., & Casey, B. J. (2010). Intersection of emotion and cognition in developmental psychopathology. In S. D. Calkins & M. A. Bell (Eds.), *Child development at the intersection of emotion and cognition*. Washington DC: American Psychological Association Press.

Nishijo, H., Ono, T., & Nishino, H. (1988). Single neuron responses in amygdala of alert monkey during complex sensory stimulation with affective significance. *Journal of Neuroscience, 8*, 3570–3583.

Nolen-Hoeksema, S., Wisco, B. E., & Lyubomirsky, S. (2008). Rethinking rumination. *Perspectives on Psychological Science, 3*, 400–424.

O'Connor, B. P., & Dvorak, T. (2001). Conditional associations between parental behavior and adolescent problems: A search for personality–environment interactions. *Journal of Research in Personality, 35*(1), 1–26.

O'Connor, T. G., Caspi, A., DeFries, J. C., & Plomin, R. (2003). Genotype–environment interaction in children's adjustment to parental separation. *Journal of Child Psychology and Psychiatry and Allied Disciplines, 44*(6), 849–856.

Oldehinkel, A. J., Hartman, C. A., De Winter, A. F., Veenstra, R., & Ormel, J. (2004). Temperament profiles associated with internalizing and externalizing problems in preadolescence. *Development and Psychopathology, 16*, 421–440.

O'Mahony, J. F. (1984) Knowing others through the self: Influence of self-perception on the perception of others: A review. *Current Psychological Research and Reviews, 3*(4), 48–62.

Ormel, J., Oldehinkel, A. J., Ferdinand, R. F., Hartman, C. A., De Winter, A. F., Veenstra, R., et al. (2005). Internalizing and externalizing problems in adolescence: General and dimension-specific effects of familial loadings and preadolescent temperament traits. *Psychological Medicine, 35,* 1825–1835.

Orobio de Castro, B., Veerman, J. W., Koops, W., Bosch, J. D., & Monshouwer, H. J. (2002). Hostile attribution of intent and aggressive behavior: A meta-analysis. *Child Development, 73*(3), 916–934.

Orth, U., Robins, R. W., & Roberts, B. W. (2008). Low self-esteem prospectively predicts depression in adolescence and young adulthood. *Journal of Personality and Social Psychology, 95*(3), 695–708.

Osofsky, J. D. (1979). *Handbook of infant development.* New York: Wiley.

Oxford, M. C., Cavell, T. A., & Hughes, J. N. (2003). Callous/unemotional traits moderate the relation between ineffective parenting and child externalizing problems: A partial replication and extension. *Journal of Clinical Child and Adolescent Psychology, 32,* 577–585.

Oyama, S. (1985). *The ontogeny of information: Developmental systems and evolution.* Cambridge, UK: Cambridge University Press.

Paine, A. B. (1912). *Mark Twain: A biography. The personal and literary life of Samuel Langhorne Clemens: Vol. 3.* New York: Harper & Brothers.

Panksepp, J. (1982). Toward a general psychobiological theory of emotions. *Behavioral and Brain Sciences, 5,* 407–467.

Panksepp, J. (1986a). The anatomy of emotions. In R. Plutchik & H. Kellerman (Eds.), *Emotion: Theory, research and experience: Vol. 3. Biological foundations of emotions* (pp. 91–124). San Diego, CA: Academic Press.

Panksepp, J. (1986b). The neurochemistry of behavior. *Annual Review of Psychology, 37,* 77–107.

Panksepp, J. (1993). Neurochemical control of moods and emotions: Amino acids to neuropeptides. In M. Lewis & J. M. Havilland (Eds.), *Handbook of emotions* (pp. 87–107). New York: Guilford Press.

Panksepp, J. (1998). *Affective neuroscience: The foundations of human and animal emotions.* New York: Oxford University Press.

Papousek, M. (2008). Disorders of behavioral and emotional regulation: Clinical evidence for a new diagnostic concept. In M. Papousek, M. Schieche, & H. Wurmser (Eds.), *Disorders of behavioral and emotional regulation in the first years of life* (pp. 53–84). Washington, DC: Zero to Three.

Papousek, M., & von Hofacker, N. (2008). Clinging, romping, throwing tantrums: Disorder of behavioral and emotional regulation in older infants and toddlers. In M. Papousek, M. Schieche, & H. Wurmser (Eds.), *Disorders of behavioral and emotional regulation in the first years of life: Early risk and intervention in the developing parent–infant relationship* (pp. 169–200). Washington, DC: Zero to Three.

Pardini, D. A., Lochman, J. E., & Frick, P. J. (2003). Callous/unemotional traits and social-cognitive processes in adjudicated youths. *Journal of the American Academy of Child and Adolescent Psychiatry, 42*(3), 364–371.

Parker, J. G., & Asher, S. R. (1987). Peer relations and later personal adjustment: Are low-accepted children at risk? *Psychological Bulletin, 102,* 357–389.

Parks, C. L., Robinson, P. S., Sibille, E., Shenk, T., & Toth, M. (1998). Increased anxiety of mice lacking the serotonin1a receptor. *Proceedings of the National Academy of Sciences of the United States of America, 95*(18), 10734–10739.

Parpal, M., & Maccoby, E. E. (1985). Maternal responsiveness and subsequent child compliance. *Child Development, 56,* 1326–1334.

Patrick, C. J. (2006). Psychophysiological correlates of aggression and violence: An integrative review. *Philosophical Transactions of the Royal Society of London: B. Biological Science, 363*(1503), 2543–2555.

Patrick, C. J., & Bernat, E. M. (2006). The construct of emotion as a bridge between personality and psychopathology. In R. F. Kreuger & J. L. Tackett (Eds.), *Personality and psychopathology*. New York: Guilford Press.

Patterson, G. R. (1979). A performance theory of coercive family interactions. In R. Cairns (Ed.), *Social interaction: Methods, analysis, and illustration* (pp. 119–162). Hillsdale, NJ: Erlbaum.

Patterson, G. R. (1980). Mothers: The unacknowledged victims. *Monographs of the Society for Research in Child Development, 45*(5).

Patterson, G. R. (1982). *Coercive family process: A social learning approach.* Eugene, OR: Castalia.

Patterson, G. R., & Capaldi, D. (1990). A mediational model for boys' depressed mood. In J. Rolf, A. S. Masten, D. Cicchetti, K. H. Nuechterlein, & S. Weintraub (Eds.), *Risk and protective factors in the development of psychopathology* (pp. 141–163). New York: Cambridge University Press.

Patterson, G. R., Littman, R. A., & Bricker, W. (1967). Assertive behavior in children: A step toward a theory of aggression. *Monographs of the Society for Research in Child Development 32*(5, Serial No. 113).

Pattij, T., Groenink, L., Hijzen, T. H., Oosting, R. S., Maes, R. A. A., van der Gugten, J., et al. (2002). Autonomic changes associated with enhanced anxiety in 5-HT-sub(1A) receptor knockout mice. *Neuropsychopharmacology, 27*(3), 380–390.

Paulus, M. P., Feinstein, J. S., Simmons, A., & Stein, M. B. (2004). Anterior cingulate activation in high trait anxious subjects is related to altered error processing during decision making. *Biological Psychiatry, 55,* 1179–1187,

Pavlov, I. P. (1935). *General types of animal and human higher nervous activity.* (Reprinted in selected works, 1955, Moscow: Foreign Language Publishing House)

Pfaff, D. W. (2007). *The neuroscience of fair play: Why we (usually) follow the Golden Rule.* Washington, DC: Dana Press.

Pfeifer, M., Goldsmith, H. H., Davidson, R. J., & Rickman, M. (2002). Continuity and change in inhibited and uninhibited children. *Child Development, 73*(5), 1474–1485.

Piaget, J. (1932). *The moral judgement of the child.* London: Routledge & Kegan Paul.

Piaget, J. (1954). *The construction of reality in the child* (M. Cook, Trans.). New York: Basic Books.

Pliszka, S. R., Carlson, C., & Swanson, J. M. (1999). *ADHD with comorbid disorders: Clinical assessment and management.* New York: Guilford Press.

Plomin, R. (1982). The concept of difficult temperament: A response to Thomas, Chess, and Korn. *Merrill–Palmer Quarterly, 28,* 25–33.

Porges, S. W., Doussard-Roosevelt, J. A., & Mati, A. K. (1994). Vagal tone and the physiological regulation of emotion. In N. A. Fox (Ed.), *Emotion regulation: Behavioral and biological considerations* (SRCD Monograph 59, Serial 240, pp. 167–186).

Posner, M. I. (1980). Orienting of attention. *Quarterly Journal of Experimental Psychology A, 32*(1), 3–25.

Posner, M. I., & Petersen, S. E. (1990). The attention system of the human brain. *Annual Review of Neuroscience, 13,* 25–42.

Posner, M. I., & Raichle, M. E. (1994). *Images of the mind*. New York: Scientific American Library.

Posner, M. I., & Rothbart, M. K. (1992). Attention and conscious experience. In A. D. Milner & M. D. Rugg (Eds.), *The neuropsychology of consciousness* (pp. 91–112). London: Academic Press.

Posner, M. I., & Rothbart, M. K. (1994). Attentional regulation: From mechanism to culture. In P. Bertelson, P. Eelen, & G. d'Ydewalle (Eds.), *International perspectives on psychological science* (Vol. 1, pp. 41–55). Hove, UK: Erlbaum.

Posner, M. I., & Rothbart, M. K. (1998). Attention, self-regulation, and consciousness. *Philosophical Transactions of the Royal Society of London, B, 353,* 1915–1927.

Posner, M. I., & Rothbart, M. K. (2000). Developing mechanisms of self-regulation. *Development and Psychopathology, 12,* 427–441.

Posner, M. I., & Rothbart, M. K. (2007a). *Educating the human brain*. Washington, DC: American Psychological Association.

Posner, M. I., & Rothbart, M. K. (2007b). Research on attention networks as a model for the integration of psychological science. *Annual Review of Psychology, 58,* 1–23.

Posner, M. I., Rothbart, M. K., & Sheese, B. E. (2007). Attention genes. *Developmental Science, 10*(1), 24–29.

Posner, M. I., Rothbart, M. K. Vizueta, N., Levy, K. N., Evans, D. E., Thomas, K. M., et al. (2002). Attentional mechanisms of borderline personality disorder. *Proceedings of the National Academy of Sciences of the United States of America, 99*(25), 16366–16370.

Preston, S. D., & de Waal, F. B. M. (2002). The communication of emotions and the possibility of empathy in animals. In S. Post, L. G. Underwood, J. P. Schloss, & W. B. Hurlburt (Eds.), *Altruistic love: Science, philosophy, and religion in dialogue* (pp. 284–308). Oxford, UK: Oxford University Press.

Prinzie, P., Onghena, P., & Hellinck, W. (2003). Parent and child personality traits and children's externalizing problem behavior from age 4 to 9 years: A cohort-sequential latent growth curve analysis. *Merrill–Palmer Quarterly, 51*(3), 335–366.

Prior, M., Smart, D., Sanson, A., & Oberklaid, F. (2000). Does shy-inhibited temperament in childhood lead to anxiety problems in adolescence? *Journal of the American Academy of Child and Adolescent Psychiatry, 39*(4), 461–468.

Puig-Antich, J. (1982). Major depression and conduct disorder in prepuberty. *Journal of the American Academy of Child and Adolescent Psychiatry, 21,* 118–128.

Pullis, M. (1985). Students' temperament characteristics and their impact on decisions by resource and mainstream teachers. *Learning Disability Quarterly, 8*, 109–122.

Putnam, S. P., Ellis, L. K., & Rothbart, M. K. (2001). The structure of temperament from infancy through adolescence. In A. Eliasz & A. Angleitner (Eds.), *Advances in research on temperament* (pp. 165–182). Lengerich, Germany: Pabst Science.

Putnam, S. P., Rothbart, M. K., & Gartstein, M. A. (2008). Homotypic and heterotypic continuity of fine-grained temperament during infancy, toddlerhood, and early childhood. *Infant and Child Development, 17*, 397–405.

Radke-Yarrow, M., & Sherman, T. (1990). Hard growing: Children who survive. In J. Rolf & A. S. Masten (Eds.), *Risk and protective factors in the development of psychopathology* (pp. 97–119). Cambridge, UK: Cambridge University Press.

Radke-Yarrow, R. M., & Zahn-Waxler, C. (1984). Roots, motives, and patterns in children's prosocial behavior. In E. Staub (Ed.), *Development and maintenance of prosocial behavior: International perspectives on positive morality* (pp. 89–99). New York: Plenum Press.

Reed, M. A., Pien, D. P., & Rothbart, M. K. (1984). Inhibitory self-control in preschool children. *Merrill–Palmer Quarterly, 30*, 131–147.

Reese, E., & Fivush, R. (1993). Parental styles for talking about the past. *Developmental Psychology, 29*, 596–606.

Reuter M., Ott U., Vaitl D., & Hennig, J. (2007). Impaired executive control is associated with a variation in the promoter region of the tryptophan hydroxylase 2 gene. *Journal of Cognitive Neuroscience, 19*, 401–408.

Rheingold, H. L., & Eckerman, C. O. (1973). Fear of the stranger: A critical examination. In H. W. Reese (Ed.), *Advances in child development and behavior* (Vol. 8, pp. 185–222). New York: Academic Press.

Riese, M. L. (1987). Temperamental stability between the neonatal period and 24 months. *Developmental Psychology, 23*, 216–222.

Roberts, B. W., Caspi, A., & Moffitt, T. (2001). The kids are alright: Growth and stability in personality development from adolescence to adulthood. *Journal of Personality and Social Psychology, 81*, 670–683.

Roberts, B. W., & DelVecchio, W. F. (2000). The rank-order consistency of personality traits from childhood to old age: A quantitative review of longitudinal studies. *Psychological Bulletin, 126*, 3–25.

Roberts, B. W., & Mroczek, D. K. (2008). Personality trait stability and change. *Current Directions in Psychological Science, 17*, 31–35.

Roberts, B. W., Walton, K., & Viechtbauer, W. (2006). Patterns of mean-level change in personality traits across the life course: A meta-analysis of longitudinal studies. *Psychological Bulletin, 132*, 1–25.

Roberts, B. W., & Wood, D. (2006). Personality development in the context of the Neo-Socioanalytic Model of personality. In D. Mroczek & T. Little (Eds.), *Handbook of personality development* (pp. 11–39). Mahwah, NJ: Erlbaum.

Robertson, J. (1952). *A two-year old goes to the hospital: A scientific film*. Retrieved July, 2010, from *www.robertsonfilms.info/2_year_old.htm*.

Robins, R. W., John, O. P., Caspi, A., Moffitt, T. E., & Stouthamer-Loeber, M. (1996).

Resilient, overcontrolled, and undercontrolled boys: Three replicable personality types. *Journal of Personality and Social Psychology, 70,* 157–171.

Robson, K. S., & Moss, H. A. (1970). Patterns and determinants of maternal attachment. *Journal of Pediatrics, 77,* 976–985.

Rosario, M., Salzinger, S., Feldman, R. S., & Ng-Mak, D. S. (2003). Community violence exposure and delinquent behaviours among youth: The moderating role of coping, *Journal of Community Psychology 31,* 489–512.

Rosch, E. (1999). Reclaiming concepts. *The Journal of Consciousness Studies, 6,* 61–77.

Rosen, J. B., & Schulkin, J. (1998). From normal fear to pathological anxiety. *Psychological Review, 105,* 325–350.

Rothbart, M., & Lewis, S. (1994). Cognitive processes and intergroup relations: A historical perspective. In P. Devine, D. Hamilton, & T. Ostrom (Eds.), *Social cognition: Impact on social psychology* (pp. 347–382). New York, Academic Press.

Rothbart, M. K. (1973). Laughter in young children. *Psychological Bulletin, 80,* 247–256.

Rothbart, M. K. (1977). Approaches to the psychological study of humor. In A. J. Chapman & H. C. Foot (Eds.), *It's a funny thing, humour* (pp. 87–94). Oxford, UK: Pergamon Press.

Rothbart, M. K. (1981). Measurement of temperament in infancy. *Child Development, 52,* 569–578.

Rothbart, M. K. (1982). The concept of difficult temperament: A critical analysis of Thomas, Chess, & Korn. *Merrill-Palmer Quarterly, 28,* 35–40.

Rothbart, M. K. (1986). Longitudinal observation of infant temperament. *Developmental Psychology, 22,* 356–365.

Rothbart, M. K. (1988). Temperament and the development of inhibited approach. *Child Development, 59,* 1241–1250.

Rothbart, M. K. (1989a). Behavioral approach and inhibition. In S. Reznick (Ed.), *Perspectives on behavioral inhibition* (pp. 139–157). Chicago: University of Chicago Press.

Rothbart, M. K. (1989b). Temperament and development. In G. A. Kohnstamm, J. E. Bates, & M. K. Rothbart (Eds.), *Temperament in childhood* (pp. 187–247). Chichester, UK: Wiley.

Rothbart, M. K. (2004). Temperament and the pursuit of an integrated developmental psychology. *Merrill-Palmer Quarterly, 50*(4), 492–505.

Rothbart, M. K. (2007a). Temperament, development, and personality. *Current Directions in Psychological Science, 16,* 207–212.

Rothbart, M. K. (2007b). [Review of Rusch, J., & Backen Jones, L., Parenting: The first three years: A group-based positive parenting program]. *Permanente Journal, 11*(3), 95.

Rothbart, M. K. (2009). *Vedantic values: A guide for living.* Unpublished manuscript. An adaptation of Swami Dayananda (1993). *The value of values.* Saylorsburg, PA: Arsha Vidya Gurukulam.

Rothbart, M. K., Ahadi, S. A., & Hershey, K. L. (1994). Temperament and social behavior in childhood. *Merrill–Palmer Quarterly, 40,* 21–39.

Rothbart, M. K., Ahadi, S. A., Hershey, K., & Fisher, P. (2001). Investigations of temperament at three to seven years: The children's behavior questionnaire. *Child Development, 72*(5), 1394–1408.

Rothbart, M. K., & Bates, J. E. (1998). Temperament. In W. Damon & N. Eisenberg (Eds.), *Handbook of child psychology (5th ed.): Vol. 3. Social, emotional and personality development* (pp. 105–176). New York: Wiley.

Rothbart, M. K., & Bates, J. E. (2006). Temperament. In W. Damon & R. Lerner (Eds.), & N. Eisenberg (Volume Ed.), *Handbook of child psychology* (6th ed.): Vol.3. Social, emotional, and personality development (pp. 99–176). New York: Wiley.

Rothbart, M. K., & Derryberry, D. (1981). Development of individual differences in temperament. In M. E. Lamb & A. L. Brown (Eds.), *Advances in developmental psychology* (Vol. 1, pp. 37–86). Hillsdale, NJ: Erlbaum.

Rothbart, M. K., & Derryberry, D. (2002). Temperament in children. In C. von Hofsten & L. Bäckman (Eds.), *Psychology at the turn of the millennium: Vol. 2. Social, developmental, and clinical perspectives* (pp. 17–35). East Sussex, UK: Psychology Press.

Rothbart, M. K., Derryberry, D., & Hershey, K. (2000). Stability of temperament in childhood: Laboratory infant assessment to parent report at seven years. In V. J. Molfese & D. L. Molfese (Eds.), *Temperament and personality development across the life span* (pp. 85–119). Hillsdale, NJ: Erlbaum.

Rothbart, M. K., Derryberry, D., & Posner, M. I. (1994). A psychobiological approach to the development of temperament. In J. E. Bates & T. D. Wachs (Eds.), *Temperament: Individual differences at the interface of biology and behavior* (pp. 83–116). Washington, DC: American Psychological Association.

Rothbart, M. K., Ellis, L. K., & Posner, M. I. (2004). Temperament and self-regulation. In R. F. Baumeister & K. D. Vohs (Eds.), *Handbook of self-regulation: Research, theory, and applications* (pp. 357–370). New York: Guilford Press.

Rothbart, M. K., Ellis, L. K., Rueda, M. R., & Posner, M. I. (2003). Developing mechanisms of temperamental effortful control. *Journal of Personality, 71*, 1113–1143.

Rothbart, M. K., & Hwang, J. (2005b). Temperament and the development of competence and motivation. In A. J. Elliot & C. S. Dweck (Eds.), *Handbook of competence and motivation* (pp. 167–184). New York: Guilford Press.

Rothbart, M. K., & Jones, L. B. (1998). Temperament, self-regulation, and education. *School Psychology Review, 27*, 479–491.

Rothbart, M. K., & Mauro, J. A. (1990). Questionnaire approaches to the study of infant temperament. In J. W. Fagen & J. Colombo (Eds.), *Individual differences in infancy: Reliability, stability, and prediction* (pp. 411–429). Hillsdale, NJ: Erlbaum.

Rothbart, M. K., & Posner, M. I. (2006). Temperament, attention, and developmental psychopathology. In D. Cicchetti & D. J. Cohen (Eds.), *Developmental psychopathology* (2nd ed., Vol. 2, pp. 465–501). New York: Wiley.

Rothbart, M. K., Posner, M. I., & Kieras, J. (2006). Temperament, attention, and the development of self-regulation. In K. McCartney & D. Philips (Eds.), *Blackwell handbook of early childhood development* (pp. 338–357). Oxford, UK: Blackwell.

Rothbart, M. K., & Rueda, M. R. (2005). The development of effortful control. In U. Mayr, E. Awh, & S. W. Keele (Eds.), *Developing individuality in the human brain: A festschrift honoring Michael I. Posner—May 2003* (pp. 167–188). Washington, DC: American Psychological Association Press.

Rothbart, M. K., & Sheese, B. (2007). Temperament and emotion regulation. In J. J. Gross (Ed.), *Handbook of emotion regulation* (pp. 331–350). New York: Guilford Press.

Rothbart, M. K., Sheese, B., & Posner, M. I. (2007). Executive attention and effortful control: Linking temperament, brain networks, and genes. *Child Development Perspectives, 1*(1), 2–7.

Rothbart, M. K., Sheese, B., Rueda, M., & Posner, M. I. (in press). Developing mechanisms of self regulation in early life. *Emotion Review.*

Rothbart, M. K., Ziaie, H., & O'Boyle, C. G. (1992). Self-regulation and emotion in infancy. In N. Eisenberg & R. A. Fabes (Eds.), *Emotion and its regulation in early development: New directions for child development, no. 55: The Jossey-Bass education series* (pp. 7–23). San Francisco, CA: Jossey-Bass.

Rotter, J. (1996). Generalized expectations for internal versus external control of reinforcement. *Psychological Monographs, 80,* 1–28.

Rubin, K. H., & Burgess, K. B. (2001). Social withdrawal and anxiety. In M. W. Vasey & M. R. Dadds (Eds.), *The developmental psychopathology of anxiety* (pp. 407–434). New York: Oxford University Press.

Rubin, K. H., Burgess, K. B., Dwyer, K. M., & Hastings, P. D. (2003). Predicting preschoolers' externalizing behaviors from toddler temperament, conflict, and maternal negativity. *Developmental Psychology, 39,* 164–176.

Rubin, K. H., Chen, X., & Hymel, S. (1993). Socioemotional characteristics of withdrawn and aggressive children. *Merrill–Palmer Quarterly, 39,* 518–534.

Rudebeck, P. H., Bannerman, D. M., & Rushworth, M. F. S. (2008). The contribution of distinct subregions of the ventromedial frontal cortex to emotion, social behavior, and decision making. *Cognitive, Affective and Behavioral Neuroscience, 8*(4), 485–497.

Rueda, M. R., Checa, P., & Rothbart, M. K. (in press). Contributions of attentional control to social emotional and academic development. *Early Education and Development.*

Rueda, M. R., Checa, P., & Santonja, M. (2008, April). *Training executive attention: Lasting effects and transfer to affective self-regulation.* Paper presented at the Annual Meeting of the Cognitive Neuroscience Society, San Francisco, CA.

Rueda, M. R., & Rothbart, M. K. (2009). The influence of temperament on the development of coping: The role of maturation and experience. In E. A. Sinner & M. J. Zimmer-Gembeck (Eds.), *Coping and the development of regulation. New directions for child and adolescent development* (Vol. 124, pp. 19–32). Hoboken, NJ: Jossey-Bass.

Rueda, M. R., Rothbart, M. K., McCandliss, B. D., Saccomanno, L., & Posner, M. I. (2005). Training, maturation, and genetic influences on the development of executive attention. *Proceedings of the National Academy of Sciences of the United States of America, 102*(41), 14931–14936.

Ruff, H. A. (1986). Components of attention during infants' manipulative exploration. *Child Development, 52,* 105–114.

Ruff, H. A., & Rothbart, M. K. (1996). *Attention in early development: Themes and variations*. New York: Oxford University Press.

Rusalov, V. M. (1987). *Questionnaire for the measurement of the structure of temperament (QST), short manual*. Moscow: Moscow University.

Rusalov, V. M., & Trofimova, I. (2007). *Structure of temperament and its measurement*. Toronto, Canada: Psychological Services Press.

Russell, A., Hart, C. H., Robinson, C., & Olsen, S. F. (2003). Children's sociable and aggressive behavior with peers: A comparison of the U.S. and Australia, and contributions of temperament and parenting styles. *International Journal of Behavioral Development, 27,* 74–86.

Rutter, M. (1979). Protective factors in children's responses to stress and disadvantage. In M. W. Kent & J. E. Rolf (Eds.), *Primary prevention of psychopathology: Vol. 3. Social competence in children* (pp. 49–74). Hanover, NH: University Press of New England.

Rutter, M. (1987). Temperament, personality, and personality disorder. *British Journal of Psychiatry, 150,* 443–458.

Rutter, M. (1989). Pathways from childhood to adult life. *Journal of Child Psychology and Psychiatry, 30,* 23–51.

Rutter, M. (1990). Psychosocial resilience and protective mechanisms. In J. E. Rolf, A. S. Masten, D. Cicchetti, K. H. Nuechterlein, & S. Weintraub (Eds.), *Risk and protective factors in the development of psychopathology* (pp. 181–214). Cambridge, UK: Cambridge University Press.

Rutter, M., & Quinton, D. (1984). Parental psychiatric disorder: Effects on children. *Psychological Medicine, 14,* 853–880.

Saarni, C., Mumme, D. L., & Campos, J. J. (1998). Emotional development: Action, communication, and understanding. In W. Damon & N. Eisenberg (Eds.), *Handbook of child psychology: Social, emotional, and personality development* (5th ed., Vol. 3, pp. 237–310). New York: Wiley.

Sagi, A., & Hoffman, M. L. (1976). Empathic distress in the newborn. *Developmental Psychology, 12,* 175–176.

Sallquist, J. V., Eisenberg, N., Spinrad, T. L., Reiser, M., Hofer, C., Zhou, Q., et al. (2009). Positive and negative emotionality: Trajectories across six years and relations with social competence. *Emotion, 9,* 15–28.

Sander, L. W. (1962). Issues in early mother–child interaction. *Journal of the American Academy of Child Psychiatry, 1,* 141–166.

Sander, L. W. (1969). The longitudinal course of early mother–child interaction: Cross case comparison in a sample of mother–child pairs. In B. M. Foss (Ed.), *Determinants of infant behavior IV* (pp. 189–228). London: Methuen.

Sander, L. W. (1977). The regulation of exchange in the infant–caretaker system and some aspects of the context–content relationship. In M. Lewis & L. Rosenblum (Eds.), *Interaction, conversation, and the development of language. The origins of behavior* (Vol. 5, pp. 133–156). New York: Wiley.

Sander, L. W. (2007). *Living systems, evolving consciousness, and the emerging person: A selection of papers from the life work of Louis Sander. Psychoanalytic inquiry book series, Vol. 26* (G. Amadei & I. Bianchi, Eds.). London: Routledge.

Sander, L. W., Julia, H. L., Stechler, G., & Burns, P. (1972). Continuous 24-hour interactional monitoring in infants reared in two caretaking environments. *Psychosomatic Medicine, 34*(3). 270–282.

Sanson, A. V., Smart, D. F., Prior, M., Oberklaid, F., & Pedlow, R. (1994). The structure of temperament from three to seven years: Age, sex, and sociodemographic influences. *Merrill-Palmer Quarterly, 40*(2), 233–252.

Sapolsky, R. L., Romero, M., & Munck, A. U. (2000). How do glucocorticoids influence stress responses? Integrating permissive, suppressive, stimulatory, and preparative actions. *Endocrine Reviews, 21,* 55–89.

Saucier, G. (2002). Orthogonal markers for orthogonal factors: The case of the Big Five. *Journal of Research in Personality, 36*(1), 1–31.

Scarr, S., & McCartney, K. (1983). How people make their own environments: A theory of genotype–environment effects. *Child Development, 54,* 242–435.

Schaffer, H. R. (1974). Cognitive components of the infant's response to strangeness. In M. Lewis, & L. A. Rosenblum (Eds.), *The origins of fear* (pp. 11–24). New York: Wiley.

Schaffer, H. R., & Emerson, P. E. (1964). Patterns of response to physical contact in early human development. *Journal of Child Psychology and Psychiatry, 5,* 1–13.

Schieche, M., Rupprecht, C., & Papousek, M. (2008). Sleep disorders: Current results and clinical experience. In M. Papousek, M. Schieche, & H. Wurmser (Eds.), *Disorders of behavioral and emotional regulation in the first years of life* (pp. 117–140). Washington, DC: Zero to Three.

Schiefele, A., Krapp, A., & Winteler, A. (1992). Interest as a predictor of academic achievement: A meta-analysis of research. In K. A. Renninger, S. Hidi, & A. Krapp (Eds.), *The role of interest learning and development* (pp. 183–212). Hillsdale, NJ: Erlbaum.

Schneider, M. L., & Suomi, S. J. (1992). Laboratory assessment of temperament and postrotary nystagmus responses in rhesus monkey infants (Macaca mulatta). *Physical and Occupational Therapy in Pediatrics, 12*(1), 37–52.

Schneirla, T. C. (1959). An evolutionary and developmental theory of biphasic processes underlying approach and withdrawal. In M. R. Jones (Ed.), *Nebraska symposium on motivation* (Vol. 7, pp. 297–339). Lincoln: University of Nebraska Press.

Schulkin, J., Morgan, M. A., & Rosen, J. B. (2005). A neuroendocrine mechanism for sustaining fear. *Trends in Neurosciences, 28,* 629–635.

Schwartz, T. (1978). Where is the culture? Personality as the distributive locus of culture. In G. D. Spindler (Ed.), *The making of psychological anthropology* (pp. 419–441). Berkeley: University of California Press.

Schwebel, D. C. (2004). Temperamental risk factors for children's unintentional injury: The role of impulsivity and inhibitory control. *Personality and Individual Differences 37,* 567–578.

Sears, R. R., Maccoby, E. E., & Levin, H. (1957). *Patterns of child rearing.* Evanston, IL: Row Peterson.

Seligman, M., & Csikszentmihalyi, M. (2000). Positive psychology. An introduction. *American Psychologist, 55*(1), 5–14.

Selman, R. (1980). *The growth of interpersonal understanding.* New York: Academic Press.

Sethi, A., Mischel, W., Aber, J. L., Shoda, Y., & Rodriguez, M. L. (2000). The role of strategic attention deployment in development of self-regulation: Predicting preschoolers' delay of gratification from mother–toddler interactions. *Developmental Psychology, 6*(6), 767–777.

Shaw, D. S., Gilliom, M., Ingoldsby, E. M., & Nagin, D. S. (2003). Trajectories leading to school-age conduct problems. *Developmental Psychology, 39*(2), 189–200.

Sheese, B. E., Voelker, P. M., Posner, M. I., & Rothbart, M. K. (2009). Genetic variation influences on the early development of reactive emotions and their regulation by attention. *Cognitive Neuropsychiatry, 14,* 332–355.

Sheese, B. E., Voelker, P. M., Rothbart, M. K., & Posner, M. I. (2007). Parenting quality interacts with genetic variation in dopamine receptor D4 to influence temperament in early childhood. *Development and Psychopathology, 19*(4), 1039–1046.

Shiner, R. L. (1998). How shall we speak of children's personalities in middle childhood? A preliminary taxonomy. *Psychological Bulletin, 124*(3), 308–332.

Shiner, R. L. (2000). Linking childhood personality with adaptation: Evidence for continuity and change across time into late adolescence. *Journal of Personality and Social Psychology, 78*(2), 310–325.

Shiner, R. L., Masten, A. S., & Roberts, J. M. (2003). Childhood personality foreshadows adult personality and life outcomes two decades later. *Journal of Personality and Social Psychology, 71*(6), 1145–1170.

Shiner, R. L., Masten, A. S., & Tellegen, A. (2002). A developmental perspective on personality in emerging adulthood: Childhood antecedents and concurrent adaptation. *Journal of Personality and Social Psychology, 83,* 1165–1177.

Shinn, M. W. (1909). *Notes on the development of a child.* Berkeley: University of California Press.

Shirley, M. (1933). *The first two years. Vol. 111: Personality manifestations.* Minneapolis: University of Minnesota Press.

Shoda, Y., Mischel, W., & Peake, P. K. (1990). Predicting adolescent cognitive and self-regulatory competencies from preschool delay of gratification: Identifying diagnostic conditions. *Developmental Psychology, 26,* 978–986.

Shulman, G. L., Astafiev, S. V., Franke, D., Pope, D. L. W., Snyder, A. Z., McAvoy, M. P., et al. (2009). Interaction of stimulus-driven reorienting and expectation in ventral and dorsal frontoparietal and basal ganglia–cortical networks. *Journal of Neuroscience, 29,* 4392–4407.

Silbersweig, D., Clarkin, J. F., Goldstein, M., Kernberg, O. F., Tuescher, O., Levy, K. N., et al. (2007). Failure of frontolimbic inhibitory function in the context of negative emotion in borderline personality disorder. *American Journal of Psychiatry, 164,* 1832–1841.

Singer, D., Golinkoff, R. M., & Hirsh-Pasek, K. (Eds.). (2006). *Play = Learning: How play motivates and enhances children's cognitive and social–emotional growth.* New York: Oxford University Press.

Singh, L., Morgan, J. L., & Best, C. T. (2002). Infants' listening preferences: Baby talk or happy talk? *Infancy, 3*(3), 365–394.

Skinner, E., Edge, K., Altman, J., & Sherwood, H. (2003). Searching for the structure of coping: A review and critique of category systems for classifying ways of coping. *Psychological Bulletin, 129*, 216–269.

Skinner, E. A. (1999). Action regulation, coping and development. In J. B. Brandtstädter & R. M. Lerner (Eds.), *Action and self-development* Thousand Oaks, CA: Sage.

Skinner, E. A., & Zimmer-Gembeck, M. J. (2007). The development of coping. *Annual Review of Psychology, 58*, 119–144.

Slabach, E. H., Morrow, J., & Wachs, T. D. (1991). Questionnaire measurement of infant and child temperament: Current status and future directions. In J. Strelau & A. Angleitner (Eds.), *Explorations in temperament: International perspectives on theory and measurement* (pp. 205–234). New York: Plenum.

Sluyter, F., van der Vlugt, J. J., van Oortmerssen, G. A., Koolhaas, J. M., Van Der Hoeven, F., & De Boer, P. (1996). Studies on wild house mice: VII. Prenatal maternal environment and aggression. *Behavior Genetics, 26*(5), 513–518.

Sluyter, F., & van Oortmerssen, G. A. (2000). A mouse is not just a mouse. *Animal Welfare, 9*(2), 193–205.

Smeets, W. J. A. J., & González, A. (2000). Catecholamine systems in the brain of vertebrates: New perspectives through a comparative approach. *Brain Research—Brain Research Reviews, 33*(2–3), 308–379.

Snow, C. (1972). Mothers' speech to children learning language. *Child Development, 43*, 549–565.

Snyder, J. A. (1997). A reinforcement analysis of interaction in problem and non-problem children. *Journal of Abnormal Psychology, 86*, 528–535.

Somerville, L. H., Jones, R. M., & Casey, B. J. (2010). A time of change: Behavioral and neural correlates of adolescent sensitivity to appetitive and aversive environmental cues. *Brain and Cognition, 72*, 124–133.

Spangler, G. (1989). Toddlers' everyday experiences as related to preceding mental and emotional disposition and their relationship to subsequent mental and motivational development: A short-term longitudinal study. *International Journal of Behavioral Development, 12*(3), 285–303.

Spencer-Booth, Y., & Hinde, R. A. (1971). The effects of 13 days maternal separation on infant rhesus monkeys compared with those of shorter and repeated separations. *Animal Behaviour, 19*(3), 595–605.

Spoont, M. R. (1992). Modulatory role of serotonin in neural information processing: Implications for human psychopathology. *Psychological Bulletin, 112*, 330–350.

Sroufe, L. A. (1979). The coherence of individual development. *American Psychologist, 34*, 834–841.

Stanovitch, K. E. (1997). *How to think straight about psychology.* Boston: Allyn & Bacon.

Stattin, H., & Kerr, M. (2000). Parental monitoring: A reinterpretation. *Child Development, 71*, 1070–1083.

Stechler, G., & Latz, E. (1966). Some observations on attention and arousal in the human infant. *Journal of the American Academy of Child Psychiatry, 5,* 517–525.

Stern, D. N. (1985). *The interpersonal world of the infant. A view from psychoanalysis and developmental psychology.* New York: Basic Books.

Stevenson-Hinde, J. (1989) Behavioral inhibition: Issues of context. In J. S. Reznick (Ed.), *Perspectives on behavioral inhibition* (pp. 125–138). Chicago: University of Chicago Press.

Stevenson-Hinde, J., & Hinde, R. A. (1986). Changes in associations between characteristics and interactions. In R. Plomin & J. Dunn (Eds.), *The study of temperament: Changes, continuities and challenges* (pp. 115–129). Hillsdale, NJ: Erlbaum.

Stevenson-Hinde, J., & Shouldice, A. (1993). Wariness to strangers: A behavior systems perspective revisited. In K. H. Rubin & J. B. Asendorpf (Eds.), *Social withdrawal, inhibition, and shyness in childhood* (pp. 101–116). New York: Erlbaum.

Stevenson-Hinde, J., & Zunz, M. (1978). Subjective assessment of individual rhesus monkeys. *Primates, 19*(3), 473–482.

Stice, E., & Gonzales, N. (1998). Adolescent temperament moderates the relation of parenting to antisocial behavior and substance use. *Journal of Adolescent Research, 13,* 5–31.

Stifter, C. A., & Braungart, J. M. (1995). The regulation of negative reactivity in infancy: Function and development. *Developmental Psychology, 31,* 448–455.

Stipek, D. (1995). The development of pride and shame in toddlers. In J. Tangney & K. Fischer (Eds.), *Self-conscious emotions* (pp. 237–252). New York: Guilford Press.

Stipek, D., Recchia, S., & McClintic, S. (1992). Self-evaluation in young children. *Monographs of the Society for Research in Child Development, 57*(1).

Stoneman, Z., & Brody, G. H. (1993). Sibling temperaments, conflict, warmth, and role asymmetry. *Child Development, 64,* 1786–1800.

Stoolmiller, M. (2001). Synergistic interaction of child manageability problems and parent-discipline tactics in predicting future growth in externalizing behavior for boys. *Developmental Psychology, 37*(6), 814–825.

Strauss, M. E., & Rourke, D. L. (1978). A multivariate analysis of neonatal behavioral assessment scale in several examples. In A. J. Sameroff (Ed.), Organization and stability of newborn behavior. A commentary on the Brazelton neonatal behavior assessment scale. *Monographs of the Society for Research in Child Development, 43*(Serial No. 177, pp. 81–91).

Strelau, J. (1972). A diagnosis of temperament by non–experimental techniques. *Polish Psychological Bulletin, 3,* 97–105.

Strelau, J. (1983). *Temperament personality activity.* New York: Academic Press.

Strelau, J. (2008). *Temperament as a regulator of behavior: After fifty years of research.* Clinton Corners, NY: Werner.

Studman, L. G. (1935). Studies in experimental psychiatry: V, W, and F factors in relation to traits of personality. *Journal of Mental Science, 81,* 107–137.

Super, C. M., Axia, G., Harkness, S., Welles-Nystrom, B., Zylicz, P. O., Parminder, P., Bonichini, S., et al. (2008). Culture, temperament, and the "difficult child":

A study in seven western cultures. *European Journal of Developmental Science,* 2(1/2), 136–157.

Swanson, J. M., Flodman, P., Kennedy, J., Spence, M. A., Moyzis, R., Schuck, S., et al. (2000). Dopamine genes and ADHD. *Neuroscience and Biobehavioral Reviews, 24*(1), 21–25.

Tamm, L., McCandliss, B. D., Liang, A., Wigal, T. L., Posner, M. I., & Swanson, J. M. (2008). Can attention itself be trained? Attention training for children at-risk for ADHD. In K. McBurnett & L. J. Pfiffner (Eds.), *Attention deficit hyperactivity disorder: Concepts, controversies, new directions* (pp. 397–410). New York: Informa Healthcare USA.

Tellegen, A. (1985). Structures of mood and personality and their relevance to assessing anxiety, with an emphasis on self-report. In A. H. Tuma & J. D. Maser (Eds.), *Anxiety and the anxiety disorders* (pp. 681–706). Hillsdale, NJ: Erlbaum.

Tellegen, A., Lykken, D. T., Bouchard, T. J., Jr., Wilcox, K. J., Segal, N. L., & Rich, S. (1988). Personality similarity in twins reared apart and together. *Journal of Personality and Social Psychology, 54,* 1031–1039.

Teplov, B. M. (1964). Problems in the study of general types of higher nervous activity in man and animals. In J. A. Gray (Ed.), *Pavlov's typology* (pp. 3–158). Oxford, UK: Pergamon.

Tessler, M. (1986). *Mother-child talk in a museum: The socialization of a memory.* Unpublished manuscript, City University of New York, Graduate Center, New York.

Thomas, A., & Chess, S. (1977). *Temperament and development.* New York: Brunner/Mazel.

Thomas, A., Chess, S., & Birch, H. G. (1968). *Temperament and behavior disorders in children.* New York: New York University Press.

Thomas, A., Chess, S., Birch, H. G., Hertzig, M. E., & Korn, S. (1963). *Behavioral individuality in early childhood.* New York: New York University Press.

Thompson, R. A. (1994). Emotion regulation: A theme in search of definition. In N. A. Fox (Ed.), The development of emotion regulation: Biological and behavioral considerations. *Monographs of the Society for Research in Child Development, 59*(Serial No. 240), 25–52.

Thurstone, L. L., & Thurstone, T. G. (1941). *Factorial studies of intelligence.* Chicago: University of Chicago Press.

Tolan, P., & Grant, K. (2009). How social and cultural contexts shape the development of coping: Youth in the inner city as an example. *New Directions for Child and Adolescent Development, 124,* 61–74.

Tooby, J., Cosmides, L., & Barrett, H. C. (2005). Resolving the debate on innate ideas: Learnability constraints and the evolved interpenetration of motivational and conceptual functions. In P. Carruthers, S. Laurence, & S. Stich (Eds.), *The innate mind: Structure and content* (pp. 305–337). New York: Oxford University Press.

Trainor, L. J., Austin, C. M., & Desjardins, R. N. (2000). Is infant-directed speech prosody a result of the vocal expression of emotion? *Psychological Science, 11,* 188–195.

Tremblay, R. E., & Nagin, D. S. (2005). The developmental origins of physical aggression in humans. In R. E. Tremblay, W. W. Hartup, & J. Archer (Eds.), *Developmental origins of aggression* (pp. 83–106). New York: Guilford Press.

Tronick, E. (2007). *The neurobehavioral and social–emotional development of infants and children*. New York: Norton Press.

Tronick, E. Z., Als, H., Adamson, L., Wise, S., & Brazelton, T. B. (1978). The infant's response to entrapment between contradictory messages in face-to-face interaction. *Journal of the American Academy of Child Psychiatry, 17,* 1–13.

Tschann, J. M., Kaiser, P., Chesney, M. A., Alkon, A., & Boyce, W. T. (1996). Resilience and vulnerability among preschool children: Family functioning, temperament, and behavior problems. *Journal of the American Academy of Child and Adolescent Psychiatry, 35*(2), 184–192.

Twain, M. (2000). The turning point of my life. In C. Neider (Ed.), *The complete essays of Mark Twain*. Cambridge, MA: Da Capo Press. (Original work published 1910)

Valentine, C. W. (1951; reprinted 1960). *The normal child and some of his abnormalities*. Baltimore: Penguin Books.

Valentine, C. W. (1956). *The normal child and some of his abnormalities*. London: Penguin Press.

Valiente, C., Eisenberg, C. L., Fabes, R., Shepard, S., Cumberland, A., & Losoya, S. (2004). Preidction of children's empathy-related responses from their effortful control and parents' expressivity. *Developmental Psychology, 40,* 911–926.

Valiente, C., Lemery-Chalfant, K. S., Swanson, J., & Reiser, M. (2008). Prediction of children's academic competence from their effortful control, relationships, and classroom participation. *Journal of Educational Psychology, 100,* 67–77.

Valiente, N., Eisenberg, C. L., Smith, M., Reiser, R. A., Fabes, R., & Losoya, S., et al. (2003). The relations of effortful control and reactive control to children's externalizing problems: A longitudinal assessment. *Journal of Personality, 71,* 1171–1196.

van den Boom, D. C. (1989). Neonatal irritability and the development of attachment. In G. A. Kohnstamm, J. E. Bates, & M. K. Rothbart (Eds.), *Temperament in childhood* (pp. 299–318). Chichester, UK: Wiley.

van den Boom, D. C. (1991). The influence of infant irritability on the development of the mother–infant relationship in the first six months of life. In J. K. Nugen, B. M. Lester, & T. B. Brazelton (Eds.), *The cultural context of infancy* (Vol. 2, pp. 63–89). Norwood, NJ: Ablex.

van den Boom, D. C. (1994). The influence of temperament and mothering on attachment and exploration: An experimental manipulation of sensitive responsiveness among lower-class mothers with irritable infants. *Child Development, 65,* 1457–1477.

van den Boom, D. C., & Hoeksema, J. B. (1994). The effect of infant irritability on mother–infant interaction: A growth-curve analysis. *Developmental Psychology, 30,* 581–590.

van Hooff, J. (1970). A component analysis of the structure of the social behaviour of a semicaptive chimpanzee group. *Experientia, 26,* 549–550.

van Lieshout, C. F. M., & Haselager, G. J. T. (1994). The Big Five personality factors in Q-sort descriptions of children and adolescents. In C. F. Halverson, G. A. Kohnstamm, & R. Martin (Eds.), *The developing structure of temperament and personality from infancy to adulthood* (pp. 293–318). Hillsdale, NJ: Erlbaum.

Vasey, M. W., Daleiden, E. L., Williams, L. L., & Brown, L. M. (1995). Biased attention in childhood anxiety disorders: A preliminary study. *Journal of Abnormal Child Psychology, 23*(2), 267–279.

Vernon-Feagans, L., Pancsofar, N., Willoughby, M., Odom, E., Quade, A., & Cox, M. (2008). Predictors of maternal language to infants during a picture book task in the home: Family SES, child characteristics and the parenting environment. *Journal of Applied Developmental Psychology, 29*(3), 213–226.

Victor, J. B., Rothbart, M. K., & Baker, S. R. (2006). *A comprehensive model for children's personality in the child temperament and personality questionnaire (CTPQ).* Manuscript in preparation.

Vogt, B. A., Finch, D. M., & Olson, C. R. (1992). Functional heterogeneity in cingulate cortex: The anterior executive and posterior evaluative regions. *Cerebral Cortex, 2*, 435–443.

Volhard, J., & Volhard, W. (2001). *Dog training for dummies—A reference for the rest of us.* Hoboken, NJ: Wiley.

Volling, B. L., Kolak, A., & Blandon, A. Y. (2009). Family subsystems and the development of self-regulation. In S. L. Olson & A. J. Sameroff (Eds.), *Biopsychosocial regulatory processes in the development of childhood behavioral problems* (pp. 238–257). New York: Cambridge University Press.

von Hofacker, N., Papousek, M., & Wurmser, H. (2008). Feeding disorders and failure to thrive in infants and toddlers. In M. Papousek, M. Schieche, & H. Wurmser (Eds.), *Disorders of behavioral and emotional regulation in the first years of life* (pp. 141–168). Washington, DC: Zero to Three.

Vygotsky, L. S. (1962). *Thought and language.* Cambridge, MA: MIT Press. (Original work published in Russian 1934)

Wachs, T. D. (2000). *Necessary but not sufficient: The respective roles of single and multiple influences on individual development.* Washington, DC: American Psychological Association.

Waldman, I. D., Singh, A. L., & Lahey, B. B. (2006). Dispositional dimensions and the causal structure of child and adolescent conduct problems. In R. F. Krueger & J. L. Tackett (Eds.), *Personality and psychopathology* (pp. 112–152). New York: Guilford Press.

Walker, D. L., Toufexis, D. J., & Davis, M. (2003). Role of the bed nucleus of the stria terminalis versus the amygdala in fear, stress, and anxiety. *European Journal of Pharmacology, 463,* 199–216.

Wallon, H. (1925). *L'enfant turbulent.* Paris: Alcan.

Wallon, H. (1934). *Les origins du caractere chez l'enfant.* Paris: Boivin.

Wang, K. J., Fan, J., Dong, Y., Wang, C., Lee, T. M. C., & Posner, M. I. (2005). Selective impairment of attentional networks of orienting and executive control in schizophrenia. *Schizophrenia Research, 78*, 235–241.

Washburn, D. A., & Rumbaugh, D. M. (1992). Testing primates with joystick-based automated apparatus: Lessons from the Language Research Center's computerized test system. Behavior research methods, instruments, & computers. *Journal of the Psychonomic Society, 24*(2), 157–164.

Watson, D. (2005). Rethinking the mood and anxiety disorders: A quantitative hierarchical model for DSM-V. *Journal of Abnormal Psychology, 114*, 522–536.

Watson, D., & Clark, L. A. (1992a). Affects separable and inseparable: On the hierarchical arrangement of the negative affects. *Journal of Personality and Social Psychology, 62*(3), 489–505.

Watson, D., & Clark, L. A. (1992b). On traits and temperament: General and specific factors of emotional experience and their relation to the five-factor model. *Journal of Personality, 60*(2), 441–476.

Watson, D., & Clark, L. A. (1997). The measurement and mismeasurement of mood: Recurrent and emergent issues. *Journal of Personality Assessment, 68*, 267–296.

Watson, D., Kotov, R., & Gamez, W. (2006). Basic dimensions of temperament in relation to personality and psychopathology. In R. Krueger & J. Tackett (Eds.), *Personality and psychopathology* (pp. 7–38). New York: Guilford Press.

Watson, J. B. (1930). *Behaviorism* (rev. ed.). Chicago: University of Chicago Press.

Watson, K. K., Matthews, B. J., & Allman, J. M. (2007). Brain activation during sight gags and language-dependent humor. *Cerebral Cortex, 17*(2), 314–324.

Webb, E. (1915). Character and intelligence. *British Journal of Psychology Monographs, 1*(3), 1–99.

Weinberg, M. K., & Tronick, E. Z. (1994). Beyond the face: An empirical study of infant affective configurations of facial, vocal, gestural, and regulatory behaviors. *Child Development, 65*(5), 1503–1515.

Welwood, J. (2006). *Perfect love, imperfect relationships*. Boston: Trumpeter.

Werner, E. E. (1985). Stress and protective factors in children's lives. In A. R. Nicol (Ed.), *Longitudinal studies in child psychology and psychiatry* (pp. 335–355). New York: Wiley.

Werner, E. E., & Smith, R. S. (1982). *Vulnerable but invincible: A longitudinal study of resilient children and youth*. New York: McGraw-Hill.

White, R. W. (1959). Motivation reconsidered: The concept of competence. *Psychological Review, 66*, 297–333.

White, R. W. (1960). Competence and the psychosexual stages of development. In M. R. Jones (Ed.), *Nebraska symposium on motivation* (Vol. 8, pp. 97–141). Lincoln: Nebraska University Press.

White, R. W. (1963). *Ego and reality in psychoanalytic theory* (Psychological Issues Series, Monograph No. 11). New York: International Universities Press.

Whiting, B. B. (1963). *Six cultures: Studies of child rearing*. New York: Wiley.

Whittle, S. L. (2007). *The neurobiological correlates of temperament in early adolescence*. Unpublished doctoral dissertation, University of Melbourne, Australia.

Wilkie, C. F., & Ames, E. W. (1986). The relationship of infant crying to parental stress in the transition to parenthood. *Journal of Marriage and the Family, 48*(3), 545–550.

Willcutt, E. G., Doyle, A. E., Nigg, J. T., Faraone, S. V., & Pennington, B. F. (2005). A meta-analytic review of the executive function theory of ADHD. *Biological Psychiatry, 57*, 1336–1346.

Willcutt, E. G., Duhamel, K., & Vaccaro, D. (1995). Activity and mood temperament as preductors of adolescent substance use: Test of a self regulation mediational model. *Journal of Personality and Social Psychology, 68*, 901–916.

Wills, T. A., Sandy, J. M., Yaeger, A., & Shinar, O. (2001). Family risk factors and adolescent substance use: Moderation effects for temperament dimensions. *Developmental Psychology, 37*, 283–297.

Wolff, P. H. (1987). *The development of behavioral states and the expression of emotions in early infancy: New proposals for investigation.* Chicago: University of Chicago Press.

Wooten, J. M., Frick, P. J., Shelton, K. K., & Silverthorn, P. (1997). Ineffective parenting and childhood conduct problems: The moderating role of callous-unemotional traits. *Journal of Consulting and Clinical Psychology, 65*, 301–308.

Wundt, W. (1903). *Grundzuge der physiologischen psychologie* (5th ed., Vol. 3). Leipzig, Germany: Engelmann.

Yeung, N., Botvinick, M. M., & Cohen, J. D. (2004). The neural basis of error-detection: Conflict monitoring and the error-related negativity. *Psychological Review, 111*, 931–959.

Young, E. A., Lopez, J. F., Murphy-Weinberg, V., Watson, S. J., & Akil, H. (1998). The role of mineralocorticoid receptors in hypothalamic–pituitary–adrenal axis regulation in humans. *Journal of Clinical Endocrinology and Metabolism, 83*(9), 3339–3345.

Zahn-Waxler, C., Cole, P., & Barrett, K. (1991). Guilt and empathy: Sex differences and implications for the development of depression. In J. Garber & K. Dodge (Eds.), *The development of emotion regulation and disregulation* (pp. 243–272). New York: Cambridge University Press.

Zahn-Waxler, C., Radke-Yarrow, M., Wagner, E., & Chapman, M. (1992). Development of concern for others. *Developmental Psychology, 28*(1), 126–136.

Zentner, M. (2008). Current trends in the study of child temperament. *European Journal of Developmental Science, 2*, 2–6.

Zentner, M., & Shiner, R. (in press). *Handbook of temperament.* New York: Guilford Press.

Zuckerman, M. (1984). Sensation seeking: A comparative approach to a human trait. *Behavioral and Brain Sciences, 7*, 413–471.

Zuckerman, M. (1991). *Psychobiology of personality.* New York: Cambridge University Press.

Zuckerman, M. (1995). Good and bad humors: Biochemical bases of personality and its disorders. *Psychological Science, 6*(6), 325–332.

Zuckerman, M. (2005). *Psychobiology of personality* (2nd ed.). New York: Cambridge University Press.

Zuckerman, M., Eysenck, S. B. G., & Eysenck, H. J. (1978). Sensation seeking in England and America: Cross-cultural, age and sex comparisons. *Journal of Consulting and Clinical Psychology, 46*, 139–149.

Author Index

Subject Index